Image-Guided High-Precision Radiotherapy

Esther G. C. Troost
Editor

Image-Guided High-Precision Radiotherapy

Springer

Editor
Esther G. C. Troost, MD, PhD
Department of Radiotherapy and Radiation Oncology
Faculty of Medicine and University Hospital Carl Gustav Carus
Dresden, Sachsen, Germany

ISBN 978-3-031-08600-7   ISBN 978-3-031-08601-4 (eBook)
https://doi.org/10.1007/978-3-031-08601-4

This Springer imprint is published by the registered company Springer Nature Switzerland AG
The registered company address is: Gewerbestrasse 11, 6330 Cham, Switzerland

Preface

Radiation therapy is one of the pillars of oncological treatment. As opposed to surgery, external beam radiation therapy requires the indirect depiction of the tumour and its surrounding structures both during the phase of treatment planning and during fractionated treatment. Historically, only pretreatment imaging was available and served as basis for the entire course of treatment, irrespective of anatomical changes caused, e.g. by tumour response or by patient's weight loss.

During the last 15 years, advances in the field of image-guided radiotherapy have been dramatic. Anatomical and functional imaging is available prior to and during the course of treatment, occasionally even during the treatment fraction. Novel, tumour type-specific radionuclides have been developed for positron emission tomography (PET) and enable depiction of small tumour deposits, which would otherwise have been overlooked. Fast, highly precise radiation therapy techniques enable the treatment of small lesions. Linear accelerators integrated with magnetic resonance imaging (MRI) have revolutionized the field since they facilitate online real-time image-guided radiation dose delivery of moving soft-tissue targets. Herewith, safety margins compensating for repeat patient positioning and target motion can be reduced or even abolished, thus reducing dose to normal tissues and hopefully subsequent side effects.

This book provides the reader with an overview of the value of PET with widely available as well as more exclusive, tumour-specific for radiation treatment planning. In-room equipment for online positioning on the linear accelerator is summarized and radiation treatment techniques relying on those imaging possibilities are explained to experts outside the field of radiotherapy. Moreover, the value of MRI for soft-tissue tumours both during the phase of target volume delineation for treatment planning as well as during MR-LINAC treatments is focused on. Brachytherapy of several tumours, such as prostate and gynaecological tumours, heavily depends on MRI, also this is exemplified in one of the chapters. The ample possibilities of ultrasonography for image-guidance are furthermore referred to. In those tumours not well visible on imaging, the use of fiducial markers may play a role—this is described for oesophageal and prostate cancer. Lastly, the use of artificial intelligence, multimodal imaging for prediction of tumour control as well as of normal-tissue side effects are topics of the remaining three chapters.

Together with the authors of the different chapters, I hope that this book will be of value to residents and senior physicians in the fields of radiotherapy, radiology, and nuclear, as well as to the physicists and radiation technologists of the respective disciplines.

Dresden, Sachsen, Germany
April 2022

Esther G. C. Troost

Contents

Part I

Target Volume Definition

Use of [^{18}F]FDG PET/CT for Target Volume Definition in Radiotherapy

1

Johanna E. E. Pouw, Dennis Vriens, Floris H. P. van Velden, and Lioe-Fee de Geus-Oei

Abbreviations

ATLAAS	Automatic decision Tree-based Learning Algorithm for Advanced Segmentation
ATP	Adenosine-5′-TriPhosphate

The original version of the chapter was revised. A correction to this chapter can be found at https://doi.org/10.1007/978-3-031-08601-4_14

J. E. E. Pouw (✉)
Section of Nuclear Medicine, Department of Radiology, Leiden University Medical Center (LUMC), Leiden, The Netherlands

HollandPTC, Delft, The Netherlands

Department of Medical Oncology, Amsterdam UMC location Vrije Universiteit Amsterdam, Amsterdam, The Netherlands
e-mail: J.E.E.Pouw@amsterdamumc.nl

D. Vriens
Section of Nuclear Medicine, Department of Radiology, Leiden University Medical Center (LUMC), Leiden, The Netherlands

HollandPTC, Delft, The Netherlands
e-mail: D.Vriens@lumc.nl

F. H. P. van Velden
Section of Nuclear Medicine, Department of Radiology, Leiden University Medical Center (LUMC), Leiden, The Netherlands
e-mail: F.H.P.van_Velden@lumc.nl

L.-F. de Geus-Oei
Section of Nuclear Medicine, Department of Radiology, Leiden University Medical Center (LUMC), Leiden, The Netherlands

Biomedical Photonic Imaging Group, University of Twente, Enschede, The Netherlands
e-mail: L.F.de_Geus-Oei@lumc.nl

E. G. C. Troost (ed.), *Image-Guided High-Precision Radiotherapy*,
https://doi.org/10.1007/978-3-031-08601-4_1

CT	X-ray Computed Tomography
CTAC	(low dose) CT performed for Attenuation- and scatter Correction of the PET-image
CT-TV	CT-only based Target Volume
CTV	Clinical Target Volume
EANM	European Association of Nuclear Medicine
EARL	EANM Research Ltd.
EORTC	European Organisation for Research and Treatment of Cancer
ESTRO	European SocieTy for Radiotherapy and Oncology
FBP	Filtered Backprojection Reconstruction Algorithm
[^{18}F]FDG	2-[^{18}F]fluoro-2-deoxy-D-Glucose
GTV	Gross Tumour Volume
HNSCC	Head-and-Neck Squamous Cell Carcinoma
LOR	Line-Of-Response
MRI	Magnetic Resonance Imaging
NSCLC	Non-Small Cell Lung Carcinoma
OAR	Organs At Risk
OSEM	Ordered Subsets Expectation Maximisation reconstruction algorithm
PET	Positron Emission Tomography
PET-AS	Automatic Segmentation of contours in PET
PET-TV	PET(/CT)-based Target Volume
Planning-CT	(High dose, contrast-enhanced) CT performed for radio therapy treatment planning purpose
PTV	Planning Target Volume
STAPLE	Simultaneous Truth and Performance Level Estimate
SUV	Standardised Uptake Value
SCLC	Small Cell Lung Carcinoma

1.1 Introduction

High-precision radiotherapy is of increasing importance in oncological treatment, by striving for higher effectiveness and decreasing side effects by more conformal dose delivery. This can be accomplished by new X-ray photon radiotherapy techniques, including volumetric-modulated arc therapy (Chap. 5) and intrafraction adaptation using the magnetic resonance-based linear accelerator (Chaps. 6 and 7), by particle therapy (protons, carbon ions; Chap. 10), or by highly precise target volume definition, which will be the focus of the current chapter.

Different phases can be distinguished in the development of a treatment plan. First, accurate information about the localisation and extension of the tumour volume, with respect to its surroundings, should be obtained, the so-called gross tumour volume (GTV). This information is obtained by a combination of different diagnostic methods, including physical examination (visual inspection, palpation), medical imaging [endoscopy, (endo)ultrasonography, computed tomography (CT), magnetic resonance imaging (MRI), and positron emission tomography (PET)], and cytology or histopathology. Second, the information of these different modalities needs to be properly co-registered to the CT scan used for treatment planning purposes. Third, the target volumes are defined on the planning CT: GTV is defined as the tumour visible (or palpable) on physical examination or imaging. The clinical target volume (CTV) takes into account the microscopic tumour extension and the planning target volume (PTV) includes additionally systematic and random setup inaccuracies, resulting in the volume to be irradiated. These margins make the planning more reliable, but also account for a smaller therapeutic window [1]. The definitions of the target volumes are defined in International Commission on Radiation Units and Measurements (ICRU) Report 50 [2]. Also, the organs at risk (OAR), in which the radiation dose is to be maximally reduced, are segmented on the images. Finally, a treatment plan is generated, taking into account geometric (e.g. motion, patient setup-variability) and physical (e.g. particle range) uncertainties.

Image contrast in the planning-CT, which is ideally acquired in radiotherapy position, is determined by differences in photon attenuation of various tissues and thereby delivers anatomical (geometrical) information. The (semi)quantitative information on photon attenuation can be used to estimate the behaviour of high-energy photons in human tissues and thus to reliably calculate radiation treatment plans. CT, however, suffers from limited soft-tissue contrast, which can for a limited extent be overcome by the addition of intravenous iodinated contrast media. Additional imaging by other imaging modalities can assist in more accurate segmentation of the target volume. MRI is based on a different physical property of tissues: its nuclear magnetic spin resonance. Conventional MRI-sequences result in anatomical images of higher soft tissue contrast, compared to CT, but might, just as CT, be flawed by artefacts including magnetic susceptibility (metal implants), geometrical distortions, motion and flow (perfusion).

PET provides biological information of the tumours and organs at risk, which can be co-registered to the anatomical domain of CT or MRI. Current standard-of-care is the combination of PET with CT. Although PET/MRI is currently available, clinical application in radiotherapy planning is not yet widely implemented due to technical challenges, such as accurate MRI-based attenuation correction of the PET-images (see later) and geometrical distortions of the MRI [3–5]. Which biological information is obtained by PET-imaging depends on the administered radiopharmaceutical ("tracer"). This chapter will cover the use of the most widely used PET-radiopharmaceutical 2-[^{18}F]fluoro-2-deoxy-D-glucose ([^{18}F]FDG). The usage of this specific radiopharmaceutical can be assumed when PET is mentioned in the remainder of this chapter. Chapter 2 will cover the use of PET tracers beyond [^{18}F]FDG.

To gain insight into the additional value of PET in target volume delineation (TVD), first, the basic principles of PET/CT and the radiopharmaceutical [^{18}F]FDG will be discussed, followed by the image acquisition and reconstruction techniques, including methods for motion control ("Technical Aspects"). The role of [^{18}F]FDG PET/CT in tumour volume and lymph node segmentation, together with its value in different disease sites will be discussed in "Target volume delineation". The influence of the applied segmentation method is discussed in "PET/CT segmentation methods" and the risks and disadvantages of the application of PET will be highlighted in section "Cons and pitfalls". The chapter will end with a future perspective on the role of [^{18}F]FDG PET/CT in treatment planning.

Out of the scope of this chapter is the established role of [^{18}F]FDG PET/CT in determining the extent of different oncological diseases (staging), the use of

[^{18}F]FDG PET/CT as prognostic biomarker and predictor of treatment response and its role in detection of tumour recurrence after treatment (follow-up).

1.2 [^{18}F]FDG PET/CT

1.2.1 PET/CT

The unstable nucleus of the isotope bound to the radiopharmaceutical, fluorine-18 in the case of [^{18}F]FDG, emits a positron ($ß^+$) when it decays. This positron will slow down in the tissue around its origin and will interact with any of the electrons (e^-) in the tissue within a few millimetres from its origin. As positrons are the anti-particles of electrons, collision of positrons and electrons will result in disappearance of both particles, so-called annihilation, releasing energy in the form of two (nearly) anti-parallel 511 keV photons. By detecting these coincident, paired photons with a PET-camera, a line can be derived on where the annihilation took place, a so-called line-of-response (LOR). When enough LORs are measured, the origin of the annihilation can be retraced using a reconstruction algorithm, resulting in the spatial distribution of the radiopharmaceutical, i.e. a PET-image (Fig. 1.1). Most current PET/CT scanners have time-of-flight capabilities that can register the arrival time of each of both photons on a detector separately, allowing further localisation (with a certain probability) of the point of annihilation on the LOR. Current clinical scanners have time-of-flight coincidence timing resolutions below 210 ps, translating to a position uncertainty of less than 31.5 mm [6].

The magnitude of the signal depends on the number of degradations observed by the camera. This in turn is dependent on the concentration of the radiopharmaceutical, thus the pharmacokinetics of the injected radiopharmaceutical and the probability that a photon-pair is detected by the PET camera. The latter is, apart from detector sensitivity and scanner geometry, mainly limited by photon absorption (attenuation) in the tissue that both annihilation photons have to traverse before reaching the detector ring, which can be measured by CT. Therefore, for the purpose of attenuation correction and anatomical localisation, a low-dose CT is performed, usually immediately prior to PET-acquisition.

In order to obtain images of acceptable image quality, sufficient LORs need to be measured and, therefore, whole-body PET-acquisition is a time-consuming process, typically in the order of 15-30 min, to keep the injected amount of radiopharmaceutical, and thus the effective radiation dose for the patient, within reasonable limits.

1.2.2 [^{18}F]FDG

The most frequently used radiopharmaceutical for PET-imaging is [^{18}F]FDG [7]. The isotope ^{18}F mainly (96.9%) decays by $ß^+$-emission, with a decay half-life of 109.7 min and a maximum (mean) positron energy of 634 (250) keV. The resulting maximum (mean) positron range in water is 2.4 (0.6) mm before the annihilation, localised by PET/CT, takes place [8].

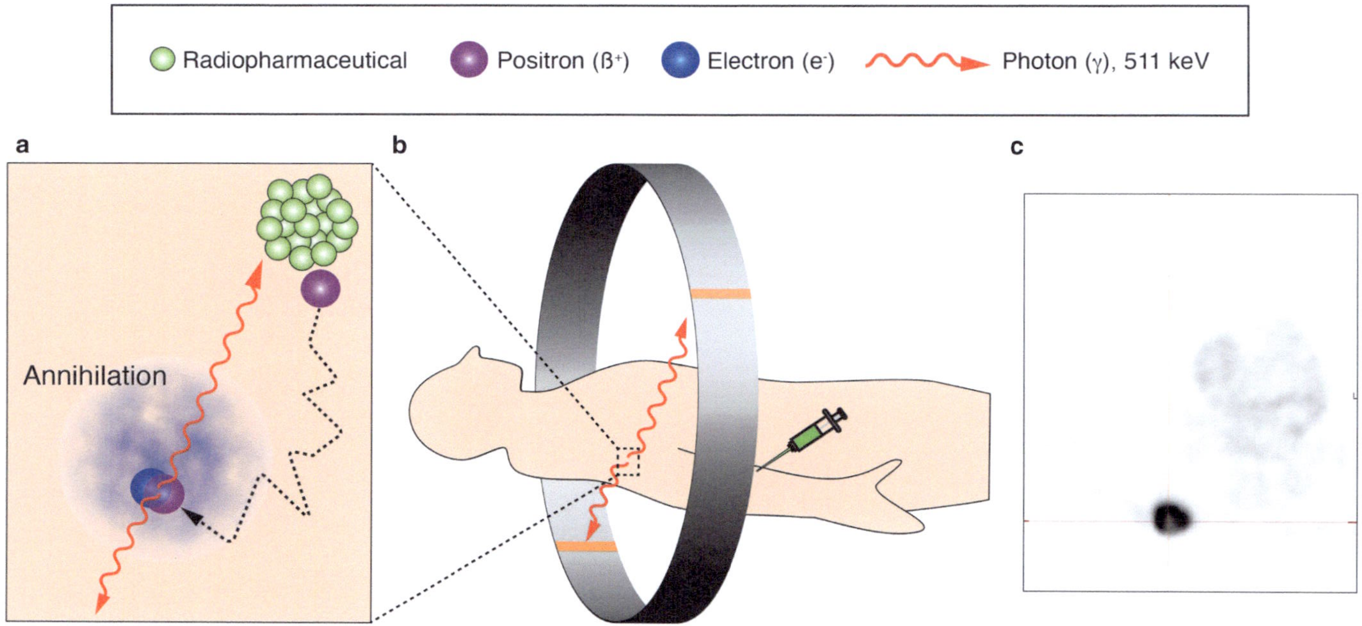

Fig. 1.1 The formation of a PET-image. (**a**) Electron–positron annihilation in the body within a few mm from the location of the radiopharmaceutical, resulting in two nearly antiparallel 511 keV photons. (**b**) Coincidence detection of the paired annihilation photons by the PET detector. (**c**) Example of an attenuation and scatter corrected PET-image, visualising a non-small cell lung carcinoma

[18F]FDG is a radiopharmaceutical analogue to glucose. [18F]FDG is transported by the blood stream, freely passes the vessel wall and extravascular extracellular space similar to D-glucose, the natural occurring form of glucose. There it is actively transported over the cellular membrane mainly by the sodium-dependent glucose transporter molecule family and is subsequently phosphorylated to [18F]FDG-6-phosphate by the hexokinase enzyme family in the cytosol. For both [18F]FDG and D-glucose the kinetics of these processes are nearly identical. Glucose-6-phosphate is catabolised to fructose-6-phosphate in the glycolysis pathway and eventually to two molecules of pyruvate. However, the enzyme responsible for this chemical reaction is not sensitive to [18F]FDG-6-phosphate. As a result, [18F]FDG-6-phosphate cannot be degraded further and, as dephosphorylation does not occur in most mammalian tissues, accumulates in the cells (Fig. 1.2). Therefore, [18F]FDG uptake is

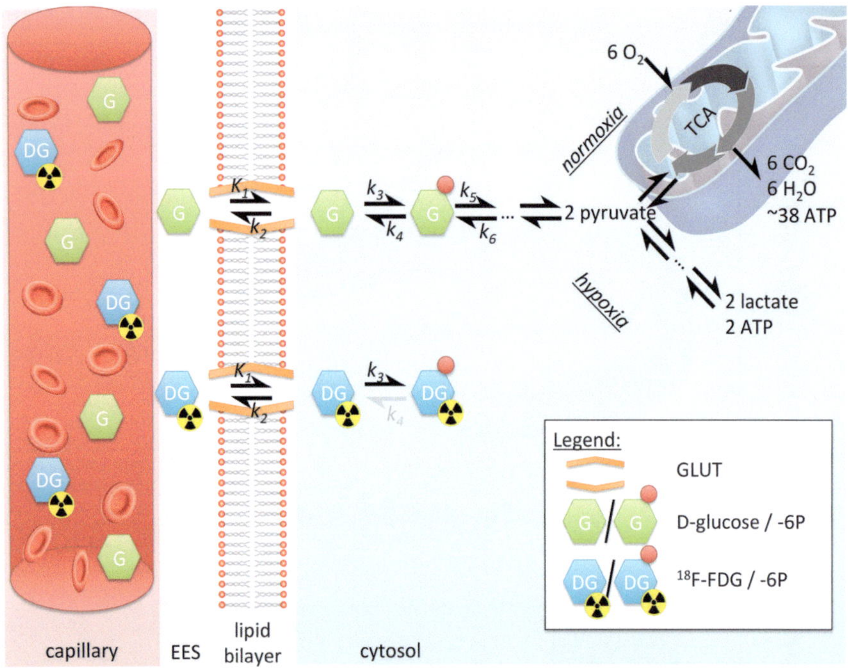

Fig. 1.2 The membrane-bound GLUT receptor family can reversibly transport both D-glucose and [18F]FDG over the lipid bilayer of the cell. In the cytosol both D-glucose and [18F]FDG are 6-phosphorylated by the hexokinase isozymes. In contrast to D-glucose-6-phosphate, [18F]FDG-6-phosphate is not a substrate for the subsequent isomerase enzyme in the glycolytic pathway and, as 6-dephosphorylation hardly occurs in most mammalian tissues, its downstream products cannot enter the TCA-cycle. As a result, [18F]FDG-6-phosphate will time-dependently accumulate in the cytosol, reflecting enzymatic activities and facilitating PET visualisation of high glucose demanding tissues. *ATP* adenosine-5′-triphosphate; CO_2 carbon dioxide; *EES* extravascular extracellular space; *[18F]FDG* 2-[18F]fluoro-2-deoxy-D-glucose; *GLUT* facilitative membrane-bound sodium-independent glucose transporters; H_2O water; K_1–k_6 equilibrium Michaelis-Menten rate constants; O_2 oxygen; *TCA* tricarboxylic acid (or Krebs) cycle. *Adapted from ISBN13/EAN 978-94-6108-927-4 (ch.1, p.xxii)* *© 2015 Dennis Vriens. All Rights Reserved*

increased in tissues with high glucose metabolism, often the case in brain and myocardium, but also in cancerous lesions and inflammatory conditions.

Tumour cells acquire their adenosine-5′-triphosphate (ATP), the energy carrier necessary for mitosis, from the inefficient anaerobic glycolysis, i.e. from pyruvate to lactate instead of mitochondrial oxidative phosphorylation, i.e. from pyruvate to carbon dioxide, even when oxygen is plentiful. The former yields 18–19x less ATP than the latter. Due to this so-called Warburg effect, higher D-glucose metabolism is required for sufficient ATP availability. This glucose demand is further increased by the high cell proliferation [9].

1.3 Technical Aspects

To obtain high-quality images and to prevent large inter-investigation variability, standardised patient preparation and image acquisition and reconstruction are of uttermost importance. To ensure high-quality images and to overcome inter-investigational variability in PET imaging, procedure guidelines are defined by the European Association of Nuclear Medicine (EANM) [10] and monitored for multicentre [^{18}F]FDG PET/CT study purposes in the EANM Research Ltd. (EARL) accreditation programme [11].

1.3.1 Patient Preparation

To ensure proper visualisation of the regions of interest, [^{18}F]FDG should specifically accumulate in the regions of interest. Uptake of [^{18}F]FDG should be prevented in non-malignant tissues, such as active muscles and brown fat, by proper patient preparation. Patients should refrain from strenuous muscle activity before [^{18}F]FDG-injection and from any muscle activity after [^{18}F]FDG-injection. To prevent uptake in thermogenic brown-adipose tissue and muscle uptake by shivering, the resting period after injection of the radiopharmaceutical takes place in a warm environment. A stable normoglycaemic, hypoinsulinaemic situation should be strived for by injecting [^{18}F]FDG only in patients who fasted for at least 4–6 h, are normoglycaemic (generally a serum glucose up to 11.1 mmol/L (i.e. 200 mg/dl) is accepted) and have not been injected with short-acting insulins for at least 4 h. Adequate hydration and voiding directly prior to PET/CT acquisition ensure fast clearance of the radiopharmaceutical and thus decrease dose to the patients, and prevent artefacts around the kidneys, ureters and urinary bladder. When the area to be imaged is located near the bladder, diuretic medication can be administered to further stimulate the emptying of the bladder during acquisition. To prevent metal artefacts, the patients are asked to remove all metal objects [10].

1.3.2 Image Acquisition and Reconstruction

After acquisition of the raw PET-data, reconstruction can be performed by mainly two methods, namely filtered backprojection (FBP) and iterative reconstruction. In FBP, the LORs are literally backprojected to recalculate the position of the [^{18}F]FDG-containing structure. Currently, the most commonly applied reconstruction technique in the clinical setting is iterative reconstruction. This method outperforms FBP by its high signal-to-noise ratio, the exclusion of counts outside the field of view and the multiple correction options within the reconstruction, e.g. time-of-flight correction.

These advantages most often outweigh the computational intensiveness of the reconstruction and the unpredictability of the nonlinear method. Iterative reconstruction is an iterative process of adjusting an estimated image, and is based on the difference between the estimated image of the projection data with the measured projection data. The most well-known example of iterative reconstruction is the ordered subsets expectation maximisation algorithm (OSEM), where the computational intensiveness is decreased by using only a subset of the projection angles in every iteration. This process is repeated over all subsets to ulimately perform one true iteration of OSEM [12]. A more extensive, but accessible, explanation of the reconstruction methods can be found in Cherry et al. [12].

Before reconstructing the raw PET-data, corrections need to be applied for several physical factors to obtain a true reflection of the radioactivity distribution of the radiopharmaceutical. The most important corrections are variations in coincidence detection efficiency between the different LORs (normalisation), dead time of the detector after a coincidence, random coincidence photons, scattered coincidence photons, and absorbed (attenuated) coincidence photons. As explained before, a low dose CT, acquired without contrast and often prior to PET-acquisition, is used for the attenuation correction of these coincidences and is also called the attenuation correction CT (CTAC). The amount of attenuation of 511 KeV annihilation photons depends on the (electron) density of the tissue. The photons will be more attenuated when passing through denser material, i.e. components with higher Hounsfield units, or when traversing more material, i.e. a larger body part [13].

1.3.3 Fusion and Registration of Treatment Planning PET/CT

1.3.3.1 Registration PET with CTAC

For correct anatomical localisation and attenuation- and scatter correction, the (low dose) CTAC and the PET need to be spatially aligned. Spatial mismatch between the PET and the CTAC results in incorrect attenuation correction and thereby scatter correction. This incorrect correction causes over- or underestimation of activity concentrations of the radiopharmaceutical (i.e. intensity), which is used to define the boundaries of the target volume on PET. Therefore, inaccurate attenuation- and scatter correction, due to spatial mismatch, also leads to inadequate information for target volume delineation.

Currently, all clinical PET/CT-scanners are dual-modality imaging devices, where the hardware accurately aligns the images of PET and CT, provided that no patient movement between the CTAC-acquisition and PET-acquisition has occurred. When (a large amount of) patient movement has occurred, PET and CT images have to be co-registered after acquisition, by translation, rotation and rescaling (rigid transformations) or by image deformation (non-rigid or elastic transformations), briefly summarised as "image registration" [14].

1.3.3.2 Registration PET(/CT) with Planning-CT

Biological information from the PET-image can be used for treatment planning by fusing either a staging PET or, preferably, a PET in treatment position with the high-dose and often contrast-enhanced planning-CT. In case of spatial mismatch between the PET and the planning-CT, improper functional-anatomical co-localisation may occur, resulting in inaccurate target volume definition. This can be overcome by manual co-registration focussing on the GTV and thus the volume planned to receive the high radiation dose. If misalignment persists, target volume coverage may be compromised, increasing the risk of geometrical miss. Therefore, the registration needs to be verified by an experienced radiation oncologist.

Imaging on different modalities increases the chance of inaccurate fusion by differences in time frames, patient position and coordinate systems [15]. Acquisition of both scans on the same machine and preferably at the same time would, therefore, minimise the spatial mismatch, but is often not realistic in clinical practice. When the planning-CT is obtained on the PET-system, this PET/CT-system needs to fulfil the quality assurance for treatment planning and thus needs to be regularly checked for its technical specifications, such as table rigidity and levelness, accurate laser alignment, and CT image matrix alignment [16]. Due to these additional, frequent quality controls on the one hand and device capacity on the other, multiple institutions use a stand-alone CT-scanner, instead of a hybrid PET/CT to perform a planning-CT.

The PET/CT for clinical diagnosis and staging purposes (*staging* PET/CT) is often one of the first steps in the clinical work-up before the decision for treatment modality has been made. Therefore, this staging PET/CT is not performed in radiotherapy position. A *staging* PET/CT is usually performed on a soft curved table top, while *treatment planning* scans are performed on a hard, rigid, flat radiotherapy table top, identical to the radiotherapy setting. The position of the patient during a staging PET/CT is optimised for both patient comfort and image quality, e.g. with a cushioned head rest and with the arms elevated, to prevent thorax imaging artefacts by beam hardening and truncation. Patient-positioning during treatment planning PET/CT is optimised for reproducibility and radiation-beam arrangement avoiding dose in body parts not belonging to the target volume, e.g. arms in thoracic tumours. Therefore, rigid transformations cannot fully compensate for the patient position differences. Software to deformably register staging PET/CTs with a planning-CT is currently commercially available and shows potential improvement in alignment, even in case of preoperative PET/CT with a postoperative CT [17–22]. The staging PET, however, can only be used for radiotherapy planning when performed shortly before start of radiotherapy. This is a pre-requisite to prevent disease progression in the meantime, resulting in understaging and undertreatment of the disease [23, 24].

1.3.4 Motion

Patient movement complicates accurate co-registration between the PET and the CTAC, and between the PET(/CT) and the planning-CT, with the above-described consequences. The effect on attenuation and thereby scatter correction, will especially be large in moving tumours at the interface of two types of tissue with large differences in Hounsfield units (photon attenuation), for example, the lower part of the lung and the liver dome around the diaphragm [25]. Motion also negatively influences the PET-image, when occurring during the relatively lengthy PET-acquisition itself, since it causes image-blurring, i.e. an overestimation of the volume of pathological radiopharmaceutical uptake and an underestimation of the concentration of radiopharmaceutical.

1.3.4.1 Types of Motion

Motion can be divided into external patient motion (e.g. rotation of the head, opening of the jaw) or internal target motion (e.g. bladder filling, diaphragm motion during breathing, bowel motion).

External patient motion is mostly non-repetitive and effectuated by skeletal muscles innervated by the somatic nervous system. It can be *bulky*, for example, when the whole body or a full extremity is moved, which can be minimised using fixation devices and patient instruction. External patient motion can be more challenging in patients who are not able to cooperate in minimising motion, e.g. very young patients, patients with reduced mental capacities, who may require sedation. External patient motion can also be *compact* such as uncontrollable tremor as a result of, e.g. Parkinson's disease.

Internal target motion is mostly involuntary, *periodic* or oscillatory in nature and is caused by autonomic (mainly sympathetic) nerve innervation of effector muscles, such as the myocardium and respiratory muscles, including the diaphragm. *Aperiodic* involuntary internal target motion, such as bowel motion, bladder filling or, at least partly, eye movement, should also be taken into account. Most forms of internal target motion are unpreventable and require special measures to deal with.

Methods to compensate for motion during the PET-acquisition will be highlighted here. Methods to compensate during the radiotherapy fraction itself are outlined elsewhere.

1.3.4.2 Motion Correction Methods

Alignment

Minimising spatial mismatch *between* scans and irradiation is achieved by performing all image acquisitions and the treatment in highly similar (i.e. reproducible), position (preferably radiotherapy position), with respect to the internal coordinate system (isocentre) of the scanners and treatment gantry. Accurate alignment can be achieved with the help of external lasers and skin (tattoo) markers. To prevent deformations, immobilising devices can be helpful. These immobilising devices can be *personalised*, for example, thermoplastics masks, bite blocks, and some headrests, or *generic*, such as overlay beds, bands, strap restraints, sand bags, shoulder depressors, head clamps, etc. Evaluation of the position directly before the start of a radiotherapy fraction and directly afterwards can be achieved by online imaging, where the 2D or 3D generated radiographic images, optional including fiducial markers, are compared with the planning-CT and its 2D digital reconstructed radiographs [26].

Minimising patient motion *during* acquisition can largely be achieved by clear patient instructions, starting with an understandable explanation of the importance of motionlessness. Moreover, immobilising devices could improve the compliance. Patients with postural pain despite adequate analgesia may be helped with reduced acquisition time, which can be compensated for with higher injected dose of the radiopharmaceutical to avoid deterioration of image quality (generally: halving acquisition time requires doubling the radiopharmaceutical dose). Alternatively, unconventional positioning can be attempted, but this will severely hamper the use of these images for radiotherapy planning. When the target volume is located near the bladder or urethra, for example, in rectum or cervix carcinoma, spatial mismatch can arise between the PET and CT, due to bladder filling between both acquisitions. For this purpose, imaging is generally performed directly after voiding and the CTAC is acquired craniocaudally followed by the PET caudocranially, to keep the time interval between PET and CT in the pelvic area as short as possible. In very anxious patients, benzodiazepines can be prescribed or even sedatives can be administered.

Respiratory motion-induced interplay effects contribute most to intra-acquisitional and intrafractional motion of breast, lung, liver and pancreatic tumours, due to the period of normal breathing (2–5 s/breath) with respect to the duration of PET-acquisition (2–5 min per bed position) or a therapeutic fraction (20–40 s per beam angle) [27]. The contemporary methods to compensate for respiratory motion will therefore be discussed separately in the next paragraph.

Compensation Methods for Respiratory Motion

Methods to control respiratory motion can be divided into four motion-encompassing categories. The first category exists of external compression methods, such as the abdominal compression technique, where an external device applies pressure on the abdomen, to minimise motion in the diaphragm. These methods are especially useful for tumours close to the diaphragm, e.g. liver dome and lower lung lobes [28].

The second category contains *controlled breathing methods*, i.e. instead of free breathing, instructions are provided to the patient to hold their breath on a specific moment in the respiratory cycle or to force shallow breathing. An automatic breath control device, used in the active breathing control-technique, can also be used to regulate the respiratory cycle.

By *respiratory gating*, being the third motion-encompassing category, the respiratory cycle is measured. The longest period in the respiratory cycle where the least thoracic volume changes occur is determined and the corresponding frames in the list-mode acquired PET-data are used for reconstruction, resulting in a 'frozen image'. This gating method generally requires longer acquisition of thorax and upper abdomen bed positions, since only a part of the acquired data is used for image reconstruction, making it a lossy technique. Newer techniques are able to only acquire PET-data at the usable moments in the respiratory cycle.

The last motion-encompassing method uses the PET-data itself for gating purposes and, therefore, requires no additional hardware. *Data-driven gating* defines an optimal binning strategy by principle component analysis. It encompasses the elastic deformation of the images post-acquisition. With this technique all acquired data are used during image reconstruction and it is, therefore, called a lossless technique [29]. Correction of lesion-specific motion seems possible by the positron emission particle tracking technique combined with time of flight information, but its clinical added value currently still needs to be determined [30].

One should keep in mind that the result of motion mitigation used for PET should match that of either CTAC and treatment-CT to prevent spatial functional-anatomical mismatch with all earlier mentioned disadvantages. Apart from the technical possibilities, one should consider the clinical value of motion compensation. When no motion compensation will be applied during the delivery of radiotherapy, motion correction during PET/CT- and treatment planning-CT-acquisition might be undesired. Therefore, some institutions use the ungated CT images for treatment planning. Using magnetic resonance-based linear accelerator for radiotherapy, intrafractional adjustment of the treatment plan to motion is possible (Chaps. 6 and 7).

1.4 Target Volume Delineation

1.4.1 PET/CT in Target Volume Delineation

Adding biological PET/CT-information, sometimes addressed to as biological or metabolic target volume, to the planning-CT could be helpful to clarify the nature (benign versus malignant) of a tumour difficult to differentiate on solely CT. It is assumed that in some tumour or scenarios tumour borders can be defined more sharply, by more clearly differentiating malignant from non-malignant tissue (e.g. post-obstructive atelectasis), by distinguishing ambiguous lymph nodes, and by differentiating residual or recurrent disease from post-treatment scar tissue [31–33]. The addition of PET/CT in TVD has shown to lower interobserver variability in several disease sites, compared to CT-based delineation [34–37]. The added value of PET/CT target volume delineation depends on, e.g., the applied segmentation

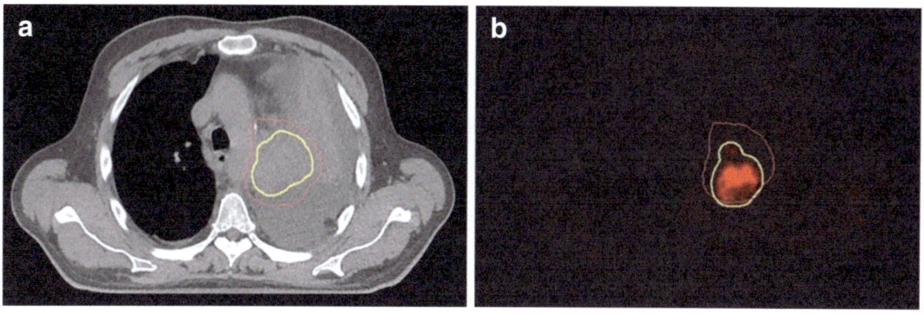

Fig. 1.3 (**a**) The target volume (GTV based on CT in yellow and CTV in red) in a non-small cell lung cancer patient delineated on CT only, (**b**) the target volume delineated with the additional information of [^{18}F]FDG PET/CT (GTV based on PET in yellow, same CTV in red)

technique and tumour location and type, which will be discussed in the following sections. In the remainder of this chapter, the PET(/CT)- and planning-CT-based target volumes are referred to as PET-TV and CT-TV, respectively. A comparison between a PET-TV and a CT-TV is provided in Fig. 1.3.

1.4.2 PET/CT Segmentation Methods

1.4.2.1 Manual, Semi-Automatic and Automatic Segmentation Methods

The contoured target volumes depend on the used segmentation method, which classifies the voxels of an image as either being malignant or non-malignant [38]. There are multiple segmentation methods under development, with different levels of complexity and intuitiveness.

Manual tumour segmentation, still most common in clinical practice, is based on visual inspection of the spatial [^{18}F]FDG-distribution, combined with the available anatomical information. This method requires interpretation, which makes it extremely prone to observer variability. Standardised instructions are therefore desired. Recommendations are given in head and neck squamous cell carcinoma (HNSCC) by Lee et al. [39] and Schinagl et al. [40].

However, since radiation treatment planning is still based on anatomical CT-imaging, PET ought to be seen as additional source of information on the GTV, not as a replacement of CT.

As PET is a quantitative imaging modality, alternative *(semi)automatic tumour segmentation* approaches have been developed which have shown to be more reproducible than manual delineation. Those methods are described next.

Thresholding is, after manual delineation, the most applied and intuitive approach in clinical practice. Multiple techniques have been proposed to determine the optimal threshold intensity value of a quantitative PET-parameter to discern benign from malignant voxels. The most often used semi-quantitative PET-parameter is the standardised uptake value (SUV). This is the activity-concentration in a voxel (in

Bq/mL) normalised for administered activity of the radiopharmaceutical per unit patient bodyweight (in Bq/g). This threshold can be set as an absolute threshold (e.g. SUV $\geq$ 2.5 g/ml) or related to the mean, peak or maximum intensity in the lesion (e.g. SUV $\geq 50\% \cdot SUV_{max}$). Alternatively, an internal reference is used, such as the lesion-to-background ratio. It is likely that the optimal threshold value depends on tumour location (background, movement) and tumour size (with respect to PET-scanner resolution). A clear outline of multiple threshold value formulas is provided by Zaidi et al. [41].

A less intuitive category of segmentation methods, *variational methods*, is based on spatial intensity variation between the foreground and the background. Examples are edge and ridge detection methods, such as Sobel operators and Watershed transformations, or active contouring methods. Drever et al. [42] provide a comprehensive comparison between the Sober, Watershed and thresholding approaches for PET TVD. An active contouring method, better known as a snake, is a spline, a function defined by multiple polynomial sub-functions, which incorporates prior knowledge, e.g. smoothness and shape, to deform around the object. Active contouring makes subpixel contouring possible [43, 44]. These variational segmentation methods are complicated due to their sensitivity to image noise, especially in case of gradient-based methods and when the lesion is surrounded by metabolic active areas [15, 45, 46].

Segmentation can also be performed by a *pattern recognition learning approach*, also known as machine learning. A distinction should be made between *classification* in case of supervised learning on the one hand, i.e. when the nature (benign vs malignant) of each voxel is known, and *clustering* by unsupervised learning on the other hand. Both techniques are based on the extraction of features from the image. Classification is widely applied in other imaging modalities, but may be hampered in PET by the large heterogeneity in tumour uptake. Clustering, on the contrary, seems valuable in target segmentation in PET. The most simple and common clustering method is the k-means-algorithm, encompassing a ‘hard’ boundary that includes every voxel in one of the two clusters, ‘tumour’ or ‘no tumour’. The centres of the clusters are initialised and updated during the algorithm, until the final clustering is retrieved. The boundaries can also be soft, allowing uncertain voxels to be probabilistic part of both clusters, which is synonymised as fuzzy. Examples of these soft boundary clustering methods are fuzzy k-means or fuzzy C-means algorithms. These computational complex learning methods, especially supervised learning, can provide much flexibility, but can also be challenging and counterintuitive [39, 47].

Within the increasingly popular field of radiomics, a large number of imaging features are extracted, which may contribute to the TVD, especially in learning segmentation [48–50]. By using a deep learning approach, features can be extracted automatically. Huang et al. [51] and Guo et al. [52] contoured the GTV of HNSCC patients on PET/CT-images accurately and with high efficiency with a deep neural network, compared to more conventional segmentation methods. The gold standard was considered manual contouring.

The last category of segmentation methods, *statistical image segmentation*, differentiates between tumour uptake and surrounding tissue by probabilistic calculation and estimation of the data. This stochastic modelling approach deals well with high noise PET-data, but is at risk of local optimal solutions in the optimisation. An example is the Gaussian mixture model, which handles the intensities as independent and Gaussian distributed. This dependency is not necessary in the usage of hidden Markov models, another statistical segmentation method [53]. Hatt et al. [54, 55] improved the segmentation of small and/or heterogeneous lesions with the statistical segmentation algorithm fuzzy locally adaptive Bayesian.

Shepherd et al. [56] performed a double-blind comparative study for 30 different and combined segmentation techniques in 2012, from manual to full automatic and concluded that up to then, manual segmentation outperformed all the (semi-)automatic delineation methods in highest overall accuracy. An overview of the PET-segmentation methods can be found in Zaidi et al. [41] and Hatt et al. [54].

1.4.2.2 Drawback of Segmentation Methods

Although manual segmentation is still most commonly performed in clinical practice, it shows a higher interobserver variability than the application of (semi-) automatic segmentation methods [41]. The accuracy of manual segmentation depends on the experience and expertise of the observer and proposes the risk of observer overrating. Rasch et al. [57] showed that updating the PET-TV defined by the treating physician with the assessment of 5–7 radiation oncologists and a radiologist leads to an alteration in 45% of the cases. Manual delineation and especially in agreement of multiple experts, preferably both radiation oncologists and medical imaging specialists, is labour-intensive and hardly feasible in current high demanding-high throughput oncology healthcare. Therefore, the development of a reliable automatic PET segmentation method (PET-AS) is desired. Automatic segmentation of PET-only data is currently under development, although automatic PET segmentation with CT-data outperforms automatic PET-only segmentation, with the disadvantage of increased complexity. For application of PET-AS, the algorithms should be accurate and precise under different clinical circumstances. Unfortunately, none of the currently existing algorithms fulfils all needs [48].

1.4.2.3 Consensus Algorithms

The success of multiple segmentation algorithms is strived to be combined by two new methods: the Majority Vote and Simultaneous Truth And Performance Level Estimate (STAPLE) method with their variances. The first method decides whether a voxel is included in the target volume, based on the outcome of the majority of the methods. The latter estimates the segmentation result, based on a probability distribution function of multiple separate segmentation methods and their performance [58]. McGurk et al. [59] compared both consensus methods in five (semi-) automatic PET segmentation algorithms and concluded that both Majority Vote and STAPLE were robust and more accurate for all separate segmentation methods in different experimental circumstances. Schaefer et al. [60] and Dewalle-Vignion et al. [61] confirmed these findings, the latter for STAPLE in semi-clinical setting, including comparison with manual segmentation.

Berthon et al. [62] developed a third consensus method: the supervised machine learning algorithm Automatic decision Tree-based Learning Algorithm for Advanced Segmentation (ATLAAS), which includes a decision tree model to select the most appropriate of 9 automatic segmentation methods, instead of combining the results like the earlier described consensus methods. ATLAAS proved robust segmentation with higher accuracy compared to each of the individual segmentation methods in phantom setting and showed promising clinical results in HNSCC PET tumour segmentation [62, 63].

For now, the International Atomic Energy Agency export report, published in 2009 and updated for non-small cell lung carcinoma (NSCLC) in 2019, recommends that target volumes, delineated by a PET-AS technique, as part of standard care, should always be visually checked by an experienced observer [64].

1.4.3 Disease Sites

1.4.3.1 NSCLC and SCLC

Several studies investigated the beneficial effect of PET(/CT) on TVD. Most evidence is available in non-small cell and small cell lung cancer (NSCLC and SCLC), for which Hallqvist et al. [65] performed a systematic review of the role of PET/CT in treatment planning. Their review shows a significant change in PET-TV, compared to CT-TV in approximately 40% of NSCLC patients. Moreover, in 20% of the patients, the intent of the treatment was changed from radical high-dose to palliative low-dose radiotherapy, as a result of upstaging of the tumour. In SCLC, target volume changed in 20% and treatment intention changed in 10% of the cases, when PET is added to the TVD [65]. For both, NSCLC and SCLC, [^{18}F]FDG PET guides the primary tumour contour, in particular in case of atelectasis, even though the tumour boundaries are drawn on the planning-CT in lung window-width/window-level setting. The PET-TV results are only applicable for target volumes defined on PET/CT-images in radiotherapy position, as discussed in 'Technical aspects' and independent of the presence of a staging PET/CT.

De Ruysscher et al. [66] compared PET-TVs with CT-TVs in mediastinal lymph nodes in a treatment planning study and subsequently treated all included NSCLC patients according to the PET-delineated treatment plan in a single-arm prospective clinical trial. The results obtained using the 3D-technique employed at the time showed a low isolated lymph node recurrence rate of 2.3%. Bradley et al. [32] published their findings of the Radiation Therapy Oncology Group study in NSCLC patients. They showed a disagreement of 51% comparing nodal PET-TV with CT-TV, mostly caused by the in- or exclusion of one or two nodal stations. Also in this study, all patients received irradiation according to the PET/CT derived treatment plan. In 2% of the patients, i.e. 1 out of 46 patients, failure occurred in [^{18}F]FDG-negative lymph nodes, not included in the PET-TV, which is stated in this study as quite low. In 2018, the MAASTRO group investigated the validity of [^{18}F]FDG PET-based selective nodal irradiation in the era of Intensity-modulated radiation therapy [67]. They, again, reported on an isolated nodal failure rate of 2.3%. So, since elective nodal irradiation is associated with lower achievable doses and higher side-effects, selective nodal irradiation is to be regarded the standard, also in the era of high conformal irradiation techniques.

In SCLC, again the MAASTRO group published their findings on 60 SCLC patients with limited disease SCLC [68]. They reported on an isolated nodal failure rate of 3%, mainly in the supraclavicular fossa. The selective nodal approach, based on [^{18}F]FDG PET/CT, was subsequently employed in the CONVERT trial, showing no detrimental effects on regional control [69].

The systematic review and meta-analysis of Hallqvist et al. [65] on [^{18}F]FDG PET in NSCLC included no studies with level I evidence, but nonetheless concluded that 'PET/CT for dose planning improves target definition and patient selection' in NSCLC patients. Only in 2020, the PET-PLAN results were published, underlining the results of the meta-analysis as well as recommendations by European Committees (see below). Nestle et al. [70] randomly assigned 205 patients with inoperable advanced stage NSCLC to PET/CT-based target volume including elective nodal irradiation versus PET-based treatment planning, including selective nodal irradiation only. At a follow-up time of 29 months at median, the locoregional progression rate of the [^{18}F]FDG PET-based group was non-inferior, and in fact even lower than that for the conventional target group anticipated in the protocol, and also the toxicity was non-inferior. Thus, the recommendation by the European Organisation for Research and Treatment of Cancer (EORTC) in 2017, that PET/CT is standard for treatment planning in lung cancer holds true, as do the guidelines adopted by the European SocieTy for Radiotherapy and Oncology Advisory Committee in Radiation Oncology Practice (ESTRO) guidelines in 2018 [71], and the Joint EANM/SNMMI/ESTRO practice recommendations for the use of 2-[^{18}F]FDG PET/CT external beam radiation treatment planning in lung cancer V1.0, which was published in March 2022 [72].

1.4.3.2 HNSCC

In HNSCC, various publications have shown the PET-TV to be smaller than those derived by CT or even MRI, when compared to histopathological resection specimen [73–80]. However, since the tumours originate from the oral mucosa and may exhibit superficial tumour spreading not visible on macroscopic imaging, the value of a thorough clinical examination is still high. Therefore, treatment planning solely based on [^{18}F]FDG PET/CT is still not standard of care.

Although Delouya et al. [75] and Chatterjee et al. [81] did not show significant changes in nodal target volume comparing PET-TV with CT-TV, Ciernik et al. [78] showed target volume changes up to approximately 20%, based on the comparison in six patients. Bearing in mind the high incidence of false-positive readings due to reactive lymph nodes in the head and neck region, though, the [^{18}F]FDG PET finding should always carefully be compared to that of the anatomical imaging modality, albeit CT or MRI [82, 83]. Instead, dose de-escalation based on the [^{18}F]FDG PET and CT finding may be investigated, which is at present the objective of a phase II clinical trial [84–86].

In HNSCC, several guidelines recommend the application of [^{18}F]FDG PET in TVD, including those of the National Comprehensive Cancer Network and the International Atomic Energy Agency [87].

1.4.3.3 Oesophageal Cancer

In a prospective study in oesophageal cancer patients, Ng et al. [88] included [^{18}F]FDG-avid disease, not identified by CT, in the PET-TV in 76% of 38 cases. This changed the intent of the treatment from curative to palliative in 24% of 57 cases. Apolle et al. [89] compared the GTV based on [^{18}F]FDG PET with that defined by fiducial markers implanted at the proximal and distal side of the tumour. They concluded that the marker locations corresponded reasonably well with metabolic tumour edges (mean: 5.4 mm more distally). The delineation of the gross nodal volume may substantially change using [^{18}F]FDG PET, as illustrated by Jimenez-Jimenez et al. [90]. The use of PET/CT in the staging and planning of radio(chemo)therapy seems to improve local recurrence-free survival in oesophageal cancer [91]. The value of [^{18}F]FDG PET in oesophageal cancer has recently been extensively reviewed [92, 93].

1.4.3.4 Gynaecological Tumours

In gynaecological oncology, the primary tumour, e.g. of the cervix, is visualised under clinical examination as well as by MRI (mainly T2-weighted imaging). MRI is used for primary staging as well as for brachytherapy planning [94, 95]. However, the value of [^{18}F]FDG PET for diagnosis and radiation treatment planning, mainly in terms of defining the nodal TV, is becoming increasingly apparent [77, 78, 88, 90, 96–99].

1.4.3.5 Lymphoma

The use of [^{18}F]FDG PET/CT for treatment response monitoring and target volume delineation in both, Hodgkin's lymphoma and non-Hodgkin's lymphoma, is unequivocally highly recommended, as described by the International Lymphoma Radiation Oncology Group [77, 100–104].

1.4.3.6 Other Tumours

The use of [^{18}F]FDG-PET/CT for TVD in case of primary brain tumours or prostate cancer is not beneficial. Tracers enabling visualisation and delineation of those solid tumours are discussed in Chap. 2.

It should be kept in mind that the success of PET TVD for nodal contouring depends on its sensitivity and specificity [66, 78, 97]. For regional lymph node detection, a high specificity between 0.90 (NSCLC) and 0.97 (cervical cancer) is typically observed, versus a moderate sensitivity between 0.66 (oesophageal cancer) and 0.84 (HNSCC) [83, 105–110].

1.5 Cons and Pitfalls

In the previous sections, the added value of PET in treatment planning is summarised. There are, however, some considerations that should be kept in mind when applying this technique.

1.5.1 Limited Spatial Resolution and High Signal-to-Noise Ratio of PET

When using PET-imaging for TVD, one must be aware of the technical shortcomings of PET in general, which is shortly discussed in section 'Technical aspects'. PET is restricted by a limited spatial resolution of around 3–5 mm full-width-at-half-maximum. Due to this low spatial resolution compared to anatomical modalities such as CT and MRI, small lesions will be underestimated in activity concentration or might even missed (i.e. false-negative), due to the resulting partial volume effects. The consequences of this effect should be considered in all small, low contrast lesions (typically <2 cm) and depend, amongst others, on the resolution of the PET/CT-scanner, the applied reconstruction algorithm, the post-reconstruction filter and the shape, size, uptake and motion of the lesion [111]. Additional post processing and/or resolution modelling reconstruction algorithms can be applied to correct for partial volume effects up to a certain extent, although the risk of introducing new artefacts should be considered [54].

PET/CT-images can have a low signal-to-noise ratio, dependent of patient- and institution-specific factors. The signal-to-noise ratio is, amongst others, negatively influenced in case of limited radiopharmaceutical uptake, when the injected dose of the radiopharmaceutical is not adjusted to acquisition time (e.g. lossy respiratory gating) or in case of large patient attenuation (high body mass index). The latter might cause lesions to go undetected or treatment planning to become less reproducible. On the contrary, the signal-to-noise ratio is enhanced by improved system geometry (longer bores, whole-body PET-scanners), advanced (digital) detectors and improved reconstruction algorithms (time-of-flight, Bayesian methods, deep learning methods, smaller voxel sizes) [112, 113].

1.5.2 Interpretation Errors Due to Limited Specificity (and Sensitivity) of the Radiopharmaceutical [18F]FDG

Although regions with high [18F]FDG-uptake represent tissues with high glucose-demand, the amount of uptake does not fully depend on the presence and the degree of malignancy. High physiological uptake in healthy tissue or low uptake in tumour tissue can be physiological (e.g. brain, liver, urinary tract) or occur by improper patient preparation (hyperglycaemia, hyperinsulinemia, some drugs, brown adipose tissue). False-positive lesions can be found on PET/CT-images due to influx of inflammatory cells (lymphocytes, macrophages), due to infection (e.g. pneumonia), inflammatory conditions (e.g. sarcoidosis) or after invasive intervention (e.g. biopsy, radiotherapy). Another frequent cause of false-positive lesions are benign lesions such as incidentalomas in the thyroid or intestines, that are misinterpreted as metastases or secondary primaries and often require additional (invasive) diagnostics, potentially leading to unnecessary delay in definite treatment.

The success of lesion detection using [^{18}F]FDG depends on the metabolic profile of the tumour histology as some subtypes are notoriously false-negative (e.g. low-grade tumours such as most neuroendocrine tumours and low-risk prostate cancer or those with much extracellular matrix such as mucinous adenocarcinomas) and its location (i.e. in regions with physiological high background including brain, liver, kidneys and bladder) are other influencing factors. Therefore, the disease-specific sensitivity and specificity of the radiopharmaceutical should be considered. The additional value of PET in nodal delineation is presumably caused by the in- or exclusion of nodal stations, which depends on the error rate. PET's high sensitivity is especially useful in the inclusion of nodal stations in the GTV.

Altogether, it can be stated that lesions for treatment planning should ideally be interpreted jointly by an experienced nuclear medicine physician and radiation oncologist to place the images into context and to minimise the consequences of false-positive or -negative findings [66]. In case of doubt, it is recommended to obtain cytological or histopathological confirmation. This is especially of importance when treatment would change from curative- to palliative intent, due to distant metastases detected by PET.

1.6 Future Outlook

Radiation treatment outcome may be improved by incorporating patient-specific tumour control probability and normal tissue complication probability in the treatment plan, based on [^{18}F]FDG-derived biological information of the tumour and the OAR.

[^{18}F]FDG uptake in lesions, to some extent, reflects sensitivity of the tumour to treatment. Less radiosensitive areas may profit from treatment intensification, e.g. hypoxia modifiers, immunotherapy, or radiation dose escalation. Personalised dose escalation may be beneficial in selected patients (stratification) and/or tumour subvolumes (subvolume boosting, dose painting by contours), even on voxel level (dose painting by numbers).

To study feasibility, toxicity and efficacy of dose escalation in stage III NSCLC patients, the PET-boost trial was initiated in 2010. In this multicentre randomised phase II clinical trial, hypofractionated dose escalation was prospectively studied in both the entire primary tumour (arm A) as in subvolumes of the GTV, defined by increased [^{18}F]FDG uptake (arm B). First, a planning study reported by van Elmpt et al. [114] demonstrated feasibility of dose escalation, both in the entire primary tumour (arm A) as well as in subvolumes of the GTV (arm B). Subsequently, toxicity was tested. Preliminary results are reported by van Diessen et al. [115]. Although increased acute and long-term toxicities were observed in the study, the dose limits of the OAR were maintained. Efficacy results were presented on the World Conference on Lung Cancer 2020 (which took place virtually in January 2021). An excellent local control rate was observed in both hypofractionated dose escalation arms, with a 2-year local failure rate of less than 20% and a regional failure of only 27% [116]. Final results are awaited.

Additional research is required into mechanisms of radioresistance, methods (radiopharmaceuticals, parameters) to adequately quantify radiosensitivity and on techniques to accurately deliver the biologically adapted dose to the patient. The relation between the imaging parameter and dose escalation should also be studied, as well as the necessity of dose escalation (prescription function) [117].

Pre-treatment [^{18}F]FDG PET/CT also provides plenty of information on the surrounding tissue. This information might be useful in predicting toxicity in the surrounding OAR, although limited studies are available yet. Van Dijk et al. [118] showed that pre-treatment high metabolic parotid gland activity is associated with lower risk of developing late xerostomia. Anthony et al. [119] demonstrated that pre-treatment [^{18}F]FDG uptake in combination with CT lung texture features in low-, medium-, and high-dose regions, could predict the risk of radiation pneumonitis in lung cancer patients. Zschaeck et al. showed that [^{18}F]FDG PET uptake in normal tissue within irradiated HNSCC [120] and oesophageal cancer [121] during treatment is a prognostic factor for local tumour control. Besides these promising studies, more research should be performed to analyse whether [^{18}F]FDG PET image biomarkers (i.e. radiomics) of non-tumorous tissue have predictive potential. The result of van Dijk et al. [118] should be verified in an independent dataset. To verify the findings of Anthony et al. [118], a larger patient population, in varying circumstances, with more positive cases is required.

When the biological information provided by PET/CT of both the tumour and the non-tumorous tissue is integrated in the treatment plan, this may result in a more personalised treatment plan with maximal tumour control probability and minimal normal tissue complication probability.

Acknowledgements We would like to thank dr. C.S. van der Vos for her valuable input, Mr. G. Kracht for the design of Fig. 1.1 and prof. dr. E.G.C. Troost for writing the paragraph on the clinical value of [^{18}F]FDG PET for various tumour sites and for providing Fig. 1.3.

References

1. Chua S. PET/CT in radiotherapy planning. In: Chua S, editor. PET/CT. 1st ed. Berlin: Springer International Publishing; 2017. 78p.
2. International Commission on Radiation UaM. ICRU report 50: prescribing, recording and reporting photon beam therapy 1993;os-26(1):3–38.
3. Winter RM, Leibfarth S, Schmidt H, Zwirner K, Monnich D, Welz S, et al. Assessment of image quality of a radiotherapy-specific hardware solution for PET/MRI in head and neck cancer patients. Radiother Oncol. 2018;128(3):485–91.
4. Thorwarth D, Leibfarth S, Monnich D. Potential role of PET/MRI in radiotherapy treatment planning. Clin Transl Imaging. 2013;1(1):45–51.
5. Paulus DH, Thorwath D, Schmidt H, Quick HH. Towards integration of PET/MR hybrid imaging into radiation therapy treatment planning. Med Phys. 2014;41(7):072505.
6. van Sluis J, de Jong J, Schaar J, Noordzij W, van Snick P, Dierckx R, Borra R, Willemsen A, Boellaard R. Performance characteristics of the digital biograph vision PET/CT system. J Nucl Med. 2019;60(7):1031–6.

7. van der Born D, Pees A, Poot AJ, Orru RVA, Windhorst AD, Vugts DJ. Fluorine-18 labelled building blocks for PET tracer synthesis. Chem Soc Rev. 2017;46(15):4709–73.
8. Conti M, Eriksson L. Physics of pure and non-pure positron emitters for PET: a review and a discussion. EJNMMI Phys. 2016;3(1):8.
9. Vander Heiden MG, Cantley LC, Thompson CB. Understanding the Warburg effect: the metabolic requirements of cell proliferation. Science. 2009;324(5930):1029–33.
10. Boellaard R, Delgado-Bolton R, Oyen WJ, Giammarile F, Tatsch K, Eschner W, et al. FDG PET/CT: EANM procedure guidelines for tumour imaging: version 2.0. Eur J Nucl Med Mol Imaging. 2015;42(2):328–54.
11. Boellaard R, Willemsen AT, Arends B, Visser EP. EARL procedure for assessing PET/CT system specific patient FDG activity preparations for quantitative FDG PET/CT studies. 2014.
12. Cherry SR, Dahlbom M. PET: physics, instrumentation, and scanners. In: Phelps ME, editor. PET: physics, instrumentation, and scanners. New York, NY: Springer; 2006. p. 1–117.
13. Cherry SR, Sorenson JA, Phelps ME. Physics in nuclear medicine. Philadelphia: Elsevier Saunders; 2012.
14. Paulino AC. PET-CT in radiotherapy treatment planning. Amsterdam: Elsevier Health Sciences; 2008.
15. Greco C, Rosenzweig K, Cascini GL, Tamburrini O. Current status of PET/CT for tumour volume definition in radiotherapy treatment planning for non-small cell lung cancer (NSCLC). Lung Cancer. 2007;57(2):125–34.
16. van de TA W, van JA D. PET-CT in radiation treatment planning. In: Database R, editor. Federatie medisch specialisten. Kloosterhof Neer Bv, Netherlands; 2016. p. 716–49. https://libris.nl/BookInfo/GetSample?guid=6df17221-0444-4ee0-b691-c84be878a2d2. https://richtlijnendatabase.nl/gerelateerde_documenten/f/17305/PET-CT%20in%20Radiation%20Treatment%20Planning.pdf
17. Kovalchuk N, Jalisi S, Subramaniam RM, Truong MT. Deformable registration of preoperative PET/CT with postoperative radiation therapy planning CT in head and neck cancer. Radiographics. 2012;32(5):1329–41.
18. Fortin D, Basran PS, Berrang T, Peterson D, Wai ES. Deformable versus rigid registration of PET/CT images for radiation treatment planning of head and neck and lung cancer patients: a retrospective dosimetric comparison. Radiat Oncol. 2014;9:50.
19. Guo Y, Li J, Zhang P, Shao Q, Xu M, Li Y. Comparative evaluation of target volumes defined by deformable and rigid registration of diagnostic PET/CT to planning CT in primary esophageal cancer. Medicine (Baltimore). 2017;96(1):e5528.
20. Hanna GG, De Koste JRVS, Carson KJ, O'Sullivan JM, Hounsell AR, Senan S. Conventional 3D staging PET/CT in CT simulation for lung cancer: impact of rigid and deformable target volume alignments for radiotherapy treatment planning. Br J Radiol. 2011;84(1006):919–29.
21. Hwang AB, Bacharach SL, Yom SS, Weinberg VK, Quivey JM, Franc BL, et al. Can positron emission tomography (PET) or PET/computed tomography (CT) acquired in a nontreatment position be accurately registered to a head-and-neck radiotherapy planning CT? Int J Radiat Oncol Biol Phys. 2009;73(2):578–84.
22. Ward G, Ramasamy S, Sykes JR, Prestwich R, Chowdhury F, Scarsbrook A, et al. Superiority of deformable image co-registration in the integration of diagnostic positron emission tomography-computed tomography to the radiotherapy treatment planning pathway for oesophageal carcinoma. Clin Oncol (R Coll Radiol). 2016;28(10):655–62.
23. Konert T, Vogel W, MacManus MP, Nestle U, Belderbos J, Gregoire V, et al. PET/CT imaging for target volume delineation in curative intent radiotherapy of non-small cell lung cancer: IAEA consensus report 2014. Radiother Oncol. 2015;116(1):27–34.
24. Everitt S, Plumridge N, Herschtal A, Bressel M, Ball D, Callahan J, et al. The impact of time between staging PET/CT and definitive chemo-radiation on target volumes and survival in patients with non-small cell lung cancer. Radiother Oncol. 2013;106(3):288–91.
25. Fin L, Daouk J, Morvan J, Bailly P, El Esper I, Saidi L, et al. Initial clinical results for breath-hold CT-based processing of respiratory-gated PET acquisitions. Eur J Nucl Med Mol Imaging. 2008;35(11):1971–80.
26. Goyal S, Kataria T. Image guidance in radiation therapy: techniques and applications. Radiol Res Pract. 2014;2014:705604.

27. Langen KM, Jones DTL. Organ motion and its management. Int J Radiat Oncol. 2001;50(1):265–78.
28. Huang TC, Wang YC, Chiou YR, Kao CH. Respiratory motion reduction in PET/CT using abdominal compression for lung cancer patients. PLoS One. 2014;9(5):e98033.
29. Kesner AL, Meier JG, Burckhardt DD, Schwartz J, Lynch DA. Data-driven optimal binning for respiratory motion management in PET. Med Phys. 2018;45(1):277–86.
30. Tumpa TR, Acuff SN, Gregor J, Lee S, Hu D, Osborne DR. Respiratory motion correction using a novel positron emission particle tracking technique: a framework towards individual lesion-based motion correction. Conf Proc IEEE Eng Med Biol Soc. 2018;2018:5249–52.
31. Schechter NR, Gillenwater AM, Buyers RM, Garden AS, Morrison WH, Nguyen LN, et al. Can positron emission tomography improve the quality of care for head-and-neck cancer patients? Int J Radiat Oncol Biol Phys. 2001;51(1):4–9.
32. Bradley J, Bae K, Choi N, Forster K, Siegel BA, Brunetti J, et al. A phase II comparative study of gross tumor volume definition with or without PET/CT fusion in dosimetric planning for non-small-cell lung cancer (NSCLC): primary analysis of radiation therapy oncology group (RTOG) 0515. Int J Radiat Oncol Biol Phys. 2012;82(1):435–41.e1.
33. Yaraghi Y, Jabbari I, Akhavan A, Ghaffarian P, Monadi S, Saeb M. Comparison of PET/CT and CT-based tumor delineation and its effects on the radiation treatment planning for non-small cell lung cancer. Iran J Nucl Med. 2018;26(1):9–15.
34. Anderson CM, Sun W, Buatti JM, Maley JE, Policeni B, Mott SL, et al. Interobserver and intermodality variability in GTV delineation on simulation CT, FDG-PET, and MR images of head and neck cancer. Jacobs J Radiat Oncol. 2014;1(1):006.
35. Metwally H, Courbon F, David I, Filleron T, Blouet A, Rives M, et al. Coregistration of prechemotherapy PET-CT for planning pediatric Hodgkin's disease radiotherapy significantly diminishes interobserver variability of clinical target volume definition. Int J Radiat Oncol*Biol*Phys. 2011;80(3):793–9.
36. Buijsen J, van den Bogaard J, van der Weide H, Engelsman S, van Stiphout R, Janssen M, et al. FDG-PET-CT reduces the interobserver variability in rectal tumor delineation. Radiother Oncol. 2012;102(3):371–6.
37. van Baardwijk A, Bosmans G, Boersma L, Buijsen J, Wanders S, Hochstenbag M, et al. PET-CT-based auto-contouring in non-small-cell lung cancer correlates with pathology and reduces interobserver variability in the delineation of the primary tumor and involved nodal volumes. Int J Radiat Oncol Biol Phys. 2007;68(3):771–8.
38. Mansoor A, Bagci U, Foster B, Xu Z, Papadakis GZ, Folio LR, et al. Segmentation and image analysis of abnormal lungs at CT: current approaches, challenges, and future trends. Radiographics. 2015;35(4):1056–76.
39. Lee JA. Segmentation of positron emission tomography images: some recommendations for target delineation in radiation oncology. Radiother Oncol. 2010;96(3):302–7.
40. Schinagl DA, Span PN, van den Hoogen FJ, Merkx MA, Slootweg PJ, Oyen WJ, et al. Pathology-based validation of FDG PET segmentation tools for volume assessment of lymph node metastases from head and neck cancer. Eur J Nucl Med Mol Imaging. 2013;40(12):1828–35.
41. Zaidi H, El Naqa I. PET-guided delineation of radiation therapy treatment volumes: a survey of image segmentation techniques. Eur J Nucl Med Mol Imaging. 2010;37(11):2165–87.
42. Drever L, Roa W, McEwan A, Robinson D. Comparison of three image segmentation techniques for target volume delineation in positron emission tomography. J Appl Clin Med Phys. 2006;8(Spring 2007):93–109.
43. Abdoli M, Dierckx RA, Zaidi H. Contourlet-based active contour model for PET image segmentation. Med Phys. 2013;40(8):082507.
44. Zhuang M, Dierckx RAJO, Zaidi H, eds. Novel active contour model-based automated segmentation of PET images. 2016 IEEE Nuclear Science Symposium, Medical Imaging Conference and Room-Temperature Semiconductor Detector Workshop (NSS/MIC/RTSD); 2016 29 Oct.-6 Nov. 2016.

45. Geets X, Lee JA, Bol A, Lonneux M, Gregoire V. A gradient-based method for segmenting FDG-PET images: methodology and validation. Eur J Nucl Med Mol Imaging. 2007;34(9):1427–38.
46. Fonti R, Conson M, Del Vecchio S. PET/CT in radiation oncology. Semin Oncol. 2019;46(3):202–9.
47. Belhassen S, Zaidi H. A novel fuzzy C-means algorithm for unsupervised heterogeneous tumor quantification in PET. Med Phys. 2010;37(3):1309–24.
48. Konert T, van de Kamer JB, Sonke JJ, Vogel WV. The developing role of FDG PET imaging for prognostication and radiotherapy target volume delineation in non-small cell lung cancer. J Thorac Dis. 2018;10(Suppl 21):S2508–S21.
49. Hatt M, Tixier F, Pierce L, Kinahan PE, Le Rest CC, Visvikis D. Characterization of PET/CT images using texture analysis: the past, the present... Any future? Eur J Nucl Med Mol Imaging. 2017;44(1):151–65.
50. Yu H, Caldwell C, Mah K, Mozeg D. Coregistered FDG PET/CT-based textural characterization of head and neck cancer for radiation treatment planning. IEEE Trans Med Imaging. 2009;28(3):374–83.
51. Huang B, Chen Z, Wu PM, Ye Y, Feng ST, Wong CO, et al. Fully automated delineation of gross tumor volume for head and neck cancer on PET-CT using deep learning: a dual-center study. Contrast Media Mol Imaging. 2018;2018:8923028.
52. Guo Z, Guo N, Gong K, Zhong S, Li Q. Gross tumor volume segmentation for head and neck cancer radiotherapy using deep dense multi-modality network. Phys Med Biol. 2019;64(20):205015.
53. Hatt M, Lamare F, Boussion N, Turzo A, Collet C, Salzenstein F, et al. Fuzzy hidden Markov chains segmentation for volume determination and quantitation in PET. Phys Med Biol. 2007;52(12):3467–91.
54. Hatt M, Lee JA, Schmidtlein CR, Naqa IE, Caldwell C, De Bernardi E, et al. Classification and evaluation strategies of auto-segmentation approaches for PET: report of AAPM task group no. 211. Med Phys. 2017;44(6):e1–e42.
55. Hatt M, Cheze le Rest C, Descourt P, Dekker A, De Ruysscher D, Oellers M, et al. Accurate automatic delineation of heterogeneous functional volumes in positron emission tomography for oncology applications. Int J Radiat Oncol Biol Phys. 2010;77(1):301–8.
56. Shepherd T, Teras M, Beichel RR, Boellaard R, Bruynooghe M, Dicken V, et al. Comparative study with new accuracy metrics for target volume contouring in PET image guided radiation therapy. IEEE Trans Med Imaging. 2012;31(11):2006–24.
57. Rasch C, Belderbos J, van Giersbergen A, De Kok I, Laura T, Boer M, et al. The influence of a multi-disciplinary meeting for quality assurance on target delineation in radiotherapy treatment preparation. Int J Radiat Oncol. 2009;75(3):S452–S3.
58. Warfield SK, Zou KH, Wells WM. Simultaneous truth and performance level estimation (STAPLE): an algorithm for the validation of image segmentation. IEEE Trans Med Imaging. 2004;23(7):903–21.
59. McGurk RJ, Bowsher J, Lee JA, Das SK. Combining multiple FDG-PET radiotherapy target segmentation methods to reduce the effect of variable performance of individual segmentation methods. Med Phys. 2013;40(4):042501.
60. Schaefer A, Vermandel M, Baillet C, Dewalle-Vignion AS, Modzelewski R, Vera P, et al. Impact of consensus contours from multiple PET segmentation methods on the accuracy of functional volume delineation. Eur J Nucl Med Mol Imaging. 2016;43(5):911–24.
61. Dewalle-Vignion AS, Betrouni N, Baillet C, Vermandel M. Is STAPLE algorithm confident to assess segmentation methods in PET imaging? Phys Med Biol. 2015;60(24):9473–91.
62. Berthon B, Marshall C, Evans M, Spezi E. ATLAAS: an automatic decision tree-based learning algorithm for advanced image segmentation in positron emission tomography. Phys Med Biol. 2016;61(13):4855–69.
63. Parkinson C, Evans M, Guerrero-Urbano T, Michaelidou A, Pike L, Barrington S, et al. Machine-learned target volume delineation of (18)F-FDG PET images after one cycle of induction chemotherapy. Phys Med. 2019;61:85–93.

64. Das SK, McGurk R, Miften M, Mutic S, Bowsher J, Bayouth J, et al. Task group 174 report: utilization of [(18) F]fluorodeoxyglucose positron emission tomography ([(18) F]FDG-PET) in radiation therapy. Med Phys. 2019;46(10):e706–e25.
65. Hallqvist A, Alverbratt C, Strandell A, Samuelsson O, Bjorkander E, Liljegren A, et al. Positron emission tomography and computed tomographic imaging (PET/CT) for dose planning purposes of thoracic radiation with curative intent in lung cancer patients: a systematic review and meta-analysis. Radiother Oncol. 2017;123(1):71–7.
66. De Ruysscher D, Wanders S, van Haren E, Hochstenbag M, Geeraedts W, Utama I, et al. Selective mediastinal node irradiation based on FDG-PET scan data in patients with non-small-cell lung cancer: a prospective clinical study. Int J Radiat Oncol Biol Phys. 2005;62(4):988–94.
67. Martinussen HM, Reymen B, Wanders R, Troost EG, Dingemans AC, Ollers M, et al. Is selective nodal irradiation in non-small cell lung cancer still safe when using IMRT? Results of a prospective cohort study. Radiother Oncol. 2016;121(2):322–7.
68. van Loon J, De Ruysscher D, Wanders R, Boersma L, Simons J, Oellers M, et al. Selective nodal irradiation on basis of (18)FDG-PET scans in limited-disease small-cell lung cancer: a prospective study. Int J Radiat Oncol Biol Phys. 2010;77(2):329–36.
69. Faivre-Finn C, Snee M, Ashcroft L, Appel W, Barlesi F, Bhatnagar A, et al. Concurrent once-daily versus twice-daily chemoradiotherapy in patients with limited-stage small-cell lung cancer (CONVERT): an open-label, phase 3, randomised, superiority trial. Lancet Oncol. 2017;18(8):1116–25.
70. Nestle U, Schimek-Jasch T, Kremp S, Schaefer-Schuler A, Mix M, Küsters A, et al. Imaging-based target volume reduction in chemoradiotherapy for locally advanced non-small-cell lung cancer (PET-plan): a multicentre, open-label, randomised, controlled trial. Lancet Oncol. 2020;21(4):581–92.
71. Nestle U, De Ruysscher D, Ricardi U, Geets X, Belderbos J, Pottgen C, et al. ESTRO ACROP guidelines for target volume definition in the treatment of locally advanced non-small cell lung cancer. Radiother Oncol. 2018;127(1):1–5.
72. Vaz SC, Adam JA, Delgado Bolton RC, et al. Joint EANM/SNMMI/ESTRO practice recommendations for the use of 2-[18F]FDG PET/CT external beam radiation treatment planning in lung cancer V1.0. Eur J Nucl Med Mol Imaging. 2022;49:1386–406. https://doi.org/10.1007/s00259-021-05624-5.
73. Gregoire V, Thorwarth D, Lee JA. Molecular imaging-guided radiotherapy for the treatment of head-and-neck squamous cell carcinoma: does it fulfill the promises? Semin Radiat Oncol. 2018;28(1):35–45.
74. Alongi P, Laudicella R, Desideri I, Chiaravalloti A, Borghetti P, Quartuccio N, et al. Positron emission tomography with computed tomography imaging (PET/CT) for the radiotherapy planning definition of the biological target volume: PART 1. Crit Rev Oncol Hematol. 2019;140:74–9.
75. Delouya G, Igidbashian L, Houle A, Belair M, Boucher L, Cohade C, et al. (1)(8)F-FDG-PET imaging in radiotherapy tumor volume delineation in treatment of head and neck cancer. Radiother Oncol. 2011;101(3):362–8.
76. Paulino AC, Koshy M, Howell R, Schuster D, Davis LW. Comparison of CT- and FDG-PET-defined gross tumor volume in intensity-modulated radiotherapy for head-and-neck cancer. Int J Radiat Oncol Biol Phys. 2005;61(5):1385–92.
77. Verma V, Choi JI, Sawant A, Gullapalli RP, Chen W, Alavi A, et al. Use of PET and other functional imaging to guide target delineation in radiation oncology. Semin Radiat Oncol. 2018;28(3):171–7.
78. Ciernik IF, Dizendorf E, Baumert BG, Reiner B, Burger C, Davis JB, et al. Radiation treatment planning with an integrated positron emission and computer tomography (PET/CT): a feasibility study. Int J Radiat Oncol Biol Phys. 2003;57(3):853–63.
79. Ligtenberg H, Willems SM, Ruiter LN, Jager EA, Terhaard CHJ, Raaijmakers CPJ, et al. Verification of HE-based CTV in laryngeal and hypopharyngeal cancer using pan-cytokeratin. Clin Transl Radiat Oncol. 2018;12:21–7.

80. Daisne JF, Duprez T, Weynand B, Lonneux M, Hamoir M, Reychler H, et al. Tumor volume in pharyngolaryngeal squamous cell carcinoma: comparison at CT, MR imaging, and FDG PET and validation with surgical specimen. Radiology. 2004;233(1):93–100.
81. Chatterjee S, Frew J, Mott J, McCallum H, Stevenson P, Maxwell R, et al. Variation in radiotherapy target volume definition, dose to organs at risk and clinical target volumes using anatomic (computed tomography) versus combined anatomic and molecular imaging (positron emission tomography/computed tomography): intensity-modulated radiotherapy delivered using a tomotherapy hi art machine: final results of the VortigERN study. Clin Oncol (R Coll Radiol). 2012;24(10):e173–9.
82. Kyzas PA, Evangelou E, Denaxa-Kyza D, Ioannidis JP. 18F-fluorodeoxyglucose positron emission tomography to evaluate cervical node metastases in patients with head and neck squamous cell carcinoma: a meta-analysis. J Natl Cancer Inst. 2008;100(10):712–20.
83. Kim SJ, Pak K, Kim K. Diagnostic accuracy of F-18 FDG PET or PET/CT for detection of lymph node metastasis in clinically node negative head and neck cancer patients; a systematic review and meta-analysis. Am J Otolaryngol. 2019;40(2):297–305.
84. Schinagl DA, Hoffmann AL, Vogel WV, van Dalen JA, Verstappen SM, Oyen WJ, et al. Can FDG-PET assist in radiotherapy target volume definition of metastatic lymph nodes in head-and-neck cancer? Radiother Oncol. 2009;91(1):95–100.
85. van den Bosch S, Dijkema T, Kunze-Busch MC, Terhaard CH, Raaijmakers CP, Doornaert PA, et al. Uniform FDG-PET guided GRAdient dose prEscription to reduce late radiation toxicity (UPGRADE-RT): study protocol for a randomized clinical trial with dose reduction to the elective neck in head and neck squamous cell carcinoma. BMC Cancer. 2017;17(1):208.
86. van den Bosch S, Vogel WV, Raaijmakers CP, Dijkema T, Terhaard CHJ, Al-Mamgani A, et al. Implications of improved diagnostic imaging of small nodal metastases in head and neck cancer: radiotherapy target volume transformation and dose de-escalation. Radiother Oncol. 2018;128(3):472–8.
87. Pedraza S, Ruiz-Alonso A, Hernandez-Martinez AC, Cabello E, Lora D, Perez-Regadera JF. (18)F-FDG PET/CT in staging and delineation of radiotherapy volume for head and neck cancer. Rev Esp Med Nucl Imagen Mol. 2019;38(3):154–9.
88. Ng SP, Tan J, Osbourne G, Williams L, Bressel MAB, Hicks RJ, et al. Follow up results of a prospective study to evaluate the impact of FDG-PET on CT-based radiotherapy treatment planning for oesophageal cancer. Clin Transl Radiat Oncol. 2017;2:76–82.
89. Apolle R, Brückner S, Frosch S, Rehm M, Thiele J, Valentini C, et al. Utility of fiducial markers for target positioning in proton radiotherapy of oesophageal carcinoma. Radiother Oncol. 2019;133:28–34.
90. Jimenez-Jimenez E, Mateos P, Aymar N, Roncero R, Ortiz I, Gimenez M, et al. Radiotherapy volume delineation using 18F-FDG-PET/CT modifies gross node volume in patients with oesophageal cancer. Clin Transl Oncol. 2018;20(11):1460–6.
91. Cooper JS, Guo MD, Herskovic A, Macdonald JS, Martenson J, James A, Al-Sarraf M, et al. Chemoradiotherapy of locally advanced esophageal CancerLong-term follow-up of a prospective randomized trial (RTOG 85-01). JAMA. 1999;281(17):1623–7.
92. Muijs CT, Beukema JC, Pruim J, Mul VE, Groen H, Plukker JT, et al. A systematic review on the role of FDG-PET/CT in tumour delineation and radiotherapy planning in patients with esophageal cancer. Radiother Oncol. 2010;97(2):165–71.
93. Muijs CT, Beukema JC, Woutersen D, Mul VE, Berveling MJ, Pruim J, et al. Clinical validation of FDG-PET/CT in the radiation treatment planning for patients with oesophageal cancer. Radiother Oncol. 2014;113(2):188–92.
94. Dimopoulos JC, Petrow P, Tanderup K, Petric P, Berger D, Kirisits C, et al. Recommendations from Gynaecological (GYN) GEC-ESTRO working group (IV): basic principles and parameters for MR imaging within the frame of image based adaptive cervix cancer brachytherapy. Radiother Oncol. 2012;103(1):113–22.

95. Petrič P, Hudej R, Rogelj P, Blas M, Tanderup K, Fidarova E, et al. Uncertainties of target volume delineation in MRI guided adaptive brachytherapy of cervix cancer: a multi-institutional study. Radiother Oncol. 2013;107(1):6–12.
96. Fiorentino A, Laudicella R, Ciurlia E, Annunziata S, Lancellotta V, Mapelli P, et al. Positron emission tomography with computed tomography imaging (PET/CT) for the radiotherapy planning definition of the biological target volume: PART 2. Crit Rev Oncol Hematol. 2019;139:117–24.
97. Gandy N, Arshad MA, Park WE, Rockall AG, Barwick TD. FDG-PET imaging in cervical cancer. Semin Nucl Med. 2019;49(6):461–70.
98. Adam JA, Arkies H, Hinnen K, Stalpers LJ, van Waesberghe JH, Stoker J, et al. 18F-FDG-PET/CT guided external beam radiotherapy volumes in inoperable uterine cervical cancer. Q J Nucl Med Mol Imaging. 2018;62(4):420–8.
99. Adam JA, Loft A, Chargari C, Delgado Bolton RC, Kidd E, Schoder H, et al. EANM/SNMMI practice guideline for [(18)F]FDG PET/CT external beam radiotherapy treatment planning in uterine cervical cancer v1.0. Eur J Nucl Med Mol Imaging. 2020;
100. Illidge T, Specht L, Yahalom J, Aleman B, Berthelsen AK, Constine L, et al. Modern radiation therapy for nodal non-Hodgkin lymphoma-target definition and dose guidelines from the international lymphoma radiation oncology group. Int J Radiat Oncol Biol Phys. 2014;89(1):49–58.
101. Specht L, Yahalom J, Illidge T, Berthelsen AK, Constine LS, Eich HT, et al. Modern radiation therapy for Hodgkin lymphoma: field and dose guidelines from the international lymphoma radiation oncology group (ILROG). Int J Radiat Oncol Biol Phys. 2014;89(4):854–62.
102. Yahalom J, Illidge T, Specht L, Hoppe RT, Li YX, Tsang R, et al. Modern radiation therapy for extranodal lymphomas: field and dose guidelines from the international lymphoma radiation oncology group. Int J Radiat Oncol Biol Phys. 2015;92(1):11–31.
103. Specht L, Berthelsen AK. PET/CT in radiation therapy planning. Semin Nucl Med. 2018;48(1):67–75.
104. Menon H, Guo C, Verma V, Simone CB 2nd. The role of positron emission tomography imaging in radiotherapy target delineation. PET Clin. 2020;15(1):45–53.
105. Sun R, Tang X, Yang Y, Zhang C. (18)FDG-PET/CT for the detection of regional nodal metastasis in patients with head and neck cancer: a meta-analysis. Oral Oncol. 2015;51(4):314–20.
106. Hu J, Zhang K, Yan Y, Zang Y, Wang Y, Xue F. Diagnostic accuracy of preoperative (18) F-FDG PET or PET/CT in detecting pelvic and para-aortic lymph node metastasis in patients with endometrial cancer: a systematic review and meta-analysis. Arch Gynecol Obstet. 2019;300(3):519–29.
107. Jiang C, Chen Y, Zhu Y, Xu Y. Systematic review and meta-analysis of the accuracy of 18F-FDG PET/CT for detection of regional lymph node metastasis in esophageal squamous cell carcinoma. J Thorac Dis. 2018;10(11):6066–76.
108. Li ZZ, Huang YL, Song HJ, Wang YJ, Huang Y. The value of 18F-FDG-PET/CT in the diagnosis of solitary pulmonary nodules: a meta-analysis. Medicine (Baltimore). 2018;97(12):e0130.
109. Schmidt-Hansen M, Baldwin DR, Hasler E, Zamora J, Abraira V, Roque IFM, PET-CT for assessing mediastinal lymph node involvement in patients with suspected resectable non-small cell lung cancer. Cochrane Database Syst Rev, 2014(11): p. CD009519. https://doi.org/10.1002/14651858. CD009519.pub2.
110. Yu W, Kou C, Bai W, Yu X, Duan R, Zhu B, et al. The diagnostic performance of PET/CT scans for the detection of para-aortic metastatic lymph nodes in patients with cervical cancer: a meta-analysis. PLoS One. 2019;14(7):e0220080.
111. Soret M, Bacharach SL, Buvat I. Partial-volume effect in PET tumor imaging. J Nucl Med. 2007;48(6):932–45.
112. Surti S. Update on time-of-flight PET imaging. J Nucl Med. 2015;56(1):98–105.

113. van der Vos CS, Koopman D, Rijnsdorp S, Arends AJ, Boellaard R, van Dalen JA, et al. Quantification, improvement, and harmonization of small lesion detection with state-of-the-art PET. Eur J Nucl Med Mol Imaging. 2017;44(Suppl 1):4–16.
114. van Elmpt W, De Ruysscher D, van der Salm A, Lakeman A, van der Stoep J, Emans D, et al. The PET-boost randomised phase II dose-escalation trial in non-small cell lung cancer. Radiother Oncol. 2012;104(1):67–71.
115. van Diessen J, De Ruysscher D, Sonke JJ, Damen E, Sikorska K, Reymen B, et al. The acute and late toxicity results of a randomized phase II dose-escalation trial in non-small cell lung cancer (PET-boost trial). Radiother Oncol. 2019;131:166–73.
116. Cooke SA. Local, regional and pulmonary failures in the randomised PET-boost trial for NSCLC patients. 2020 World Conference on Lung Cancer: International Association for the Study of Lung Cancer; 2021.
117. Thorwarth D. Biologically adapted radiation therapy. Z Med Phys. 2018;28(3):177–83.
118. van Dijk LV, Noordzij W, Brouwer CL, Boellaard R, Burgerhof JGM, Langendijk JA, et al. (18)F-FDG PET image biomarkers improve prediction of late radiation-induced xerostomia. Radiother Oncol. 2018;126(1):89–95.
119. Anthony GJ, Cunliffe A, Castillo R, Pham N, Guerrero T, Armato SG 3rd, et al. Incorporation of pre-therapy (18) F-FDG uptake data with CT texture features into a radiomics model for radiation pneumonitis diagnosis. Med Phys. 2017;44(7):3686–94.
120. Zschaeck S, Lock S, Leger S, Haase R, Bandurska-Luque A, Appold S, et al. FDG uptake in normal tissues assessed by PET during treatment has prognostic value for treatment results in head and neck squamous cell carcinomas undergoing radiochemotherapy. Radiother Oncol. 2017;122(3):437–44.
121. Zschaeck S, Hofheinz F, Zophel K, Butof R, Jentsch C, Schmollack J, et al. Increased FDG uptake on late-treatment PET in non-tumour-affected oesophagus is prognostic for pathological complete response and disease recurrence in patients undergoing neoadjuvant radiochemotherapy. Eur J Nucl Med Mol Imaging. 2017;44(11):1813–22.

2 Specific PET Tracers for Solid Tumors and for Definition of the Biological Target Volume

Constantin Lapa, Ken Herrmann, and Esther G. C. Troost

2.1 Introduction

As highlighted in Chap. 1, positron emission tomography (PET) is a key component of primary disease staging in numerous solid tumors. For this means, mainly 2-[^{18}F]fluorodeoxyglucose-(FDG) is used, and [^{18}F]FDG-PET-scans are in general

C. Lapa
Nuclear Medicine, Medical Faculty, University of Augsburg, Augsburg, Germany
e-mail: constantin.lapa@uk-augsburg.de

K. Herrmann
Department of Nuclear Medicine, University of Duisburg-Essen, and German Cancer Consortium (DKTK)-University Hospital Essen, Essen, Germany
e-mail: ken.herrmann@uk-essen.de

E. G. C. Troost (✉)
Department of Radiotherapy and Radiation Oncology, Faculty of Medicine and University Hospital Carl Gustav Carus, Technische Universität Dresden, Dresden, Germany

OncoRay—National Center for Radiation Research in Oncology, Faculty of Medicine and University Hospital Carl Gustav Carus, Technische Universität Dresden, Helmholtz-Zentrum Dresden-Rossendorf, Dresden, Germany

Helmholtz-Zentrum Dresden—Rossendorf, Institute of Radiooncology—OncoRay, Dresden, Germany

National Center for Tumor Diseases (NCT), Partner Site Dresden, Dresden, Germany: German Cancer Research Center (DKFZ), Heidelberg, Germany; Faculty of Medicine and University Hospital Carl Gustav Carus, Technische Universität Dresden, Dresden, Germany; Helmholtz Association / Helmholtz-Zentrum Dresden-Rossendorf (HZDR), Dresden, Germany

German Cancer Consortium (DKTK), Partner Site Dresden, and German Cancer Research Center (DKFZ), Heidelberg, Germany
e-mail: esther.troost@uniklinikum-dresden.de

E. G. C. Troost (ed.), *Image-Guided High-Precision Radiotherapy*,
https://doi.org/10.1007/978-3-031-08601-4_2

fused with anatomical imaging modalities, such as computed tomography (CT) and magnetic resonance imaging (MRI). In radiation oncology, the entire [^{18}F]FDG-positive tumor volume is most commonly included in the irradiated target volume, not taking into account underlying intratumoral heterogeneity regarding radiation sensitivity or resistance.

In 2000, Ling et al. [1] introduced the concept of the biological target volume (BTV). They postulated that different imaging modalities may unravel the underlying tumor microenvironment and enable—by including this information—the definition of different tumor subvolumes believed to require different radiation doses or other forms of treatment. Already at that time, PET was postulated to be one of the key imaging modalities for defining the BTV. Thus, in this chapter, PET tracers beyond [^{18}F]FDG, which depict (1) specific metabolic pathways of the primary solid tumors, e.g., in primary brain tumors or prostate adenocarcinoma, and/or (2) characteristics of tumor subvolumes, in head and neck squamous cell carcinoma and non-small cell lung cancer will be presented.

2.2 Brain Tumors

Anatomical MRI, with its high soft-tissue contrast and spatial resolution, is the cornerstone of delineating the tumor extent in primary brain tumors. However, MRI is incapable of accurately depicting the tumor boundaries due to the tumors' infiltrative behavior. [^{18}F]FDG cannot be reasonably used due to the physiological glucose consumption of the healthy brain [2].

The proliferation marker [^{18}F]-3′-deoxy-3′-fluorothymidine ([^{18}F]-FLT), that accumulates in cerebral gliomas, is related to the grade of malignancy and prognosis [3, 4]. It may thus constitute a suitable alternative to [^{18}F]FDG. However, it is unable to identify the full extent of a glioma, because it is not capable of passing the intact blood–brain barrier (BBB) and thus usually accumulates in tumor parts that show disruption of the BBB, i.e., higher grade tumor subvolumes, as indicated by contrast enhancement on MRI after application of paramagnetic contrast media [5].

In contrast to [^{18}F]FDG, the uptake of radiolabelled amino acids is low in normal brain tissue, rendering them appealing in brain tumors since tumor detection by radiolabelled amino acid PET tracers is feasible with a high tumor-to-background contrast. The increased uptake of amino acids seems to be predominantly caused by increased transport of large neutral amino acids through the plasma membrane of glioma cells via the L-type amino acid transporter (LAT) system subtypes LAT1 and LAT2 [6–8]. In addition, common amino acid PET tracers pass through the intact BBB, which enables the depiction of the tumor mass beyond contrast enhancement on MRI [9].

The longest-established amino acid tracer for PET is [^{11}C]-methyl-L-methionine ([^{11}C]-MET), but [^{11}C]-MET–PET is restricted to only few neuro-oncology centers because of the short half-life of [^{11}C] (20 min) that necessitates an on-site cyclotron. Consequently, amino acids labeled with [^{18}F] (with the logistic advantage of a half-life of 109.8 min), such as *O*-(2-^{18}F-fluoroethyl)-L-tyrosine ([^{18}F]-FET) and

3,4-dihydroxy-6-^{18}F-fluoro-L-phenylalanine ([^{18}F]-FDOPA), have been developed [10, 11]. Several studies investigating the role of pre-treatment [^{18}F]-FET-PET either after surgery or after postoperative chemo/radiotherapy in glioblastoma demonstrated amino acid PET-derived BTV to be highly prognostic for outcome, providing a rationale for the incorporation of amino acid PET in radiotherapy planning [12–16].

Beyond MRI-based morphologic gross tumor volume (GTV) delineation, the BTV may be defined by radiotracer uptake on amino acid PET that identifies tumor beyond standard MRI [17, 18]. Several studies examining primary tumor material on a histopathological level have shown that amino acid PET may be more sensitive to detect the true tumor extent (Fig. 2.1) [19–24]. The BTV defined by [^{18}F]FET-PET has been shown to extend beyond the MRI-defined GTV in a considerable number of cases [25, 26] and the spatial congruence of MRI and [^{18}F]FET-PET for the identification of glioma GTV has been poor [27]. In addition, the metabolic information provided by PET may identify subregions of tumor at higher risk of recurrence, which can be included in the radiation boost volume in order to improve the therapeutic ratio of radiation treatment. In this setting, PET-guided radiation dose escalation to metabolically active foci in newly diagnosed glioblastoma patients could be demonstrated to be feasible and safe; however, overall survival was not prolonged so far [28].

Small studies analyzing patterns of failure following conventional radiochemotherapy based on standard MRI-defined tumor volumes suggest that amino acid PET–defined tumor volumes may yield a more appropriate radiation target volume [29, 30]. In these investigations, a proportionate increase in marginal or non-central tumor recurrences was noted when regions of PET abnormality were not adequately

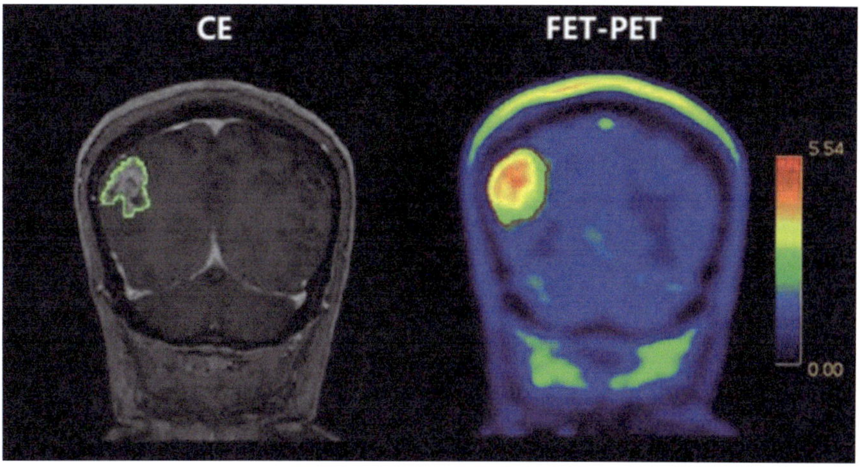

Fig. 2.1 Example of increased amino acid PET-derived BTV as compared to contrast-enhancement as detected by standard magnetic resonance imaging. In a patient with newly diagnosed glioblastoma, biologic tumor volume derived by [^{18}F]-FET-PET/CT is considerably larger than the volume with contrast enhancement on conventional MRI. Modified from [18]

covered by high-dose radiation. Recently, a prospective trial investigating the association of time to recurrence in glioblastoma with [^{11}C]-MET uptake before postoperative radiochemotherapy demonstrated a negative prognostic value of increased tracer accumulation [31]. Of note, regions of PET positivity were often not detected by MRI and exploratory analysis suggested a spatial correlation of the glioma recurrence region with pre-radiochemotherapy PET tracer accumulation in the majority of patients, hinting at an added value of metabolic imaging beyond anatomical information.

The impact of PET-based radiation treatment planning in recurrent high-grade glioma was evaluated in a prospective single-institution trial [32], which showed a significantly improved overall survival when the target volume was delineated on both amino acid PET and CT/MRI compared with CT/MRI alone. In 2016, the PET/RANO report concluded that—in the setting of relapsed glioma—biological target volumes may be more accurately depicted using amino acid PET tracers and that metabolically more active tumor sub-volumes may be amenable for dose-painting [7]. In this light, the current statement by the same group regarding the contribution of PET imaging to radiotherapy planning and monitoring in glioma patients confirmed that the most frequently used radiolabeled amino acids MET, FET, and FDOPA may improve the delineation of radiotherapy target volumes beyond conventional MRI and identify additional tumor parts that should be targeted by irradiation [13].

Currently, a multicenter phase II trial (GLIAA, NOA-10, ARO2013/1) is testing the hypothesis that [^{18}F]FET-PET-based re-irradiation is superior to radiotherapy only based on conventional MRI [33]. However, the inclusion of amino acid PET-based tumor volumes in standard-dose radiation therapy and re-irradiation protocols continue to demonstrate a predominance of in-field tumor recurrences, highlighting the need for more effective therapies [28]. Additionally, the impact of amino acid PET in comparison with advanced MRI techniques has not been proven yet and warrants further investigation.

After radiotherapy, amino acid PET has consistently proven a useful tool in radiotherapy response assessment in glioma patients with changes in tumor metabolism harboring prognostic value for both progression-free and overall survival [12, 14]. Of note, this technique is particularly valuable in the differentiation between radiation-related injury and glioma progression with a diagnostic accuracy between 80 and 90% [34, 35].

2.2.1 Glioma Hypoxia and Activated Microglia

Tumor hypoxia is characterized by an oxygen concentration below critical O_2 levels and triggers several molecular, biological, and clinical effects, making it a negative prognostic marker in nearly all solid tumors, including GBM. Hypoxia is a very important tumor characteristic when considering tumor aggressiveness, leading to the overexpression of the hypoxia inducible factor (HIF)-1 alpha, which enhances a number of genes related to proliferation, thus making the tumor more radioresistant

[36]. Identifying hypoxia within gliomas may highlight the areas, which could potentially benefit from a radiation dose escalation.

Several PET radiopharmaceuticals have been developed to target hypoxia, including the nitroimidazole-based compounds [^{18}F]-fluoromisonidazole ([^{18}F]FMISO) and [^{18}F]-fluoroazomycin arabinoside ([^{18}F]FAZA). [^{18}F]FMISO and [^{18}F]FAZA are tracers that penetrate the cell by passive diffusion, and under low oxygen concentration ($pO_2 < 10$ mmHg), are progressively reduced, leading to the production of reactive radicals that bind covalently and irreversibly, to intracellular molecules. Thus, both vectors accumulate in severely hypoxic tumor cells, which are reported to be found mainly in high-grade glioma [37, 38]. Hypoxia PET has been used pre-clinically to guide radiation treatment in a rat glioblastoma model [39]. However, only a few clinical experiences are available on patients with high-grade glioma undergoing hypoxia PET scans before and after radiotherapy [40, 41], and this interesting approach has not achieved clinical relevance in brain tumor diagnosis or treatment planning yet.

Another promising target for brain tumor imaging is the mitochondrial translocator protein (TSPO) [42]. Accumulation of TSPO ligands might extend beyond the tumor margins on amino acid PET and indicate an infiltration zone with activated microglia as a marker of further tumor spread [43]. Further research to demonstrate the suitability of this approach for radiotherapy planning is warranted.

2.2.2 Meningioma

Meningioma constitutes the most common primary brain tumor, with about 80% being classified as WHO grade I, whereas WHO grade II and III meningioma are less common [44]. If indicated, microsurgical resection is generally the therapy of choice. Radiotherapy, including radiosurgery, which is predominantly used in the recurrent situation, may be preferred in small WHO grade I meningioma or in locations not eligible for complete neurosurgical resection. Standard MRI is the imaging method of choice and usually shows a homogeneous contrast enhancement and a characteristic attachment to the dura mater [45].

On the molecular level, meningioma may express specific somatostatin receptors (SSTR) [46]. SSTR expression can be non-invasively visualized using radiolabeled SSTR ligands, usually compounds containing SSTR agonists, such as tyrosine3-octreotate (TATE) or the octapeptide octreotide (TOC) and a chelator, e.g., tetraxetane (DOTA), coupled to the short-lived radionuclide gallium ([^{68}Ga]). Since their development in the 1990s, SSTR agonists have been increasingly used in meningioma imaging. The main indication for SSTR-PET is identifying meningioma tissue, including the delineation of meningioma extent, especially in complex anatomical regions, such as the skull base or the orbital region, and with a special focus on the diagnosis of intraosseous infiltration [47].

Exact tumor delineation in complex anatomical regions, such as the skull base, is not only crucial for surgical considerations but also of crucial importance for radiotherapy planning, as the MRI-based morphologic GTV delineation may be

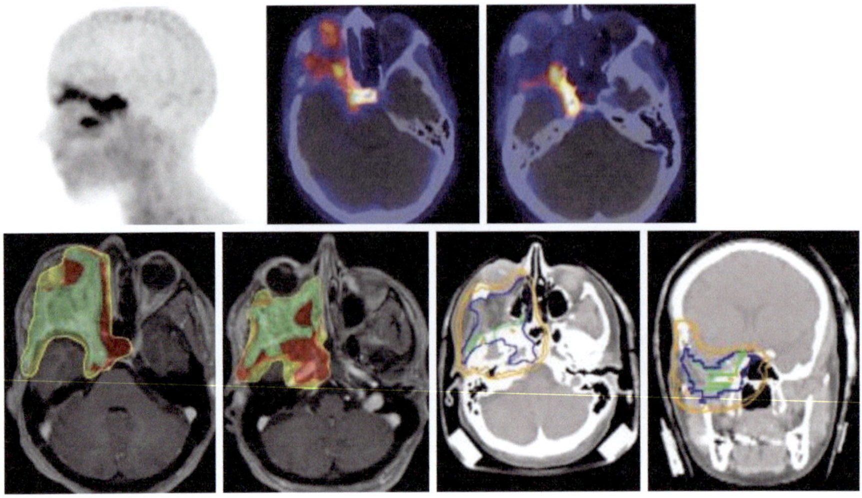

Fig. 2.2 Improved meningioma delineation using somatostatin receptor-directed (SSTR) positron emission tomography/computed tomography (PET/CT). Beyond physiological tracer uptake of the pituitary gland, SSTR-PET/CT facilitates tumor contouring in radiotherapy planning. Adapted from [48]

insufficient to truly address the entire tumor volume. Particularly for the detection of intra-osseous meningioma infiltration or for the tumor delineation at the skull base, PET using SSTR ligands has been shown to strongly complement anatomical information from MRI and CT [47–49]. Inclusion of PET imaging for stereotactic radiation treatment planning was not only able to identify infiltrated tissue and provide information beyond bone windowing on CT and contrast enhancement on MRI, but also has led to a preservation of critical areas, such as the pituitary gland and the optic chiasm [50, 51].

Subsequent studies confirmed that an improved target volume delineation for fractionated radiation therapy in patients with benign, atypical, and even anaplastic meningiomas (WHO grades I–III) can be obtained by DOTATOC PET (Fig. 2.2) [47, 48, 50].

Following treatment, SSTR-directed PET is reliably able to differentiate between scar tissue and vital remnants or tumor recurrence [52].

2.3 Head and Neck Squamous Cell Carcinomas (HNSCC)

In recent years, significant improvements in radio(chemo)therapy of head and neck squamous cell carcinomas (HNSCC) have been achieved. In part, this is due to improved imaging for accurate tumor staging and radiation treatment planning. Apart from [^{18}F]FDG-PET, eluded to in Chap. 1, PET tracers targeting the distinct tumor microenvironment have been studied in prospective imaging trials regarding their potential predictive and/or prognostic potential. These tracers include those depicting tumor cell hypoxia, tumor cell proliferation, and other distinct tumor characteristics.

Acute and chronic hypoxia originating from acute occlusion of blood vessels and from insufficient diffusion of oxygen from the vessel to the tumor cell, respectively, are known tumor characteristics adversely affecting outcome after surgery, chemotherapy, and also after radiotherapy [53]. These conclusions have been drawn from studies including invasive measurement of the oxygenation status, e.g., using an Eppendorff electrode, or from immunohistochemical staining of tumor biopsies taken from HNSCC accessible for this invasive procedure [54–58]. However, both this invasive nature of the assessment as well as the geometrical limitations of immunohistochemical staining of tumor sections hampered the repeat use of this procedure. PET imaging is capable of depicting tumor characteristics of the entire tumor and owing to its non-invasive nature it can also be performed at several time-points prior to and during treatment. Finally, a review on hypoxia imaging supported the correlation with treatment outcome [59].

The PET-tracers most widely used to image tumor cell hypoxia in HNSCC are [^{18}F]FMISO, [^{18}F]FAZA, [^{18}F]fluoro flortanidazole ([^{18}F]HX4), [^{18}F]fluorerythronitroimidazole ([^{18}F]FETNIM), and diacetylbis(4-methylthiosemicarbazonato)copperII ([^{62}Cu]Cu-ATSM), of which the first has been most widely studied. The underlying idea was and is that those tracers can be incorporated in defining the biological target volume, ideally in the primary tumor and lymph nodes, and to identify changes over time indicative of tumor changes requiring adaptation of the treatment plan or even the form of treatment.

For [^{18}F]FMISO, the entire chain from pre-clinical imaging of xenograft tumors to inclusion in clinical studies and modeling efforts had been followed by a few dedicated research sites. In Nijmegen, [^{18}F]FMISO imaging of xenograft HNSCC tumor models was correlated with levels of hypoxia identified by immunohistochemical staining of the nitroimidazole pimonidazol on tumor sections. Overall, the crude level of hypoxia correlated between micro- and macroscopic imaging, however, not on an individual xenograft tumor basis [60]. Also the signal of autoradiography was found to correlate with levels of hypoxia under ambient conditions, after carbogen breathing, and tumor clamping, again in three different xenograft tumor lines [61].

In a modeling study on HNSCC and non-small cell lung cancer (NSCLC), Eschmann et al. [62] were the first to assess the prognostic value of [^{18}F]FMISO imaging prior to radiochemotherapy on both dynamic and static scans. A tracer kinetic characterized by accumulation as well as high SUV 4 h after injection were correlated with poor response to treatment. Refined kinetic models as well as a correlation of [^{18}F]FMISO with [^{18}F]FDG were subsequently performed by the same group [63–65].

Since then, several prospective clinical trials have assessed the value of (repeat) [^{18}F]FMISO-PET-imaging for patient stratification. The largest study to date was initiated in 2005, performing [^{18}F]FMISO-PET not only prior to treatment, but also at several time-points during treatment, i.e., weeks 1, 2, and 5, as well as [^{18}F]FDG-PET scanning prior to, after completion and during follow-up visits. The study consisted of a planned exploratory and validation cohort, each including 25 patients with advanced-stage HNSCC of varying origin. In both parts of the study, the hypoxia status, determined on the [^{18}F]FMISO-PET of the second week of treatment was found to be highly predictive for locoregional control [66, 67] (Fig. 2.3). Recently, a prospective clinical phase II study in oropharyngeal cancer patients only suggests that the radiation dose may be deescalated from the conventional dose of 70 to 30 Gy in tumors exhibiting no hypoxia on [^{18}F]FMISO-PET prior to or with a re-oxygenating tumor during radiation treatment [68].

Thorwarth et al. [69] were the first to incorporate [^{18}F]FMISO and [^{18}F]FDG information into a treatment planning study in 13 HNSCC. They found dose painting my numbers to deliver the radiation dose more effectively than an additional uniform boost to [^{18}F]FDG-positive areas. Based on the findings of the [^{18}F]FMISO studies, both test and validation, performed in Dresden, Zschaeck et al. [70] came to the conclusion that dose painting by numbers on [^{18}F]FMISO-positive tumor subvolumes prior to treatment is insufficient to represent the ever-changing distribution of [^{18}F]FMISO, which became apparent by repeat [^{18}F]FMISO imaging throughout the course of treatment. The intra-tumoral stability of [^{18}F]FMISO update was insufficient for such an approach, and moreover, the site of local failure was in many patients not within the [^{18}F]FMISO-positive areas. Thus, the authors supported the idea of utilizing [^{18}F]FMISO as surrogate of tumor hypoxia per se and to rather increase the radiation dose to the entire tumor, an approach, which is included in the INDIRA-MISO (in preparation). This study design is also pursued in the phase III

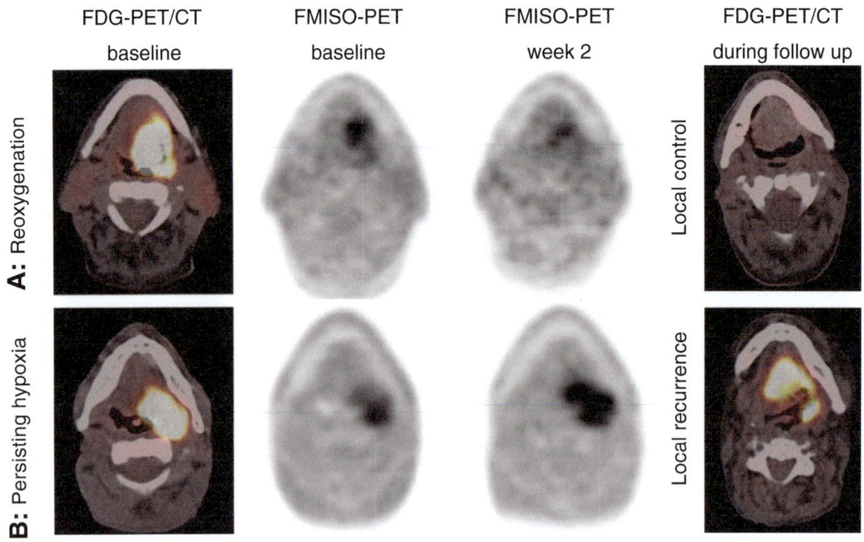

Fig. 2.3 FDG-PET/CT at baseline and FMISO-PET at baseline and after week two of treatment for two patients with tumors of similar size and location at the base of the tongue. While patient A showed substantial reoxygenation after 2 weeks of treatment and was locally controlled despite worse initial tumor stage (cT4 cN1), patient B (cT3 cN0) showed persisting hypoxia and an early local recurrence developed. Reprinted with permission from [66]

randomized ESCALOX trial, supported by the German Research Council (DFG), which tests the hypothesis whether radiation dose escalation to the GTV improves 2-year locoregional control and overall survival after concurrent radiochemotherapy in HNSCC patients [71]. Radiation will be delivered to a total dose of 80.5 Gy using a simultaneous integrated boost and cisplatin is administered either weekly or three-weekly. In the translational part of this study, 100 patients will undergo [^{18}F]FMISO-PET twice in the week before treatment start in order to assess the presence of and possible changes in tumor hypoxia.

The metabolic target volume (MTV) and hypoxic volume (HV) were assessed based on [^{18}F]FDG-PET and [^{18}F]FMISO-PET imaging in 20 primary HNSCC tumors and 19 metastatic lymph nodes [72]. When considering the intra-tumor MTV of the [^{18}F]FDG-PET and [^{18}F]FMISO-PET, only 26% of the primary tumors and 15% of the lymph nodes were found to strongly correlate. For the HV, only 19% of the primary tumors and 12% of the lymph nodes were strongly correlated. On a quantitative level, correlations between both tracers were present for the primary tumors, but not for the lymph node metastases. Since high levels of both [^{18}F]FDG-PET and [^{18}F]FMISO-PET can be found in selected tumors only, [^{18}F]FDG-PET is no surrogate to identify or predict intra-tumor hypoxia, the authors concluded.

In the context of the EORTC 1219 clinical trial, the value of [^{18}F]FAZA-PET is being assessed in patients treated with radiochemotherapy and randomized to also receive the hypoxia-modifying agent nimorazole, to evaluate [^{18}F]FAZA-PET/CT as a prognostic factor of the loco-regional control rate at 2 years in HNSCC patients receiving radiochemotherapy ± nimorazole. Following their initial study on [^{18}F]FAZA-PET, Imaizumi et al. [73] published a comparative analysis on [^{18}F]FAZA-PET and diffusion-weighted magnetic resonance imaging (DWI-MRI). In 11 patients investigated, the authors reported on a significant positive correlation between [^{18}F]FAZA-PET and the slow compartment of a two/compartment model for DWI, whereas diffusional kurtosis had a significant negative correlation.

As part of the TROG 02.02 phase III clinical study, 41 HNSCC patients were imaged using [^{18}F]FDG-PET and [^{18}F]FAZA-PET, both of which were assessed qualitatively and quantitatively [74]. Using multivariate analysis, the hypoxic volume derived from [^{18}F]FAZA-PET was found to significantly correlate with the T-stage, not with HPV-status or other adverse characteristics. Moreover, hypoxic tumors treated with cisplatin had a significantly worse treatment outcome relative to oxic tumors as defined by [^{18}F]FAZA-PET or hypoxic tumors treated with tirapazamine.

Interestingly, a multicenter individual patient database meta-analysis of 163 hypoxia PET-scans ([^{18}F]FMISO, N = 102; [^{18}F]FAZA, N = 51) correlated PET readings with locoregional control and overall survival [75]. Even though the baseline characteristics significantly differed between the cohorts, the commonly used hypoxic parameters, i.e., maximum tumor-to-background radio (TMR_{max}) and hypoxic volume with a 1.6 threshold (HV1.6) strongly correlated with locoregional control and overall survival. It was thus concluded that both tracers appeared robust and seemed equivalent in multicenter trials.

[^{18}F]HX4-PET has been studied to a lesser extent in HNSCC patients. First, the reproducibility and spatial stability of the marker was assessed in HNSCC [76]. Subsequently, in 2016, Zegers et al. [77] assessed changes of the tracer as well as of blood biomarkers in 20 HNSCC patients. Within the GTV, the hypoxic fraction and hypoxic volume were found to significantly decrease in 69% of the analyzed GTVs ($N = 32$). Conversely, the levels of the blood biomarkers, i.e., carbonic anhydrase IX (CAIX), osteopontin and vascular endothelial growth factor (VEGF), did not change or increased (osteopontin). A recent publication by the same group, first author Sanduleanu et al. [78], summarized results on the prognostic value of repeat [^{18}F]HX4-PET in 34 HNSCC patients included in two prospective clinical trials. Patients were scanned prior to radio(chemo)therapy ($N = 33$) as well as during treatment ($N = 28$). Noteworthy, the interval between the start of treatment and the per-treatment scan varied from 3 to 17 days with a median of 13 days. Based on [^{18}F]HX4-PET, the hypoxic fraction and hypoxic volume were analyzed and correlated with treatment outcome. The static [^{18}F]HX4-PET images were not of prognostic value, whereas the dynamic changes revealed a significantly shorter local progression-free survival and overall survival (OS) in patients with an increase in the hypoxic volume and also a shorter OS in patients with residual hypoxia on the per-treatment scan. Thus, these findings are in line with reports on [^{18}F]FMISO findings.

For completion, also the two hypoxia-related PET-tracers [^{18}F]FETNIM and [^{62}Cu]Cu-ATSM should also be eluded to here, even though it has only been studied in a limited number of publications [79–83]. In the early 2000s, Lehtiö et al. [81, 82] performed initial assessments of [^{18}F]FETNIM-PET and established analytical methods. In 2019, 32 patients with locoregionally advanced HNSCC undergoing concurrent radiochemotherapy underwent [^{18}F]FETNIM-PET imaging prior to and per-treatment after 5 weeks of treatment [83]. On multivariate analysis, maximum SUV (SUV_{max}) of the primary tumor prior to treatment was correlated with worse local control, whereas a high mid-treatment SUV_{max} was associated with worse distant-metastasis free survival and overall survival. On multivariate analysis, tumor grade and mid-SUV_{max} were significant predictors of worse overall survival.

Besides hypoxia imaging, [^{18}F]FLT-PET as imaging biomarker of tumor cell proliferation in HNSCC was of interest in the early 2010s. Troost et al. [84, 85] showed in two comparative analyses between immunohistochemical staining of tumor and lymph node resection specimen on the one hand, and [^{18}F]FLT-PET on the other hand, that Ki-67 and IdUrd staining correlated well with [^{18}F]FLT-PET in 17 primary tumors, but that [^{18}F]FLT-PET was not capable of distinguishing metastatic from reactive lymph nodes in 10 HNSCC patients. Subsequent studies by the same group proved that [^{18}F]FLT-PET holds high prognostic value regarding locoregional control [85–87]. However, since the synthesis of the tracer is complicated, it has not yet found its way into routine clinical practice, neither for oropharyngeal tumors, esophageal carcinoma, nor for NSCLC [88, 89].

The fibroblast activation protein (FAP), which is highly expressed on the fibroblasts of tumor stroma, is a relatively new biological target, which can be addressed with suitable FAP inhibitors (FAPI) that can be labeled with several radionuclides such as [^{68}Ga] and [^{18}F]. Syed et al. [90] have shown a high tumor-to-background-ratio of the FAP-ligand along with significant alteration of TV-delineation in HNSCC patients. The value of PET using [^{18}F]FAPI is being evaluated for a variety of tumors in the context of a prospective register (NCT04571086). The value of this novel radiotracer PET for radiotherapy planning is to be assessed in prospective clinical studies with relevant oncological endpoints.

2.4 Non-small Cell Lung Cancer

[^{18}F]FDG-PET/CT has been recognized as the key imaging method for staging of (non-)small cell lung cancer [(N)SCLC], for radiation treatment planning, for response monitoring during radio(chemo)therapy, and for detection of recurrent disease [91–94], see Chap. 1.

Similar to HNSCC, other PET tracers apart from [^{18}F]FDG, which reflect tumor characteristics, such as hypoxia, proliferation, or immune status, have been investigated in (N)SCLC. This stems from the fact that glycolysis, depicted by [^{18}F]FDG, is not concordant to other parameters, e.g., hypoxia [95]. In this paragraph, therefore, the PET-tracers used in NSCLC will be briefly mentioned.

In terms of hypoxia, the same tracers reported for HNSCC have also been used in NSCLC, i.e., [^{18}F]FMISO, [^{18}F]FAZA, or [^{18}F]HX4. In a multicenter, phase II clinical trial, [^{18}F]FMISO-PET was used to determine the hypoxia status in NSCLC patients [96, 97]. In this study, [^{18}F]FMISO-positive patients received a boost of 70–84 Gy, depending on the dose to surrounding organs at risk, while the other patients received the standard dose of 66 Gy. The overall and progression-free survival rates of the 54 patients included were 48.5 and 28.8%, respectively, at 3 years after treatment. The median overall survival in [^{18}F]FMISO-positive patients was 25.8 months, whereas it was not reached in the [^{18}F]FMISO-negative patients. Owing to the small number of patients, no dose-effect relationship could be established in the [^{18}F]FMISO-positive patient subset. So, also this phase II study underlines the fact that [^{18}F]FMISO-uptake is strongly associated with poor prognosis in NSCLC.

In a recent publication, hypoxia represented by both [^{18}F]FMISO- and [^{18}F]FAZA-PET was compared to immunohistochemical analyses (GLUT-1, CAIX, LDH-5, and HIF-1alpha) in 18 NSCLC patients undergoing primary tumor resection [98]. The SUV_{max} of [^{18}F]FMISO was found to be higher than that of [^{18}F]FAZA, but to correlate well. Noteworthy, the results of PET-imaging were not correlated with immunohistochemical results, regardless of the staining.

For [^{18}F]HX4, the group from MAASTRO clinic performed subsequent studies on the performance of the tracer, quantified the hypoxic status in NSCLC patients prior to and during radio(chemo)therapy, and employed it in radiation treatment planning studies [76, 99–101]. In 2013, Zegers et al. [101] defined the optimal time-point of imaging [^{18}F]HX4 statically, as being 4 h post injection. Subsequently, the authors [100] compared [^{18}F]HX4 with [^{18}F]FDG-PET imaging in NSCLC patients prior to radio(chemo)therapy. They found hypoxic tumor volumes to be smaller than metabolically active volumes, with half of the tumors exhibiting a good overlap between the two PET-tracers. In the other patients, there was a (partial) mismatch. In a radiation treatment planning study, Even et al. [99] created radiation treatment plans for 10 NSCLC patients. Dose escalation based on metabolic subvolumes, hypoxic subvolumes, or on the entire tumor volume was found to be feasible, with doses ranging as high as 107 ± 20 Gy for metabolic subvolumes and 117 ± 15 Gy for hypoxic subvolumes. Since the PET-Boost trial, referred to in Chap. 1, escalating the radiation dose on ^{18}F]FDG-PET subvolumes was still recruiting patients and the tracer [^{18}F]HX4 is not amply available, no dose escalation trial has been initiated.

Finally, [^{18}F]FLT-PET representing tumor cell proliferation has only been tested in a few studies. It has been used to monitor treatment response during radiochemotherapy as well as during targeted therapy [102–104].

2.5 Prostate Cancer

Molecular imaging is widely used for detecting, staging, and restaging of prostate cancer patients. While previously mainly FDG and cellular membrane lipogenesis markers such as [^{18}F]- and [^{11}C]-Choline-PET contributed to the patient management of prostate cancer patients this has nowadays almost completely shifted to radiolabelled PSMA inhibitors. In contrast to the historically used metabolic PET tracers, PSMA-PET visualizes the expression of the glutamate carboxypeptidase PSMA (prostate-specific membrane antigen) representing a trans-membrane protein, which is highly expressed in the majority of prostate cancers [105]. Due to its excellent performance PSMA-PET is currently implemented in the major clinical guidelines for detection of biochemical recurrence, primary staging of high-risk disease, in case of PSA persistence after primary treatment as well as for selecting patients for PSMA radioligand therapy [106].

Another important aspect is the availability and accessibility of novel PET tracers. Currently, FDA approvals for both [^{68}Ga]Ga-PSMA and [^{18}F]F-DCFPyL are in place, whereas in Europe so far only [^{18}F]F-PSMA 1007 has a local market authorization in France. However, within the next months EMA approvals for both [^{68}Ga]Ga-PSMA, [^{18}F]F-PSMA 1007 and potentially [^{18}F]F-DCFPyL are expected. To help navigate among the ever-increasing number of PSMA PET tracers, it is important to state that the clinically best developed PSMA PET tracers diagnostic is overall probably very similar justifying the overarching term of a "class of PSMA PET tracers". Major discriminators are routes of production and batch sizes (and accordingly cost of goods) and pathways of excretion (predominantly renal vs. predominantly hepatic-biliary). Hepatic-biliary dominant excreted PSMA PET tracers such as [^{18}F]F-PSMA 1007 seem to have a certain advantage for local staging in the prostate and prostate bed due to the lower activity in the surrounding urinary bladder; however, a higher rate of so-called unspecific bone uptake might negatively affect the overall performance [107]. In summary, the novel class of PSMA PET tracers plays an important role for the management of prostate cancer patients. In the following part, the impact of the "class of PSMA PET tracers" on radiation therapy planning will be discussed in more detail.

2.5.1 PET in Primary Staging

In the primary setting, PSMA-PET/CT imaging can be applied for initial staging in patients with high-risk prostate cancer [108]. The recently published prospective randomized phase III study proPSMA showed that PSMA-PET/CT favorably impacts patient management since the accuracy for lymph node and bone metastases is higher as compared to conventional imaging changing subsequently also the radiation treatment plan [109]. Moreover, PSMA-PET/CT significantly reduced the number of equivocal findings at an overall lower radiation dose compared to conventional imaging. Several additional retrospective analyses have also addressed this issue. Dewes et al. [110] reported on a change in TNM stage in 8 of 15 patients or modifications of clinical target volumes (CTVs) and changes in prescribed radiation dose in 5 and 12 patients, respectively. In another retrospective analysis, PSMA-PET/CT led to major changes in the radiotherapy plan in approximately one-third of the patients, especially when no elective radiation to the pelvic lymphatic drainage system was initially planned [111].

Recently, an academically driven prospective phase III trial randomizing patients with unfavorable, intermediate, and high-risk profiles to groups with or without PSMA-PET prior to definitive radiotherapy planning (NCT04457245) has been initiated. The primary endpoint of this study is the progression-free survival after initiation of definite radiotherapy aiming for improvement in oncological outcome for the PSMA PET arm.

Interestingly, a clear dose-response relationship was shown for prostate cancer patients. The prospective multicenter phase III study "FLAME" reported that dose escalation to intraprostatic MRI-derived tumor lesions resulted in a significant improvement in recurrence-free survival [112]. However, it can be assumed from previous publications that the contouring of the intraprostatic tumor mass determined taking account the potential additional information of PSMA-PET might lead to a further improvement [113–116]. Recently, Zamboglou et al. [117] reported in 10 patients on the feasibility to escalate the tumor dose to 95 Gy while contouring the intraprostatic tumor lesions based on [^{68}Ga]Ga-PSMA PET. Based on this very promising data, a prospective multicenter phase II study is currently investigating focal dose escalation to intraprostatic tumor volumes derived by PSMA-PET/CT and MRI (HypoFocal; DRKS00017570).

2.5.2 Salvage Radiotherapy in Recurrent Prostate Cancer

In patients with biochemical recurrence (BCR) salvage radiotherapy (SRT) represents the most important therapeutic option. Since the introduction of PSMA and its implementation into all major clinical guidelines, BCR patients are offered—if

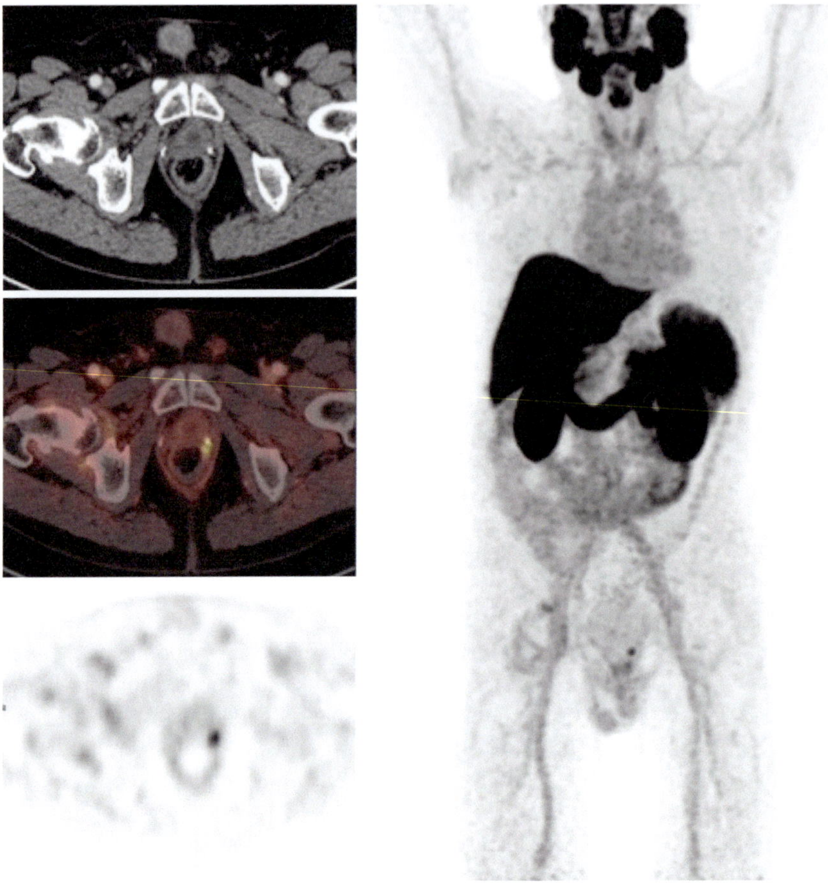

Fig. 2.4 Prostate cancer patient having undergone primary radical prostatectomy (pT2c pN0 L0 R0; Gleason 3 + 4). [^{18}F]-PSMA 1007 PET/CT performed in setting of biochemical recurrence (PSA 1.05 ng/ml) shows a local recurrence in the prostate bed guiding salvage radiation treatment planning (miTNM score: mi Tr N0 M0)

available and reimbursed—a PSMA-PET/CT scan. Despite its high effectiveness at low PSA levels, the current German S3 guideline clearly states to take into account the information provided by PSMA PET/CT for SRT planning, but not to delay SRT in case of a negative PSMA scan.

Including PSMA-PET/CT into the workup of patients with BCR led to significant impact on patient management decisions, such as by identifying patients with recurrence confined to the prostate or pelvic nodes [118, 119]. Even at low PSMA values of less than 0.5 ng/ml, PSMA-PET/CT detects lymph node metastases in approximately 20% of patients [120]. Accordingly, PSMA-PET/CT led in almost half of the patients with low PSA values to patient management changes as shown in a recently published scoping review including 45 studies in the BCR setting [120]. Important relevance is attributed to the detection of distant metastases, mostly to the bone, which was even found in patients with low PSA levels (10% if PSA <0.5 ng/ml) relevantly impacting therapy choice. This gains even relevance in case of oligometastatic disease as here the success and failure highly depends on the accurate delineation of recurrent disease [121]. PSMA PET also affected the radiation target volume leading to a field extension due to inclusion of PSMA-positive suspicious lymph nodes or in case of atypically localized recurrences at the border of the standard target volume [122–124].

Stimulated by the overall promising date radiation therapy, experts currently also discuss the possibility of PSMA-PET-guided SRT with a dose-escalated simultaneous integrated boost directed to the PSMA-positive local recurrence hoping for a positive impact on the clinical outcome and improved PSA response rates (Fig. 2.4). However, the ultimate clinical value of PSMA-PET-guided SRT and therefore prolongation of progression survival or even overall survival is not yet known. Multiple prospective randomized studies are currently intending to address this question (Clinicaltrials.gov NCT01666808, NCT03762759, NCT03525288) including a phase III study (NCT03582774) in the setting of biochemical failure following radical prostatectomy comparing the current standard of care (salvage RT to prostatic fossa) with PSMA-PET/CT-guided SRT.

2.6 Future Prospects

In recent years, a novel group of promising tracers targeting the fibroblast activation protein (FAP) on the so-called cancer-associated fibroblasts (CAFs), such as [^{68}Ga]Ga-FAPI, has been developed [125]. Due to its high tumor to background contrast in many malignancies, which often is superior to that for [^{18}F]FDG, there is also rising interest in the use of FAP-specific PET for radiation treatment planning [126, 127]. Promising first preliminary results in HNSCC with [^{68}Ga]Ga-FAPI and PET suggest it might help in accurately assessing the extent of tumor spread prior to treatment start to reduce the area exposed to radiation and thereby reduce toxicities [127]. An optimized radiation therapy planning and reduction of the treatment field is also reported in lung cancer where differentiating tumor from normal tissue is often difficult with [^{18}F]FDG in particular when the lung is affected by inflammatory conditions or chronic obstructive pulmonary disease [128]. However, large prospective trials are necessary to define the future role of FAPI-PET for radiation therapy planning [129].

There has also been significant progress in imaging with radiolabelled antibodies and antibody fragments. Labeling of these proteins with ^{89}Zr via the chelator DFO is a routine process, which only rarely affects their ligand-binding properties. Clinical studies have shown that radiolabelled antibodies allow for imaging of a variety of important targets including, for example, human epidermal growth factor receptor 2 (HER2), carbohydrate antigen 19–9 (CA19–9), and programmed death ligand 1 (PD-L1) [130–132]. Using these antibodies PET imaging may therefore reveal biological changes during radiotherapy, e.g., the up- or down-regulation of PD-L1. Broader clinical use of radiolabelled antibodies is currently limited by the significantly higher radiation dose from the long-lived isotope [^{89}Zr]. However, PET/CT systems with several fold higher sensitivity than existing scanners are currently entering the clinic. These systems allow imaging with radiolabelled antibodies at radiation doses similar to FDG-PET/CT [133].

References

1. Ling CC, Humm J, Larson S, et al. Towards multidimensional radiotherapy (MD-CRT): biological imaging and biological conformality. Int J Radiat Oncol Biol Phys. 2000;47(3):551–60.
2. Chen W. Clinical applications of PET in brain tumors. J Nucl Med. 2007;48(9):1468–81.
3. Idema AJ, Hoffmann AL, Boogaarts HD, et al. 3′-Deoxy-3′-18F-fluorothymidine PET-derived proliferative volume predicts overall survival in high-grade glioma patients. J Nucl Med Dec 2012;53(12):1904–1910.
4. Collet S, Valable S, Constans J, et al. [18F]-fluoro-L-thymidine PET and advanced MRI for preoperative grading of gliomas. NeuroImage Clin. 2015;8:448–54.
5. Nowosielski M, DiFranco MD, Putzer D, et al. An intra-individual comparison of MRI,[18F]-FET and [18F]-FLT PET in patients with high-grade gliomas. PLoS One. 2014;9(4):e95830.
6. Habermeier A, Graf J, Sandhöfer B, Boissel J-P, Roesch F, Closs EI. System L amino acid transporter LAT1 accumulates *O*-(2-fluoroethyl)-L-tyrosine (FET). Amino Acids. 2015;47(2):335–44.
7. Okubo S, Zhen H-N, Kawai N, Nishiyama Y, Haba R, Tamiya T. Correlation of L-methyl-11 C-methionine (MET) uptake with L-type amino acid transporter 1 in human gliomas. J Neuro Oncol. 2010;99(2):217–25.
8. Youland RS, Kitange GJ, Peterson TE, et al. The role of LAT1 in 18 F-DOPA uptake in malignant gliomas. J Neuro Oncol 2013;111(1):11–18.
9. Rapp M, Heinzel A, Galldiks N, et al. Diagnostic performance of 18F-FET PET in newly diagnosed cerebral lesions suggestive of glioma. J Nucl Med. 2013;54(2):229–35.
10. Albert NL, Weller M, Suchorska B, et al. Response assessment in neuro-oncology working group and European Association for neuro-Oncology recommendations for the clinical use of PET imaging in gliomas. Neuro-Oncol. 2016;18(9):1199–208.
11. Galldiks N, Langen K-J, Albert NL, et al. PET imaging in patients with brain metastasis—report of the RANO/PET group. Neuro-Oncol. 2019;21(5):585–95.
12. Galldiks N, Langen KJ, Holy R, et al. Assessment of treatment response in patients with glioblastoma using *O*-(2-18F-fluoroethyl)-L-tyrosine PET in comparison to MRI. J Nucl Med Jul 2012;53(7):1048–1057.
13. Galldiks N, Niyazi M, Grosu AL, et al. Contribution of PET imaging to radiotherapy planning and monitoring in glioma patients-a report of the PET/RANO group. Neuro Oncol. 2021;23(6):881–93.
14. Piroth MD, Pinkawa M, Holy R, et al. Prognostic value of early [18F]fluoroethyltyrosine positron emission tomography after radiochemotherapy in glioblastoma multiforme. Int J Radiat Oncol Biol Phys. 2011;80(1):176–84.
15. Poulsen SH, Urup T, Grunnet K, et al. The prognostic value of FET PET at radiotherapy planning in newly diagnosed glioblastoma. Eur J Nucl Med Mol Imaging. 2017;44(3):373–81.
16. Suchorska B, Jansen NL, Linn J, et al. Biological tumor volume in 18FET-PET before radiochemotherapy correlates with survival in GBM. Neurology. 2015;84(7):710–9.
17. Grosu A-L, Weber WA, Riedel E, et al. L-(methyl-11C) methionine positron emission tomography for target delineation in resected high-grade gliomas before radiotherapy. Int J Radiat Oncol Biol Phys. 2005;63(1):64–74.
18. Song S, Cheng Y, Ma J, et al. Simultaneous FET-PET and contrast-enhanced MRI based on hybrid PET/MR improves delineation of tumor spatial biodistribution in gliomas: a biopsy validation study. Eur J Nucl Med Mol Imaging. 2020;47:1458–67.

19. Kracht LW, Miletic H, Busch S, et al. Delineation of brain tumor extent with [11C]l-methionine positron emission tomography. Clin Cancer Res. 2004;10(21):7163.
20. Pauleit D, Floeth F, Hamacher K, et al. *O*-(2-[18F]fluoroethyl)-L-tyrosine PET combined with MRI improves the diagnostic assessment of cerebral gliomas. Brain J Neurol. 2005;128(3):678–87.
21. Pafundi DH, Laack NN, Youland RS, et al. Biopsy validation of 18F-DOPA PET and biodistribution in gliomas for neurosurgical planning and radiotherapy target delineation: results of a prospective pilot study. Neuro Oncol. 2013;15(8):1058–67.
22. Roodakker KR, Alhuseinalkhudhur A, Al-Jaff M, et al. Region-by-region analysis of PET, MRI, and histology in en bloc-resected oligodendrogliomas reveals intra-tumoral heterogeneity. Eur J Nucl Med Mol Imaging. 2019;46(3):569–79.
23. Verburg N, Koopman T, Yaqub MM, et al. Improved detection of diffuse glioma infiltration with imaging combinations: a diagnostic accuracy study. Neuro Oncol. 2019;22(3): 412–22.
24. Schön SCJ, Liesche-Starnecker F, Molina-Romero M, Eichinger P, Metz M, Karimov I, Preibisch C, Keupp J, Hock A, Meyer B, Weber W, Zimmer C, Pyka T, Yakushev I, Gempt J, Wiestler B. Imaging glioma biology: spatial comparison of amino acid PET, amide proton transfer, and perfusion-weighted MRI in newly diagnosed gliomas. Eur J Nucl Med Mol Imaging. 2020;47(6):1468–75.
25. Niyazi M, Geisler J, Siefert A, et al. FET-PET for malignant glioma treatment planning. Radiother Oncol. 2011;99(1):44–8.
26. Weber DC, Zilli T, Buchegger F, et al. [(18)F]Fluoroethyltyrosine- positron emission tomography-guided radiotherapy for high-grade glioma. Radiat Oncol. 2008;3(1):44.
27. Lohmann P, Stavrinou P, Lipke K, et al. FET PET reveals considerable spatial differences in tumour burden compared to conventional MRI in newly diagnosed glioblastoma. Eur J Nucl Med Mol Imaging. 2019;46(3):591–602.
28. Piroth M, Pinkawa M, Holy R, et al. Integrated boost IMRT with FET-PET-adapted local dose escalation in glioblastomas. Strahlenther Onkol. 2012;188(4):334–9.
29. Lee IH, Piert M, Gomez-Hassan D, et al. Association of 11C-methionine PET uptake with site of failure after concurrent temozolomide and radiation for primary glioblastoma multiforme. Int J Radiat Oncol Biol Phys. 2009;73(2):479–85.
30. Mahasittiwat P, Mizoe J-e, Hasegawa A, et al. L-[methyl-11C] methionine positron emission tomography for target delineation in malignant gliomas: impact on results of carbon ion radiotherapy. Int J Radiat Oncol Biol Phys. 2008;70(2):515–22.
31. Seidlitz A, Beuthien-Baumann B, Löck S, et al. Final results of the prospective biomarker trial PETra:[11C]-MET-accumulation in postoperative PET/MRI predicts outcome after radiochemotherapy in glioblastoma. Clin Cancer Res. 2021;27(5):1351–60.
32. Grosu AL, Weber WA, Franz M, et al. Reirradiation of recurrent high-grade gliomas using amino acid PET (SPECT)/CT/MRI image fusion to determine gross tumor volume for stereotactic fractionated radiotherapy. Int J Radiat Oncol Biol Phys. 2005;63(2):511–9.
33. Oehlke O, Mix M, Graf E, et al. Amino-acid PET versus MRI guided re-irradiation in patients with recurrent glioblastoma multiforme (GLIAA)–protocol of a randomized phase II trial (NOA 10/ARO 2013-1). BMC Cancer. 2016;16:769.
34. Galldiks N, Dunkl V, Stoffels G, et al. Diagnosis of pseudoprogression in patients with glioblastoma using *O*-(2-[18 F] fluoroethyl)-L-tyrosine PET. Eur J Nucl Med Mol Imaging. 2015;42(5):685–95.
35. Werner J-M, Stoffels G, Lichtenstein T, et al. Differentiation of treatment-related changes from tumour progression: a direct comparison between dynamic FET PET and ADC values obtained from DWI MRI. Eur J Nucl Med Mol Imaging. 2019;46(9):1889–901.
36. Harada H. Hypoxia-inducible factor 1–mediated characteristic features of cancer cells for tumor radioresistance. J Radiat Res. 2016;57(S1):i99–i105.
37. Hirata K, Terasaka S, Shiga T, et al. 18 F-Fluoromisonidazole positron emission tomography may differentiate glioblastoma multiforme from less malignant gliomas. Eur J Nucl Med Mol Imaging. 2012;39(5):760–70.

38. Koch CJ, Evans SM. Non-invasive PET and SPECT imaging of tissue hypoxia using isotopically labeled 2-nitroimidazoles. Adv Exp Med Biol. Oxygen Transport to Tissue XXIII. 2003;510:285–92.
39. Verhoeven J, Bolcaen J, De Meulenaere V, et al. Technical feasibility of [18F]FET and [18F]FAZA PET guided radiotherapy in a F98 glioblastoma rat model. Radiat Oncol. 2019;14(1):89.
40. Mapelli P, Zerbetto F, Incerti E, et al. 18F-FAZA PET/CT hypoxia imaging of high-grade glioma before and after radiotherapy. Clin Nucl Med. 2017;42(12):e525–6.
41. Narita T, Aoyama H, Hirata K, et al. Reoxygenation of glioblastoma multiforme treated with fractionated radiotherapy concomitant with temozolomide: changes defined by 18F-fluoromisonidazole positron emission tomography: two case reports. Jpn J Clin Oncol. 2012;42(2):120–3.
42. Albert NL, Unterrainer M, Fleischmann DF, et al. TSPO PET for glioma imaging using the novel ligand 18F-GE-180: first results in patients with glioblastoma. Eur J Nucl Med Mol Imaging. 2017;44(13):2230–8.
43. Unterrainer M, Fleischmann DF, Diekmann C, et al. Comparison of 18F-GE-180 and dynamic 18F-FET PET in high grade glioma: a double-tracer pilot study. Eur J Nucl Med Mol Imaging. 2019;46(3):580–90.
44. Whittle IR, Smith C, Navoo P, Collie D. Meningiomas. Lancet. 2004;363(9420):1535–43.
45. Goldbrunner R, Minniti G, Preusser M, et al. EANO guidelines for the diagnosis and treatment of meningiomas. Lancet Oncol. 2016;17(9):e383–91.
46. Reubi J, Maurer R, Klijn J, et al. High incidence of somatostatin receptors in human meningiomas: biochemical characterization. J Clin Endocrinol Metabol. 1986;63(2):433–8.
47. Nyuyki F, Plotkin M, Graf R, et al. Potential impact of 68Ga-DOTATOC PET/CT on stereotactic radiotherapy planning of meningiomas. Eur J Nucl Med Mol Imaging. 2010;37(2):310–8.
48. Gehler B, Paulsen F, Öksüz MÖ, et al. [68Ga]-DOTATOC-PET/CT for meningioma IMRT treatment planning. Radiat Oncol. 2009;4(1):56.
49. Kunz WG, Jungblut LM, Kazmierczak PM, et al. Improved detection of transosseous meningiomas using 68Ga-DOTATATE PET/CT compared with contrast-enhanced MRI. J Nucl Med. 2017;58(10):1580.
50. Graf R, Nyuyki F, Steffen IG, et al. Contribution of 68Ga-DOTATOC PET/CT to target volume delineation of skull base meningiomas treated with stereotactic radiation therapy. Int J Radiat Oncol Biol Phys. 2013;85(1):68–73.
51. Milker-Zabel S, Zabel-du Bois A, Henze M, et al. Improved target volume definition for fractionated stereotactic radiotherapy in patients with intracranial meningiomas by correlation of CT, MRI, and [68Ga]-DOTATOC-PET. Int J Radiat Oncol Biol Phys. 2006;65(1):222–7.
52. Rachinger W, Stoecklein VM, Terpolilli NA, et al. Increased ^{68}Ga-DOTATATE uptake in PET imaging discriminates meningioma and tumor-free tissue. J Nucl Med. 2015;56(3):347–53.
53. Brizel DM, Sibley GS, Prosnitz LR, Scher RL, Dewhirst MW. Tumor hypoxia adversely affects the prognosis of carcinoma of the head and neck. Int J Radiat Oncol Biol Phys. 1997;38(2):285–9.
54. Hoogsteen IJ, Lok J, Marres HA, et al. Hypoxia in larynx carcinomas assessed by pimonidazole binding and the value of CA-IX and vascularity as surrogate markers of hypoxia. Eur J Cancer. 2009;45(16):2906–14.
55. Nordsmark M, Bentzen SM, Rudat V, et al. Prognostic value of tumor oxygenation in 397 head and neck tumors after primary radiation therapy. An international multi-center study. Radiother Oncol. 2005;77(1):18–24.
56. Nordsmark M, Loncaster J, Aquino-Parsons C, et al. The prognostic value of pimonidazole and tumour pO_2 in human cervix carcinomas after radiation therapy: a prospective international multi-center study. Radiother Oncol. 2006;80(2):123–31.
57. Nordsmark M, Loncaster J, Aquino-Parsons C, et al. Measurements of hypoxia using pimonidazole and polarographic oxygen-sensitive electrodes in human cervix carcinomas. Radiother Oncol. 2003;67(1):35–44.

58. Rademakers SE, Hoogsteen IJ, Rijken PF, et al. Pattern of CAIX expression is prognostic for outcome and predicts response to ARCON in patients with laryngeal cancer treated in a phase III randomized trial. Radiother Oncol. 2013;108(3):517–22.
59. Horsman M, Mortensen LS, Petersen JB, Busk M, Overgaard J. Imaging hypoxia to improve treatment outcome. Nat Rev Clin Oncol. 2012;9(12):674–87.
60. Troost EG, Laverman P, Philippens ME, et al. Correlation of [(18)F]FMISO autoradiography and pimonodazole immunohistochemistry in human head and neck carcinoma xenografts. Eur J Nucl Med Mol Imaging. 2008;35(10):1803–11.
61. Troost EG, Laverman P, Kaanders JH, et al. Imaging hypoxia after oxygenation-modification: comparing [18F]FMISO autoradiography with pimonidazole immunohistochemistry in human xenograft tumors. Radiother Oncol. 2006;80(2):157–64.
62. Eschmann SM, Paulsen F, Reimold M, et al. Prognostic impact of hypoxia imaging with 18F-misonidazole PET in non-small cell lung cancer and head and neck cancer before radiotherapy. J Nucl Med. 2005;46(2):253–60.
63. Thorwarth D, Eschmann SM, Holzner F, Paulsen F, Alber M. Combined uptake of [18F]FDG and [18F]FMISO correlates with radiation therapy outcome in head-and-neck cancer patients. Radiother Oncol. 2006;80(2):151–6.
64. Thorwarth D, Eschmann SM, Paulsen F, Alber M. A kinetic model for dynamic [18F]-Fmiso PET data to analyse tumour hypoxia. Phys Med Biol. 2005;50(10):2209–24.
65. Thorwarth D, Eschmann SM, Scheiderbauer J, Paulsen F, Alber M. Kinetic analysis of dynamic 18F-fluoromisonidazole PET correlates with radiation treatment outcome in head-and-neck cancer. BMC Cancer. 2005;5:152.
66. Löck S, Perrin R, Seidlitz A, et al. Residual tumour hypoxia in head-and-neck cancer patients undergoing primary radiochemotherapy, final results of a prospective trial on repeat FMISO-PET imaging. Radiother Oncol. 2017;124(3):533–40.
67. Zips D, Zophel K, Abolmaali N, et al. Exploratory prospective trial of hypoxia-specific PET imaging during radiochemotherapy in patients with locally advanced head-and-neck cancer. Radiother Oncol. 2012;105(1):21–8.
68. Riaz N, Sherman E, Pei X, et al. Precision radiotherapy: reduction in radiation for oropharyngeal cancer in the 30 ROC trial. J Natl Cancer Inst. 2021;113(6):742–51.
69. Thorwarth D, Eschmann SM, Paulsen F, Alber M. Hypoxia dose painting by numbers: a planning study. Int J Radiat Oncol Biol Phys. 2007;68(1):291–300.
70. Zschaeck S, Haase R, Abolmaali N, et al. Spatial distribution of FMISO in head and neck squamous cell carcinomas during radio-chemotherapy and its correlation to pattern of failure. Acta Oncol. 2015;54(9):1355–63.
71. Pigorsch SU, Wilkens JJ, Kampfer S, et al. Do selective radiation dose escalation and tumour hypoxia status impact the loco-regional tumour control after radio-chemotherapy of head & neck tumours? The ESCALOX protocol. Radiat Oncol. 2017;12:45.
72. Nehmeh SA, Moussa MB, Lee N, et al. Comparison of FDG and FMISO uptakes and distributions in head and neck squamous cell cancer tumors. Eur J Nucl Med Mol Imaging. 2021;11:38.
73. Imaizumi A, Obata T, Kershaw J, et al. Imaging of hypoxic tumor: correlation between diffusion-weighted MR imaging and 18F-fluoroazomycin Arabinoside positron emission tomography in head and neck carcinoma. Magn Reson Med Sci. 2020;19(3):276–81.
74. Graves EE, Hicks RJ, Binns D, et al. Quantitative and qualitative analysis of [18F]FDG and [18F]FAZA positron emission tomography of head and neck cancers and associations with HPV status and treatment outcome. Eur J Nucl Med Mol Imaging. 2016;43(4):617–25.
75. Zschaeck S, Löck S, Hofheinz F, et al. Individual patient data meta-analysis of FMISO and FAZA hypoxia PET scans from head and neck cancer patients undergoing definitive radio-chemotherapy. Radiother Oncol. 2020;149:189–96.
76. Zegers CM, van Elmpt W, Szardenings K, et al. Repeatability of hypoxia PET imaging using [18F]HX4 in lung and head and neck cancer patients: a prospective multicenter trial. Eur J Nucl Med Mol Imaging. 2015;42(12):1840–9.

77. Zegers CM, Hoebers FJ, van Elmpt W, et al. Evaluation of tumour hypoxia during radiotherapy using [18F]HX4 PET imaging and blood biomarkers in patients with head and neck cancer. Eur J Nucl Med Mol Imaging. 2016;43(12):2139–46.
78. Sanduleanu S, Hamming-Vrieze O, Wesseling FWR, et al. [18F]-HX4 PET/CT hypoxia in patients with squamous cell carcinoma of the head and neck treated with chemoradiotherapy: prognostic results from two prospective trials. Clin Transl Radiat Oncol. 2020;23:9–15.
79. Ballegeer EA, Madrill NJ, Berger KL, Agnew DW, McNiel EA. Evaluation of hypoxia in a feline model of head and neck cancer using ^{64}Cu-ATSM positron emission tomography/computed tomography. BMC Cancer. 2013;13:218.
80. Chao KS, Bosch WR, Miutic S, et al. A novel approach to overcome hypoxic tumor resistance: cu-ATSM-guided intensity-modulated radiation therapy. Int J Radiat Oncol Biol Phys. 2001;49(4):1171–82.
81. Lehtio K, Oikonen V, Gronroos T, et al. Imaging of blood flow and hypoxia in head and neck cancer: initial evaluation with [(15)O]H(2)O and [(18)F]fluoroerythronitroimidazole PET. J Nucl Med. 2001;42(11):1643–52.
82. Lehtiö K, Oikonen V, Nyman S, et al. Quantifying tumour hypoxia with fluorine-18 fluoroerythronitroimidazole ([18F]FETNIM) and PET using the tumour to plasma ratio. Eur J Nucl Med Mol Imaging. 2003;30(1):101–8.
83. Hu M, Peng X, Lee NY, et al. Hypoxia with 18F-fluoroerythronitroimidazole integrated positron emission tomography and computed tomography (18F-FETNIM PET/CT) in locoregionally advanced head and neck cancer: hypoxia changes during chemoradiotherapy and impact on clinical outcome. Medicine (Baltimore). 2019;98(40):e17067.
84. Troost EG, Bussink J, Slootweg PJ, et al. Histopathologic validation of 3′-deoxy-3'-18F-fluorothymidine PET in squamous cell carcinoma of the oral cavity. J Nucl Med. 2010;51(5):713–9.
85. Troost EG, Vogel WV, Merkx MA, et al. 18F-FLT PET does not discriminate between reactive and metastatic lymph nodes in primary head and neck cancer patients. J Nucl Med. 2007;48(5):726–35.
86. Hoeben BA, Troost EG, Span PN, et al. 18F-FLT PET during radiotherapy or chemoradiotherapy in head and neck squamous cell carcinoma is an early predictor of outcome. J Nucl Med. 2013;54(4):532–40.
87. Troost EG, Bussink J, Hoffmann AL, Boerman OC, Oyen WJ, Kaanders JH. 18F-FLT PET/CT for early response monitoring and dose escalation in oropharyngeal tumors. J Nucl Med. 2010;51(6):866–74.
88. Han D, Yu J, Yu Y, et al. Comparison of (18)F-fluorothymidine and (18)F-fluorodeoxyglucose PET/CT in delineating gross tumor volume by optimal threshold in patients with squamous cell carcinoma of thoracic esophagus. Int J Radiat Oncol Biol Phys. 2010;76(4):1235–41.
89. Liu J, Li C, Hu M, et al. Exploring spatial overlap of high-uptake regions derived from dual tracer positron emission tomography-computer tomography imaging using 18F-fluorodeoxyglucose and 18F-fluorodeoxythymidine in nonsmall cell lung cancer patients: a prospective pilot study. Medicine (Baltimore). 2015;94(17):e678.
90. Syed M, Flechsig P, Liermann J, et al. Fibroblast activation protein inhibitor (FAPI) PET for diagnostics and advanced targeted radiotherapy in head and neck cancers. Eur J Nucl Med Mol Imaging. 2020;47(12):2836–45.
91. Machado Medeiros T, Altmayer S, Watte G, et al. 18F-FDG PET/CT and whole-body MRI diagnostic performance in M staging for non–small cell lung cancer: a systematic review and meta-analysis. Eur Radiol. 2020;30(7):3641–9.
92. Madsen PH, Holdgaard PC, Christensen JB, Høilund-Carlsen PF. Clinical utility of F-18 FDG PET-CT in the initial evaluation of lung cancer. Eur J Nucl Med Mol Imaging. 2016;43(11):2084–97.
93. Nestle U, Schimek-Jasch T, Kremp S, et al. Imaging-based target volume reduction in chemoradiotherapy for locally advanced non-small-cell lung cancer (PET-plan): a multicentre, open-label, randomised, controlled trial. Lancet Oncol. 2020;21(4):581–92.

94. Vaz S, Adam JA, Delgado Bolton RC, et al. Joint EANM/SNMMI/ESTRO practice recommendations for the use of 2-[18 F]FDG PET/CT external beam radiation treatment planning in lung cancer V1.0. Eur J Nucl Med Mol Imaging. 2022;49(4):1386–406.
95. Sachpekidis C, Thieke C, Askoxylakis V, et al. Combined use of (18)F-FDG and (18) F-FMISO in unresectable non-small cell lung cancer patients planned for radiotherapy: a dynamic PET/CT study. Am J Nucl Med Mol Imaging. 2015;5(2):127–42.
96. Vera P, Thureau S, Chaumet-Riffaud P, et al. Phase II study of a radiotherapy Total dose increase in hypoxic lesions identified by 18 F-Misonidazole PET/CT in patients with non-small cell lung carcinoma (RTEP5 study). J Nucl Med. 2017;58(7):1045–53.
97. Vera P, Muhailescu S-D, Lequesne J, et al. Radiotherapy boost in patients with hypoxic lesions identified by 18 F-FMISO PET/CT in non-small-cell lung carcinoma: can we expect a better survival outcome without toxicity? [RTEP5 long-term follow-up]. Eur J Nucl Med Mol Imaging. 2019;46(7):1448–56.
98. Thureau S, Piton N, Gouel P, et al. First comparison between [18f]-FMISO and [18f]-Faza for preoperative pet imaging of hypoxia in lung cancer. Cancers (Basel). 2021;13(16):4101.
99. Even AJG, van der Stoep J, Zegers CML, et al. PET-based dose painting in non-small cell lung cancer: comparing uniform dose escalation with boosting hypoxic and metabolically active sub-volumes. Radiother Oncol. 2015;116(2):281–6.
100. Zegers CM, van Elmpt W, Reymen B, et al. In vivo quantification of hypoxic and metabolic status of NSCLC tumors using [18F]HX4 and [18F]FDG-PET/CT imaging. Clin Cancer Res. 2014;20(24):6389–97.
101. Zegers CM, van Elmpt W, Wierts R, et al. Hypoxia imaging with [(1)(8)F]HX4 PET in NSCLC patients: defining optimal imaging parameters. Radiother Oncol. 2013;109(1):58–64.
102. Everitt S, Ball D, Hicks RJ, et al. Prospective study of serial imaging comparing fluorodeoxyglucose positron emission tomography (PET) and fluorothymidine PET during radical chemoradiation for non-small cell lung cancer: reduction of detectable proliferation associated with worse survival. Int J Radiat Oncol Biol Phys. 2017;99(4):947–55.
103. Everitt SJ, Ball DL, Hicks RJ, et al. Differential (18)F-FDG and (18)F-FLT uptake on serial PET/CT imaging before and during definitive Chemoradiation for non-small cell lung cancer. J Nucl Med. 2014;55(7):1069–74.
104. Kairemo K, Santos EB, Macapinlac HA, Subbiah V. Early response assessment to targeted therapy using 3′-deoxy-3′[(18)F]-Fluorothymidine (18F-FLT) PET/CT in lung cancer. Diagnostics. 2020;10(1):26.
105. Farolfi A, Calderoni L, Mattana F, et al. Current and emerging clinical applications of PSMA PET diagnostic imaging for prostate cancer. J Nucl Med. 2021;62(5):596–604.
106. Perera M, Papa N, Roberts M, et al. Gallium-68 prostate-specific membrane antigen positron emission tomography in advanced prostate cancer-updated diagnostic utility, sensitivity, specificity, and distribution of prostate-specific membrane antigen-avid lesions: a systematic review and meta-analysis. Eur Urol. 2020;77(4):403–17.
107. Grünig H, Maurer A, Thali Y, et al. Focal unspecific bone uptake on [18 F]-PSMA-1007 PET: a multicenter retrospective evaluation of the distribution, frequency, and quantitative parameters of a potential pitfall in prostate cancer imaging. Eur J Nucl Med Mol Imaging. 2021;48(13):4483–94.
108. Cappel CC, Dopcke D, Dunst J. PSMA PET-CT for primary staging in patients with advanced prostate cancer. Strahlenther Onkol. 2021;197(3):257–60.
109. Hofman MS, Lawrentschuk N, Francis RJ, et al. Prostate-specific membrane antigen PET-CT in patients with high-risk prostate cancer before curative-intent surgery or radiotherapy (proPSMA): a prospective, randomised, multicentre study. Lancet. 2020;395(10231):1208–16.
110. Dewes S, Schiller K, Sauter K, et al. Integration of (68)Ga-PSMA-PET imaging in planning of primary definitive radiotherapy in prostate cancer: a retrospective study. Radiat Oncol. 2016;11:73.
111. Calais J, Kishan AU, Cao M, et al. Potential impact of 68Ga-PSMA-11 PET/CT on the planning of definitive radiation therapy for prostate cancer. J Nucl Med. 2018;59(11):1714.

112. Kerkmeijer LGW, Groen VH, Pos FJ, et al. Focal boost to the Intraprostatic tumor in external beam radiotherapy for patients with localized prostate cancer: results from the FLAME randomized phase III trial. J Clin Oncol. 2021;39(7):787–96.
113. Bettermann AS, Zamboglou C, Kiefer S, et al. [68Ga-]PSMA-11 PET/CT and multiparametric MRI for gross tumor volume delineation in a slice by slice analysis with whole mount histopathology as a reference standard—implications for focal radiotherapy planning in primary prostate cancer. Radiother Oncol. 2019;141:214–9.
114. Kosztyla R, Raman S, Moiseenko V, Reinsberg SA, Toyota B, Nichol A. Dose-painted volumetric modulated arc therapy of high-grade glioma using 3, 4-dihydroxy-6-[18F] fluoro-l-phenylalanine positron emission tomography. Br J Radiol. 2019;92(1099):20180901.
115. Zamboglou C, Wieser G, Hennies S, et al. MRI versus (6)(8)Ga-PSMA PET/CT for gross tumour volume delineation in radiation treatment planning of primary prostate cancer. Eur J Nucl Med Mol Imaging. 2016;43(5):889–97.
116. Zamboglou C, Schiller F, Fechter T, et al. (68)Ga-HBED-CC-PSMA PET/CT versus histopathology in primary localized prostate cancer: a voxel-wise comparison. Theranostics. 2016;6(10):1619–28.
117. Zamboglou C, Sachpazidis I, Koubar K, et al. Evaluation of intensity modulated radiation therapy dose painting for localized prostate cancer using 68Ga-HBED-CC PSMA-PET/CT: a planning study based on histopathology reference. Radiother Oncol. 2017;123(3):472–7.
118. Schiller K, Stöhrer L, Düsberg M, et al. PSMA-PET/CT-based lymph node atlas for prostate cancer patients recurring after primary treatment: clinical implications for salvage radiation therapy. Eur Urol Oncol. 2021;4(1):73–83.
119. Slevin F, Beasley M, Cross W, Scarsbrook A, Murray L, Henry A. Patterns of lymph node failure in patients with recurrent prostate cancer postradical prostatectomy and implications for salvage therapies. Adv Radiat Oncol. 2020;5(6):1126–40.
120. Valle L, Shabsovich D, de Meerleer G, et al. Use and impact of positron emission tomography/computed tomography prior to salvage radiation therapy in men with biochemical recurrence after radical prostatectomy: a scoping review. Eur Urol Oncol. 2021;4(3):339–55.
121. Hurmuz P, Onal C, Ozyigit G, et al. Treatment outcomes of metastasis-directed treatment using ^{68}Ga-PSMA-PET/CT for oligometastatic or oligorecurrent prostate cancer: Turkish Society for Radiation Oncology group study (TROD 09-002). Strahlenther Onkol. 2020;196(11):1034–43.
122. Bluemel C, Krebs M, Polat B, et al. 68Ga-PSMA-PET/CT in patients with biochemical prostate cancer recurrence and negative 18F-choline-PET/CT. Clin Nucl Med. 2016;41(7):515–21.
123. Habl G, Sauter K, Schiller K, et al. 68Ga-PSMA-PET for radiation treatment planning in prostate cancer recurrences after surgery: individualized medicine or new standard in salvage treatment. Prostate. 2017;77(8):920–7.
124. Schmidt-Hegemann N-S, Fendler WP, Ilhan H, et al. Outcome after PSMA PET/CT based radiotherapy in patients with biochemical persistence or recurrence after radical prostatectomy. Radiat Oncol. 2018;13(1):37.
125. Loktev A, Lindner T, Mier W, et al. A tumor-imaging method targeting cancer-associated fibroblasts. J Nucl Med. 2018;59(9):1423.
126. Lindner T, Loktev A, Altmann A, et al. Development of quinoline-based theranostic ligands for the targeting of fibroblast activation protein. J Nucl Med. 2018;59(9):1415.
127. Syed M, Flechsig P, Liermann J, et al. Fibroblast activation protein (FAPI) specific PET for advanced target volume delineation in head and neck cancer. Int J Radiat Oncol Biol Phys. 2019;105(1):E383.
128. Giesel FL, Adeberg S, Syed M, et al. FAPI-74 PET/CT using either ^{18}F-AlF or cold-kit ^{68}Ga labeling: biodistribution, radiation dosimetry, and tumor delineation in lung cancer patients. J Nucl Med. 2021;62(2):201.
129. Windisch P, Zwahlen DR, Koerber SA, et al. Clinical results of fibroblast activation protein (FAP) specific PET and implications for radiotherapy planning: systematic review. Cancers. 2020;12(9):2629.

130. Bensch F, Brouwers AH, Lub-de Hooge MN, et al. 89 Zr-trastuzumab PET supports clinical decision making in breast cancer patients, when HER2 status cannot be determined by standard work up. Eur J Nucl Med Mol Imaging. 2018;45(13):2300–6.
131. Lohrmann C, O'Reilly EM, O'Donoghue JA, et al. Retooling a blood-based biomarker: phase I assessment of the high-affinity CA19-9 antibody HuMab-5B1 for immuno-PET imaging of pancreatic cancer. Clin Cancer Res. 2019;25(23):7014–23.
132. Sanchez-Vega F, Hechtman JF, Castel P, et al. EGFR and MET amplifications determine response to HER2 inhibition in ERBB2-amplified Esophagogastric cancer. Cancer Discov. 2019;9(2):199–209.
133. Badawi RD, Shi H, Hu P, et al. First human imaging studies with the EXPLORER Total-body PET scanner. J Nucl Med. 2019;60(3):299–303.

3 Use of Anatomical and Functional MRI in Radiation Treatment Planning

Angela Romano, Luca Boldrini, Antonio Piras, and Vincenzo Valentini

3.1 Introduction

The application of magnetic resonance imaging (MRI) in radiotherapy (RT) is being widely used in contemporary planning techniques, owing to its superior soft contrast tissue resolution compared to computed tomography (CT) [1], especially in anatomical sites such as brain, head and neck, abdomen and pelvis [2–4]. With the introduction of modern radiotherapy techniques, such as intensity-modulated radiation therapy (IMRT) and stereotactic body radiation therapy (SBRT), in which steep dose gradients are delivered to small target volumes, the accurate definition and precise delineation of the target volumes and of the organs at risk (OARs) has become crucial [5]. To this end, the use of MRI in treatment planning was proposed as early as 1987 [6], since MRI is a multiparametric imaging modality that can provide both anatomical and functional information. For its characteristics, MRI can be very useful not only in the treatment planning phase but also in evaluating the response to radiotherapy [5].

The use of MRI sequences for RT planning purposes has been boosted in the last years thanks to the development of always more reliable image fusion algorithms (e.g. rigid, affine, piecewise affine and elastic), and to the ability to co-register the MRI dataset with the planning CT, which contains the electron density information necessary for dose calculation [7]. In the following years, several authors have

A. Romano · A. Piras
Dipartimento di Diagnostica per Immagini, Radioterapia Oncologica ed Ematologia, Fondazione Policlinico Universitario "A. Gemelli" IRCCS, Rome, Italy

L. Boldrini (✉) · V. Valentini
Dipartimento di Diagnostica per Immagini, Radioterapia Oncologica ed Ematologia, Fondazione Policlinico Universitario "A. Gemelli" IRCCS, Rome, Italy

Istituto di Radiologia, Università Cattolica del Sacro Cuore, Rome, Italy
e-mail: Luca.boldrini@unicatt.it; luca.boldrini@policlinicogemelli.it; vincenzo.valentini@policlinicogemelli.it

E. G. C. Troost (ed.), *Image-Guided High-Precision Radiotherapy*, https://doi.org/10.1007/978-3-031-08601-4_3

shown that the use of MRI in radiotherapy is advantageous also for segmentation quality, as it reduces the inter- and intra-observer contouring variations [8]. In addition, MRI has the potential to increase the quality of the radiation treatments, allowing for an MRI-assisted dose escalation [9–11].

This chapter is separated into the different disease sites, which are of potential interest to an MR-based RT workflow and radiation delivery.

3.2 Brain

3.2.1 High-Grade Gliomas

MRI represents the gold standard diagnostic technique for the diagnosis and RT planning of primary brain tumours and metastases [12]. The current clinical use and possible new fields of application of MRI in the most frequent brain tumours in adults are discussed below.

3.2.1.1 What Is the MR's Standard Acquisition Protocol for RT Planning?

Glioblastoma multiforme (GBM), a high-grade, WHO grade IV, primary brain tumour, is characterized by its infiltrative nature and its tendency to recur locally: precise target delineation results enhance treatment quality, reducing RT-induced toxicity and improving quality of life. Any effort should therefore be made to identify the optimal imaging approach in order to ensure an effective and safe delivery. The standard diagnostic examination for GBM should include multiple sequences (in 3D acquisition): T2-weighted images (T2w), T2 Fluid-attenuated inversion recovery (FLAIR), native T1-weighted images (T1w) and contrast-enhanced T1w (CI-T1w) images using gadolinium.

Diffusion-weighted imaging (DWI) sequences, offering an insight into the diffusion of water molecules in tissues, should also be provided with the apparent diffusion coefficient (ADC) map calculation [13]. ADC values have been shown to decrease in highly cellular tumours (e.g. CNS lymphoma, medulloblastoma, high-grade glioma) and have been reported to correlate with prognosis [14–16]. High-resolution 3D T2w gradient echo sequences, such as susceptibility-weighted imaging (SWI), which prove to be very sensible to blood products and calcifications, are also routinely performed [17, 18].

3.2.1.2 Which Are the MRI Studies Currently Available?

Diffusion tensor imaging (DTI) sequences provide additional insights beyond DWI into the microstructure and integrity of the white matter. DTI is mostly used in the context of DTI-tractography, through the three-dimensional visualization of white matter fibres for navigation purposes [19]. The main methods for perfusion imaging include T2w dynamic susceptibility contrast-enhanced (DSC) perfusion and T1w dynamic contrast-enhanced (DCE) perfusion. Perfusion cerebral blood volume (CBV) and relative cerebral blood volume (rCBV), a parameter able to describe tumoural neoangiogenesis, can be extracted from the DSC images and Ktrans, a microvascular permeability parameter, from the DCE images [20, 21]. MR spectroscopy provides insights into the metabolic profile of analysed tissues. The obtained graph is a function of the presence and quantitative distribution of the metabolites of interest. It can be very useful in monitoring the response to chemotherapy and radiotherapy and the differentiation between tumour recurrence and radionecrosis, especially in the frame of reirradiation [22]. Functional MRI (fMRI) uses relative changes in the blood oxygen level-dependent (BOLD) signal to infer brain activity. In particular, task-based fMRI can be used for preoperative planning purposes [23]. The use of diffusion-weighted images (DWI) and MRI perfusion for contouring is being considered in contemporary clinical practice, but further studies are awaited to validate its use [24].

3.2.1.3 How Can MRI Be Used in Treatment Planning Workflow in High-Grade Glioma Radiotherapy?

The ESTRO-ACROP guidelines of "target delineation of glioblastomas" [25] provide recommendations for the radiotherapy workflow management and foresee the co-registration of the contrast-enhanced MRI with the planning CT to guide target delineation.

3.2.1.4 Which MRI Sequences Can Be Used?

Contrast-enhanced thin-slice (3 mm or less) T1w and FLAIR sequences should be co-registered with the planning CT (Fig. 3.1a,b). The use of 1-mm isotropic MPRAGE images could help in organs at risk (OARs) contouring, especially for

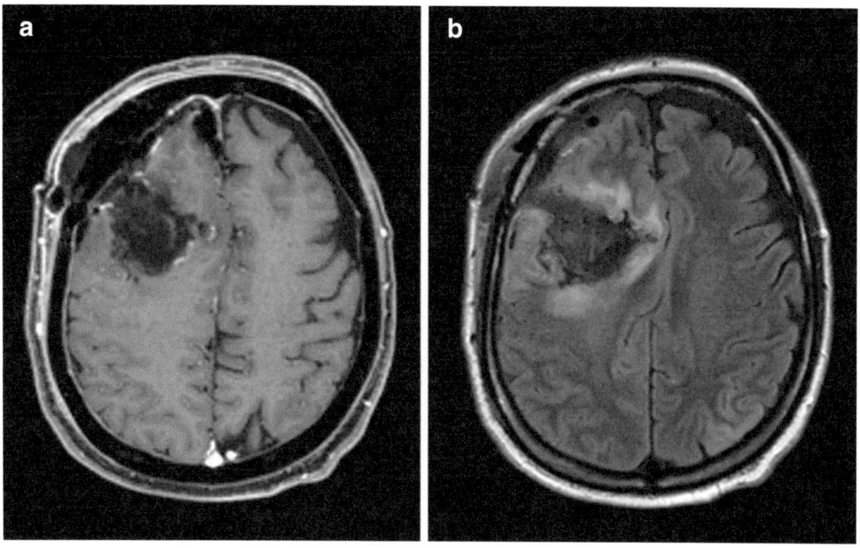

Fig. 3.1 Surgical cavity resulting from right fronto-parietal craniotomy for the removal of an expansive-infiltrative glioblastoma lesion. Brain parenchyma along the cranial margins of the surgical cavity shows contrast enhancement (**a**: contrast-enhanced T1w scan, left) and appears hyperintense in FLAIR images. This finding can be referred either to edemigenous phenomena or to probable infiltrative component of disease (**b**: FLAIR scan, right)

small anatomical structures (hippocampus, optical pathway). The use of advanced functional techniques, such as DWI, DTI, and other diagnostic techniques, such as PET-CT, remains investigational, as this is still not supported by robust scientific studies.

3.2.1.5 What Are the Recommendations for Contouring?

Referring to the ESTRO-ACROP guidelines mentioned above, the tumour bed volume (TBV) in the postoperative setting should encompass surgical cavity plus any evidence of contrast-enhancing residual tumour on contrast-enhanced T1w [25]. Comparing the postoperative MRI with the preoperative one and especially using DWI images is always suggested, in order to better identify any residual disease. All areas with contrast-enhancement must be included in the target volume, while possible areas of hyperintensity in T2w/FLAIR should not. The clinical target volume (CTV), which includes the microscopic tumour extension, is generally obtained with an expansion of 20 mm from the TBV or gross tumour volume (GTV), taking into account the surrounding anatomical barriers and avoiding overlaps with them (i.e. bones).

If low-grade disease infiltration is suspected based on T2w- or FLAIR-images, these should be included in the CTV. In case of secondary glioblastomas originated from previously lower grade gliomas (WHO grades II or III), the areas without contrast-enhancement may also represent disease components. In these cases, high-signal T2w/FLAIR areas should also be included in GTV. The planning target volume (PTV) is generally obtained with a 3–5 mm expansion from the CTV.

3.2.1.6 Which Characteristics Should an MRI Have for Adjuvant Radiotherapy Planning?

The execution of a post-surgical MRI, which is usually performed within 48 h after the surgical procedure, is fundamental to quantify the possible residual tumour extension, but its use for segmentation guidance could underestimate the real extent of the disease. The ideal condition would be to use an MRI obtained around the time of radiation treatment planning.

3.2.2 Low-Grade Gliomas

3.2.2.1 Can MRI Be Useful in Contouring of Low-Grade Gliomas?

Surgery generally represents the first choice of treatment for these diseases and post-operative radiotherapy is indicated when negative prognostic factors are present. Then, MRI also plays a key role in the management of radiation treatment planning [26, 27]. Low-grade gliomas generally do not show enhancement in T1w (which represents a possible index of focal transformation in high-grade gliomas), while they appear hyperintense in T2w/FLAIR sequences. The use of post-operative MRI to be co-registered with the RT simulation CT scan is recommended in radiotherapy planning of these malignancies.

In case of low-grade gliomas, the GTV includes the surgical bed (TBV), the macroscopically visible disease hyperintense on T2w of the post-operative MRI and any areas with contrast enhancement on T1w-MRI.

The CTV is obtained by adding a 10–15 mm expansion margin to the GTV, taking into account the anatomical barriers, as previously described [28]. The PTV is generally obtained with a 3–5 mm expansion from the CTV.

3.2.3 Brain Metastases

3.2.3.1 Can MRI Be Useful in Radiotherapy Workflow for Brain Metastases?

Brain metastases represent the most frequent malignant tumour of the central nervous system. It is estimated that brain metastases can be developed in 20–40% of cancer patients, regardless of primary disease site. The use of MRI in this setting is to date well-known in clinical practice both for the diagnosis and radiation treatment planning [29]. MRI has a higher sensitivity in detecting metastases as well as identifying leptomeningeal spread compared to other techniques. In brain metastases, which are often small in size and volume, the acquisition of an MRI on thin-slice planning is recommended [30].

3.2.3.2 How Can MRI Help in Defining GTV?

Brain metastases usually appear iso- or hypointense on T1w, hyperintense on T2w, and exhibit avid enhancement. Some metastases are hyperintense on T1w, such as those originating from melanoma, due to the presence of melanin and/or haemorrhagic areas. ADC values are high in peritumoural vasogenic oedema on T2w/FLAIR, if compared to the aspect of the oedema surrounding infiltrative lesions, such as it is the case in high-grade gliomas. The GTV can be identified with the enhancement area on T1w. The CTV is generally considered equal to the GTV, and PTV is obtained by adding an expansion margin of 1–3 mm. This small margin can be achieved by employing highly rigid immobilization devices as is common practice in stereotactic treatment or radiosurgery. With regard to this issue, the thin slice spoiled gradient-recalled echo (SPGR) post-contrast MRI performed in a head frame for gamma knife treatment planning has been demonstrated to be more sensitive in identifying small lesions than standard T1w [31].

3.2.3.3 Is the Use of Co-Registration with MRI Also Recommended in Whole-Brain Treatment?

The use of MRI in whole-brain treatments (WBRT) is recommended whenever pursuing a heterogeneous dose prescription, e.g. dose boosting protocols or specific organs at risk avoidance. Hippocampal-sparing WBRT, with the aim of reducing toxicity and cognitive impairment in patients undergoing WBRT, represents a good example of this approach. In this setting MRI results particularly useful as it guides hippocampal contouring on T1WwMRI axial sequences [32].

3.2.4 Meningiomas

3.2.4.1 Does MRI Play a Role in the Contouring of Meningiomas?

Radiotherapy is indicated in case of partial resection, surgical contraindications, or of atypical or malignant meningiomas. Meningiomas appear as extra-axial masses with signal intensity similar to cortex on T1w and T2w, avid and homogeneous enhancement after administration of gadolinium and the classical "dural tail" sign, reflecting infiltration and/or vascular congestion in the adjacent dura. The distinguishing characteristic of meningiomas, not typical of other neoplasms, is the tendency not to respect dural boundary [33]. As for the definition of the target volume, contrast-enhanced CT with a slice thickness of less than 3 mm and contrast-enhanced T1w-MRI represent the recommended diagnostic scans.

3.2.4.2 What Are the Recommendations for Contouring?

For patients who did not undergo surgery, the GTV includes the entire tumour volume identified on CT and MRI, its insertion into the dura up to the first 3 mm and all bone abnormalities visible on the CT scan using the bone window. For operated or relapsed patients, the CTV is defined by evaluating the tumour residual shown on contrast-enhancement T1w, including microscopic areas of disease based on surgical and pathological reports. As for the adjuvant setting, therapy volumes reflect the WHO classification score. In case of a WHO I meningioma, the GTV must include only the residual disease, while for WHO grade II and III meningiomas, an expansion to CTV is recommended, which can be up to 30 mm (especially in grade III).

For benign meningiomas, the CTV is equivalent to the GTV and does not include areas of oedema [34, 35]. The inclusion of the "dural tail" in the target volume is still a controversial topic and object of debate [33].

3.3 Head and Neck Cancer

Radiotherapy plays a key role in the management of head and neck cancers (HNC), and with the introduction of highly conformed irradiation techniques (such as intensity-modulated radiation therapy or volumetric modulated arc therapy) as standard of care, a highly accurate and precise definition of treatment volumes is mandatory.

3.3.1 How Can MRI Be Integrated into Treatment Planning for HNC?

To this end, MRI has significant advantages in soft tissue discrimination and does not suffer from artefacts caused by bone or dental fillings or implants [36]. The co-registration of the simulation CT-scan and the diagnostic MRI can be useful in treatment planning, both in the primary and in the post-operative settings, in order to provide more accurate definition of target volumes and organs at risk, which are generally poorly visualized on CT imaging (i.e. optic nerves, chiasm, brainstem, spinal cord, parotid glands and brachial plexus). Magnetic resonance imaging can also guide the segmentation of cervical lymph nodes. In metastatically affected lymph nodes, their shape progressively changes from oval to round, and the MRI is able to clearly show infiltration into the perinodal fat and desmoplastic reaction causing irregularities in the profile [37, 38]. A proper evaluation of image co-registration protocols is recommended, including deformable co-registration, in order to take into account possible anatomical changes relative to mandible or cervical spine position [39]. Ideally, the MRI scan is acquired in the radiation treatment position.

3.3.2 What Sequences Does the Standard MRI Acquisition Protocol Provide?

The MRI protocol for HNC includes contrast-enhanced T1w and T2w in at least two different planes.

3.3.3 How Can MRI Be Used for Nasopharyngeal Cancer Segmentation?

Compared to CT scans, MRI provides superior diagnostic performance of involvement of the base of skull, in particular in the description of cortical bone involvement, and of tumour invasion into soft tissue structures. A careful alignment of the skull-base is therefore needed when co-registering the two image datasets (simulation CT and diagnostic MRI) [40]. T2w fast spin-echo sequences proved to be useful in visualizing the involvement of the parapharyngeal space, paranasal sinuses, pterygopalatine fossa and retropharyngeal nodes [41]. T1w imaging determines the involvement of the clivus (sagittal plane) and the base of skull, with tumour marrow invasion typically appearing hypointense in relation to surrounding normal marrow [42]. Contrast-enhanced T1w allows the visualization of perineural invasion and intracranial involvement, which is of particular interest in adenoid cystic carcinomas. Intracranial extension can be recognized particularly on coronal planes on contrast-enhanced T1w-images acquired with fat suppression, thanks to the higher contrast resolution. These sequences can be also useful in assessing cavernous sinus infiltration and nodular dural thickening and disease relations with the adjacent normal structures [43].

3.3.4 How Can MRI Be Used for Segmentation of Oropharyngeal Cancer?

MRI improves delineation of the GTV and normal tissues in oropharyngeal tumours, adding complementary information to the ones obtained from CT and 18FDG-PET imaging. More specifically, T2w with fat saturation sequences give information about the possible involvement of the retropharyngeal lymph nodes, as well as of the parapharyngeal and pre-epiglottic space [41]. T1w sequences are used primarily for the evaluation of parapharyngeal fat space for asymmetries and for bone marrow involvement assessment [44, 45]. For the adequate contouring of the GTV, it is essential to use information obtained by clinical examination, derived from contrast-enhanced T1w, and to combine it with the functional information of 18FDG-PET, whenever available. Contrast-enhanced T1w sequences also give information about possible perineural invasion, and this may be reflected in larger GTVs, as it has been reported in the case of the base of the tongue tumours [46].

3.3.5 How MRI Be Used in Segmentation of Tumours of the Oral Cavity?

MRI is useful in the delineation of both primary tumours and postoperative recurrences in the oral cavity. It may also be helpful in the evaluation of perineural spread in this particularly challenging anatomical site. In the T1w MRI, the contrast between the hypointensity of the tumour and the hyperintensity of the surrounding fatty tissue and bone marrow is clearly visible. Reliability of the GTV segmentation in T1w could be hampered by the isointensity of squamous cell carcinomas of the tongue when compared to the surrounding muscles. In contrast-enhanced T1w, tumour appears hyperintense, in contrast to the hypointense surrounding oedema. In T2w-MRI, tumours appear slightly hyperintense to muscle [47, 48].

3.3.6 How Can MRI Be Used in Glottic Cancer Segmentation?

MRI is used as staging imaging in larynx cancer when there is suspicion of cartilage invasion. The obtained information can be included in treatment planning for the correct definition of GTV, especially in case of extralaryngeal disease and cartilage invasion [49]. Laryngeal cancer in glottic, subglottic, and supraglottic presentations appears as a hypointense lesion in T1w, showing homogeneous enhancement in post-contrast T1w and hyperintense in T2w (Fig. 3.2a,b) [50].

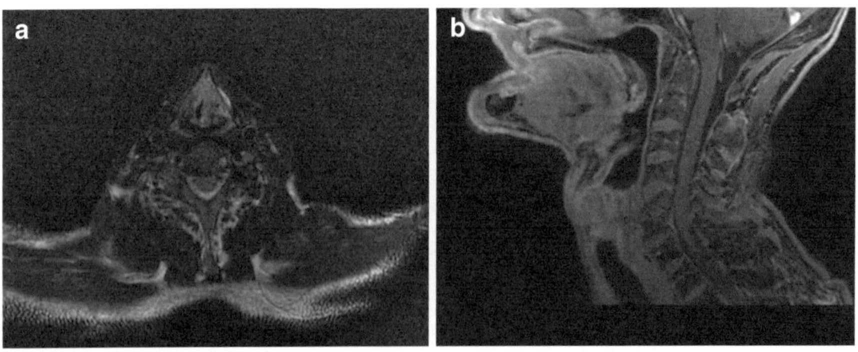

Fig. 3.2 Evidence of a solid heteroformative expansive and infiltrative lesion of the larynx with trans-glottic development. Lesion's core is located in the left true vocal cord, characterized by altered and inhomogeneous signal hyperintensity in T2w sequences (**a**: T2w axial scan, left) and marked enhancement after gadolinium administration (**b**: contrast-enhanced T1w sagittal scan, right)

3.3.7 How Can MRI Be Used in Hypopharyngeal Cancer Segmentation?

MRI may be of support in the segmentation of tumour borders, describing possible cartilage or oesophageal invasion and assessing of perineural spread. Hypopharyngeal cancers present with intermediate to low signal in T1w sequences and intermediate to high signal in T2w; enhancement in T1w after contrast injection is generally present. MRI can also be useful in lymph node contouring, thanks to its ability to present rapid lymph node enhancement [51].

3.3.8 How Can MRI Be Used in Paranasal Sinus Cancer Segmentation?

MRI is pivotal for the definition of the GTV, especially in the case of tumour extension towards the foramen and cranial nerves, skull base, brainstem and optic chiasm. Malignant tumours usually exhibit nonspecific hyperintensity on T2w and hypo- to isointensity on T1w. When there is high cellularity or high mucin or cartilage content, marked hyperintensity in T2w can be observed. Otherwise, hypointensity is shown, especially when calcifications or fibrosis are present. Squamous cell carcinoma (SCC) is the most common histology of paranasal sinus cancer: typical and non-specific findings of SCCs are isointensity on T1w, slight hyperintensity on T2w and moderate enhancement on contrast-enhanced T1w [52]. Hyperintensity on T1w could be indicative of the presence of met-haemoglobin, melanin, lipid, protein, and mineral elements. Contrast-enhanced MRI sequences are fundamental for the definition of perineural diffusion and invasion of the dura. Nerve enhancement secondary to thickening, widening of the neural foramen and loss of perineural fat can suggest perineural spread of disease.

3.3.9 How Can MRI Be Used in Major Salivary Glands Cancer Segmentation?

MRI is highly recommended to support the segmentation of salivary gland tumours. Several authors have in fact pointed out the importance of T2w in determining malignancy [53–55]. Parotid glands appear hyperintense in T1w, with a signal intensity intermediate between fat and muscle, while in T2w they show a signal intensity close to fat. The submandibular glands present with an intensity similar to the muscle one, both in T1w and T2w. T1w gives a clear assessment of tumour margins, tumour extent and infiltration pattern [56]. The fat-saturated contrast-enhanced T1w gives information about the depth of invasions, neural spread, bone invasion, or meningeal infiltration. Benign and malignant masses may have overlapping characteristics, although benign masses show hyperintensity in T2w, whereas masses with low-moderate signal are malignant.

3.3.10 Can DWI Sequences Be Used in Segmentation in HNC?

DWI sequences are a very promising imaging tool, with the potential to improve target volume delineation in HNC. Cardoso et al. [57] demonstrated that the GTVs obtained using DWI and T2w as a support for delineation are larger than those obtained using CT or 18FDG PET/CT in HNC patients. For the assessment of lymph node metastases, DWI has shown a high negative predictive value with a potential impact on organ sparing and tumour control, allowing the radiation oncologists to identify nodal volumes in a more reliable way. More supporting validation studies and guidelines release are required to better described this issue.

3.3.11 How Can Functional MRI Imaging Be Used in HNC?

Functional imaging methods are very promising to guide dose painting approaches in radiation treatment planning. Dynamic contrast-enhanced (DCE) sequences allow for a non-invasive definition of hypoxic areas of the disease that could be the target of treatment strategies to identify and successfully manage hypoxia-induced radio-resistance niches [39, 58].

3.3.12 Are New MRI Imaging Methods Evolving to Support Segmentation in HNC?

Hybrid PET/MRI-guided GTV delineation has been evaluated for SCC of the tongue. It has been shown that this new image modality may represent an important support in target volume delineation compared to traditional imaging, but further studies are needed to validate its clinical use [59].

3.4 Liver

Radiotherapy and, more specifically, stereotactic body radiation therapy (SBRT), is considered an effective and safe therapeutic approach in the treatment of hepatocellular carcinoma (HCC) and of liver metastases [60, 61]. As such, SBRT is a valid therapeutic alternative to surgery. Due to the poor performances of CT-based simulation imaging, complementary MRI tools for correct target delineation and treatment guidance are required to ensure precise treatment delivery [61–63].

3.4.1 What Is the Role of MRI in the Radiotherapy Workflow for Hepatic Lesions?

MRI is rapidly evolving into the method of choice for the detection of malignant liver lesions, as CT is often inadequate for the correct target definition, especially when the use of fiducial markers is logistically difficult or clinically contraindicated [64, 65]. MRI can be successfully incorporated into the radiation treatment planning workflow to correctly identify both, the target and residual healthy liver parenchyma.

Pech et al. [66] reported that MRI identifies substantially larger tumour volumes compared to CT-based delineation. The authors recommended the use of MRI for target definition, especially to ensure that the target volume does not only contain the macroscopically visible lesions, but also the surrounding satellite inflammatory reaction and microscopic tumour spread. In particular, the treatment volumes obtained using T2w-MRI (i.e. tumour including the surrounding oedema) or by contrast-enhanced T1w are larger compared to non-enhanced T1w. Both CT and MRI should therefore be considered for a reliable target definition, as they provide complementary information [65]. When necessary, fiducial markers can also be implanted in proximity of the tumour to be irradiated using the MRI setting: platinum markers provide superior visualization on planning MRI and allow for a reliable image co-registration [67].

3.4.2 What Do Liver Metastases and HCC Lesions Look Like in the Different MRI Sequences?

The imaging characteristics of liver metastases depend on the primary tumour and the MRI study needs to be done in the different contrast-enhancing phases in order to achieve a complete characterization of the lesion. Metastases originating from adenocarcinomas are usually hypointense in T1w-imaging, moderately hyperintense in T2w and show restricted diffusion in DWI and low ADC values (Fig. 3.3a,b) [68]. In dynamic studies, after the injection of contrast agents, they show a hypovascularized central area and may present a hypervascularized peripheral rim [69].

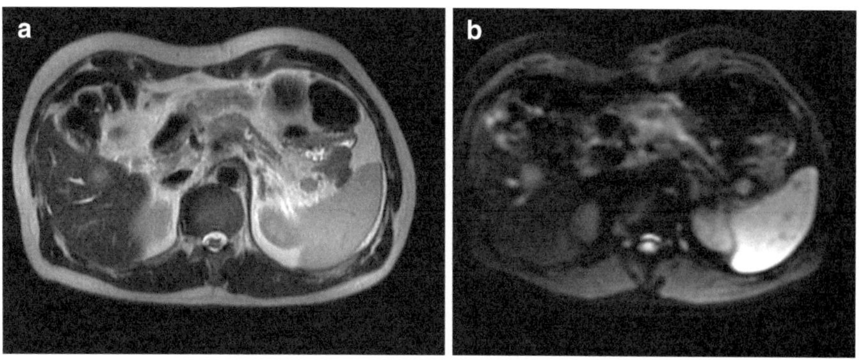

Fig. 3.3 Hepatic metastasis from pancreatic adenocarcinoma between the V and VI segments. The lesion measures 22 mm, appears moderately hyperintense in T2w sequences (**a**: T2w axial scan, left) and shows abnormal restricted diffusion (**b**: DWI axial scan, right)

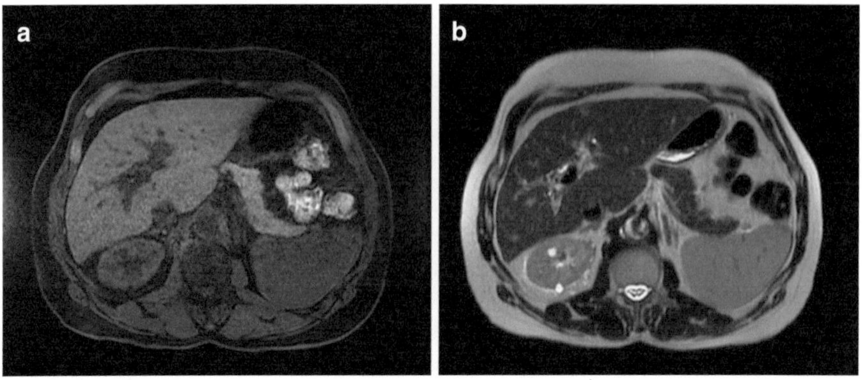

Fig. 3.4 HCC nodule (13 mm) in anterior subcapsular site, between III and IV hepatic segments. The lesion appears hypointense in T1w images (**a**: T1w axial scan, left) and mildly hyperintense in T2w images (**b**: T2w axial scan, right)

Conversely, metastases originating from neuroendocrine tumours (NETs), thyroid cancer, melanoma and renal cancer more often show a hypervascularized aspect [70–72]. Metastases originating from melanomas are generally hyperintense on T1w, due to the presence of melanin and extracellular methaemoglobin.

HCC shows great variability in malignancy characteristics and tissue architecture, both in the stromal component and in the content of substances such as fat, glycogen or metal ions. For these reasons, the signal on T1w- and T2w-imaging can be very variable and dynamic acquisition is mandatory to support a reliable imaging diagnosis (Fig. 3.4a,b) [73].

Hypervascularized liver metastases originating from NETs, renal cell carcinoma, melanoma and thyroid carcinoma generally show peak enhancement in images of the hepatic arterial phase. Hypovascularized liver metastases appear hypointense when compared to the enhancing normal liver parenchyma in the portal venous phase. This behaviour is typical for metastases of colorectal (CRC), lung and breast cancer, although occasionally breast cancer metastases may be hypervascularized. CRC metastases typically show rim enhancement in the arterial phase while they appear hypointense in the venous phase [74].

It has to be noted that papillary cystic ovarian tumours can generate cystic metastases with no enhancement [68]. Hepatobiliary contrast agents (e.g. gadolinium-eth oxybenzyldiethylenetriaminepentaacetic acid Gd-EOB-DTPA) allow the visualization of delayed hepatocyte uptake and have partial excretion in the biliary system, as clearly visible in the hepatobiliary phase (HBP) (also called liver-specific phase) [75]. In the HBP, liver metastases appear clearly hypointense with respect to the brightly enhanced healthy liver parenchyma due to cellular substitution phenomena [76].

HCC typically shows early arterial phase intratumoural enhancement with rapid washout in the portal venous phase or delayed phases, as well demonstrated in dynamic MRI studies [77].

HCC lesions appear hypointense in the HBP: very rarely HCC lesions described as hyperintense in this phase, need to be studied also in on other sequences, such as T2w and DWI, in order to distinguish hyperintense HCC from benign lesions, such as focal nodular hyperplasia.

3.5 Pancreatic Cancer

The role of RT in pancreatic cancer is evolving rapidly in recent years thanks to the successful introduction of SBRT in clinical practice. In this setting, target delineation is a crucial step, especially considering the relative radiosensitivity of the surrounding organs at risk (i.e. duodenum and small bowel) [78, 79].

3.5.1 How Can MRI Be Used in Pancreatic Cancer Segmentation?

Historically, high-resolution contrast-enhanced CT has been used for staging and radiotherapy planning in pancreatic cancer. Some working groups analysed the role of MRI in the target delineation, showing that its use reduces local observer variation when compared to standard CT, resulting in smaller and more precise volumes. However, the authors pointed out the need for detailed instructions in order to further improve delineation in such a complex anatomical site [80, 81].

3.5.2 How Can MRI Be Included in the Pancreatic RT Treatment Planning Workflow?

The MRI to be used for planning support should be ideally acquired on the same day or a few days before or after the simulation CT. Thereby, the patients' positioning and organ filling conditions should be as reproducible as possible (i.e. dietary instructions for reproducible stomach filling). Co-registration of the MRI on the planning CT should be based on GTV, or when present on fiducial markers, making manual adjustments, basing the alignment directly on target volumes rather than organs at risk [82].

3.5.3 What Does Pancreatic Cancer and Surrounding Organs at Risk Look like in MRI?

Pancreatic adenocarcinoma is visualized as a hypointense area surrounded by healthy pancreatic tissue, characterized by bright/high signal in morphological sequences. Considering post-contrast sequences, in the arterial phase, the tumour enhances less than the surrounding parenchyma, while in the venous phase, it shows increasing enhancement, especially for small tumours. The portal venous phase can be useful to assess venous involvement and to visualize suspicious lymph nodes

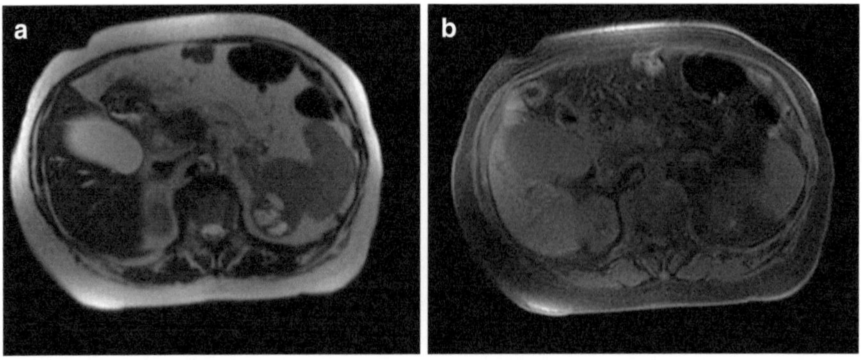

Fig. 3.5 Hypointense pancreatic adenocarcinoma lesion in all pulse sequences (**a**: T2w axial scan, left and **b**: T1w axial scan, right) of the pancreatic head. The lesion infiltrates the main pancreatic duct, extends to the peripancreatic adipose tissue, encases the superior mesenteric vein and obliterates more than half of superior mesenteric artery circumference

[83, 84]. On T2w-imaging tumour may appear from isointense to moderately hypointense (Fig. 3.5a,b). Even if not reliable in effectively distinguishing the margins of the lesion, T2w may be of help in highlighting tumoural cystic areas [85].

Organs at risk are better visualized on T2w-MRI, and using MRI to guide their segmentation generally results in smaller volumes when compared to CT-based segmentation. In particular, T2w-images are very useful in case of suspected duodenal invasion, while both T1w and T2w may be of help for stomach segmentation [86]. Vessels are better defined in arterial and venous phases of the contrast-enhanced sequences and can support the delineation of nodal volumes [85].

3.5.4 Are There Any Recommendations to Follow in the Different Segmentation Steps?

Hall et al. [81] presented a systematic MRI-based method for GTV contouring, while Heerkens et al. [85] proposed practical recommendations for contouring pancreatic volumes. The aforementioned authors recommended to start contouring using T1w-MRI to identify the GTV. Next, the delineation has to be optimized using post-contrast sequences and T2w-imaging. It is suggested to use DWI sequences only at the end of segmentation process, as DWI alone does not allow for discrimination of pancreatitis from tumour and of pathological lymph nodes from benign ones [83].

3.6 Prostate Cancer

MRI represents the imaging modality of choice for RT target delineation in prostate cancer (PC).

Multiparametric magnetic resonance imaging (mpMRI) allows the acquisition of multiplanar images and is recommended for the diagnosis and staging of PC, the detailed study of biochemical recurrence after radical prostatectomy to support treatment choice (surgery, standard radiotherapy, focal therapies or salvage radiotherapy).

The complete MRI study for PC combines a morphological study (T1w- and T2w-imaging) with functional DWI sequences and dynamic contrast-enhanced imaging (DCE) with gadolinium [87]. MRI has indeed proven to be the most reliable imaging support for prostatic volume segmentation, especially in the apex and seminal vesicles, avoiding over- or under-estimation of the volumes that are commonly obtained on CT-based segmentations [88, 89]. Furthermore, the improved definition of the anatomic structures involved in erection, such as internal pudendal artery, the periprostatic nerve fibres and penile bulb, may lead to higher rates of erectile function preservation and better quality of life [90]. The use of MRI allows for smaller treatment volumes and fewer inter-observer variations in prostate delineation, suggesting that MRI-based contouring can reduce treatment-related toxicity, with the possibility to perform more safe and effective focal treatments and dose-escalation protocols [91–94].

The use of MRI scanners with field strength of 1.5 T or more is strongly suggested, and the diagnostic scan should be performed at least 8 weeks following biopsy to allow for post-procedure changes to resolve, such as secondary hematomas that could hamper the correct tumour identification.

3.6.1 What Are the Recommendations for the Use of MRI in the Simulation Phase of Radiotherapy Planning?

Planning CT and support MRI should ideally be simulated under similar conditions, both regarding patient positioning and organ filling (i.e. voiding instructions, endorectal ballon) [95].

mpMRI is to date not mandatory for RT treatment planning: T2w-imaging in transverse plan is therefore sufficient to obtain the necessary anatomical information. However, mpMRI should be performed if focal treatments are to be performed or when the use of escalation dose protocols is foreseen.

The target volume delineation in primary PC has been the object of several guidelines, such as those formulated by the European Organisation for Research and Treatment of Cancer (EORTC) group [96].

More recently, a consensus on CT-MRI-based contouring for primary prostate cancer has been formulated by the European Society for Radiotherapy and Oncology (ESTRO) together with the Advisory Committee on Radiation Oncology Practice (ACROP) [97]. It is recommended to perform CT-MRI co-registration based on bone anatomy. If present, alignment on implanted fiducial markers can increase the accuracy of registration [98]. As reported by the recent ESTRO-ACROP consensus, MRI allows a better discrimination between the posterior prostate edge and the anterior rectal wall, as the prostate capsule is displayed as a sharply demarcated dark rim on T2w-imaging. Moreover, the low intensity of the rectum well contrasts with the high signal intensity of the normal prostatic peripheral zone in this sequence.

The external urethral sphincter and distal urethra can be visualized as they contrast with the prostatic apex, visible as a triangular area. This area is also generally well distinguishable from the prostatic sphincter, from the urogenital diaphragm and from the lateral levator ani muscle, characterized by low signal intensity.

The anterior edge of the prostate is difficult to delineate on CT, as the anterior surface of the prostate consists of the anterior fibromuscular stroma (AFMS), characterized by the same density of the adjacent venous plexus and therefore hardly distinguishable. Noteworthy, AFMS shows low signal intensity as opposed to high signal intensity of the venous plexus on T2w-imaging. This can prevent unnecessary inclusion of this structure in the target volume. The correct visualization of the prostate base must take into account the possible presence of benign hyperplasia protruding into the bladder, which will be easily displayed on T2w-MRI thanks to the significant intensity difference with the urine. Seminal vesicles are characterized by high signal intensity on T2w-imaging [97].

3.6.2 How Does Prostate Cancer Show Up on MRI Images?

Malignant lesions appear as nodules or hypointense areas on T2w-imaging, with less-defined margins at the transitional zone. According to the Prostate Imaging Reporting and Data System (PI-RADS v2) model, the T2w-imaging sequence is key to the diagnosis of PC in transition zones. T1w-imaging is useful for detecting the presence of post-biopsy bleedings (a common cause of false-positive PC diagnosis), nodal disease and bone metastasis in the pelvic area.

According to the PI-RADS v2 model, DWI is crucial to the diagnosis of PC in peripheral zone and in characterising indeterminate lesions in the transitional zone, while DCE sequences have a secondary value in the characterization of indeterminate lesions in the peripheral zone (Fig. 3.6a,b).

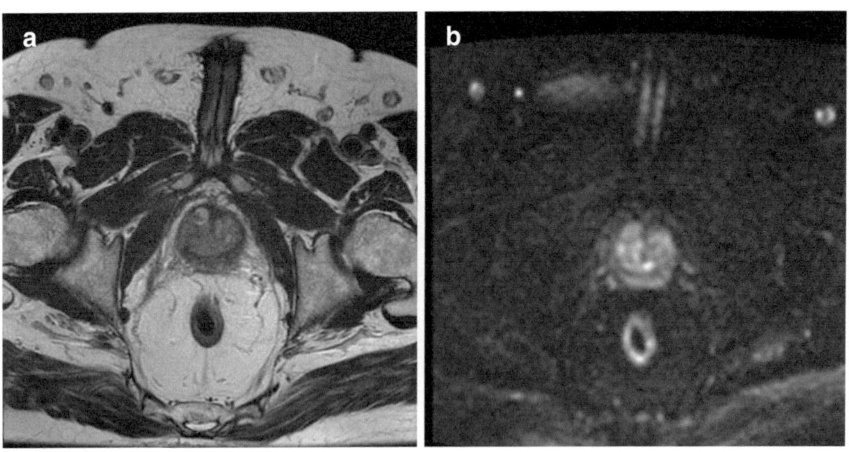

Fig. 3.6 Area of hypointensity in T2w images (**a**: axial T2w scan, left), with signal restriction in DWI (**b**, axial DWI scan, right) referable to prostate adenocarcinoma of the right central region

Extracapsular extension is displayed on MRI as irregular capsule margins or periprostatic fat infiltration. If suspected, it should always be included in the target volume, while the decision to include seminal vesicles, regardless of their involvement, depends on the biological characteristics and staging of the disease [99, 100].

3.6.3 Can MRI Help in Identifying Intraprostatic Tumour Lesions to Guide the Definition of a Radiotherapy Boost?

Local recurrences often occur at the site of the primary macroscopic tumour, and boosting the macroscopic tumour might therefore increase local control [101, 102]. The precise delineation of the intraprostatic lesion is a topic of ongoing research and several studies showed that it should be based on functional imaging. mpMRI plays an important role in this setting even if its use is still limited to clinical trials [103–107].

3.6.4 What Is the Use of MRI in Salvage Radiation Therapy after Radical Prostatectomy and for Local Recurrence?

There is no consensus on the target volume delineation in adjuvant or salvage radiotherapy and great variability can be observed when comparing the different existing guidelines [108]. The principal reason can be identified in the common anatomical changes in postoperative setting that can significantly alter the target definition. The combination of MRI and CT for planning purposes tends to decrease the target volume and its variations ensuring a more reliable target identification [109, 110]. Local recurrence generally appears as an early-enhancing area relatively to the surrounding tissues in the surgical bed, including fibrosis and/or scars. It can also appear as a slightly hyperintense nodule on T2w-imaging, showing restricted diffusion [111]. The precision in the target delineation becomes even more important when deciding to adopt protocols of hypofractionated radiotherapy at the relapse site, especially in the retreatment setting, with the aim of minimizing the dose to healthy tissues to reduce side-effects [112, 113].

3.6.5 What Is the Role of MRI in PC Brachytherapy?

This aspect of imaging is in lengthy discussed in "Image-Guided Adaptive Brachytherapy" of this book. In short, MRI can be used to guide focal therapies in both primary and salvage settings, due to the better visualization of the prostate apex, external urinary sphincter, vascular structures and interface with rectum and bladder [114]. More specifically, T2w-imaging can be used to adequately display the tumour nodule in the context of online image guidance for interstitial catheters insertion for high dose rate brachytherapy (HDR-BRT) [115, 116]. Despite the good image quality, this approach is not widely used because it is associated with logistical difficulties, extensive use of resources and long duration of the procedure.

More frequently, a T2w-MRI is acquired before the implantation and co-registered with trans-rectal ultrasound images (TRUS) to drive either permanent source positioning or HDR catheter insertion [114, 117, 118]. Alternatively, MRI can be acquired after completing TRUS-guided implant procedure, to improve target delineation and for dosimetric optimization purposes. In this case, the use of T1w-sequences for implant reconstruction is recommended even if significant signal distortion can be observed in the applicator site, thus decreasing treatment accuracy [119].

As for low dose rate BRT (LDR-BRT) post-implant imaging for seed reconstruction is generally CT-based: the integration of MRI can make the dosimetry phase more accurate by compensating for the worse contrast resolution of CT and co-registration between CT and T1w-MRI is recommended, in order to better visualize the seeds [120]. The use of proton-weighted sequences, the implementation of specific reconstruction methods and the use of contrast agents may improve the entire workflow in the future [121–123].

3.6.6 What Are the Perspectives of MRI for PC in the Future?

The recent large-scale use of 3 T scanners and the introduction of multichannel surface coils may represent a significant advantage in the use of MRI in PC in the near future. The use of hybrid PET/MRI imaging, especially for its ability in detecting biochemical relapse and bone metastases with the use of new tracers, will open new scenarios in patient management. Monitoring the response to therapies will benefit from the increasing use of more advanced and reliable ADC sequences and mpMRI tools.

Above all, MRI will not only be used only as a traditional tool for staging and treatment planning, but will increasingly be used in the context of hybrid radiotherapy units to online guide radiotherapy treatments, opening new perspectives of medical technology and clinical knowledge [124–128]. Several experiences have described prostate motion using electromagnetic tracking, based on fiducial markers, and evaluating data derived from prostate treatment with MR hybrid units, concluding that prostate motion is irregular and not predictable. This new technology therefore allows effective motion management, through the possibility of real-time soft-tissue tracking and gating and adaptive RT protocols [128].

3.7 Cervical Cancer

According to the "Gyn GEC-ESTRO" working group of the Groupe Européen de Curiethérapie (GEC) and the European SocieTy for Radiotherapy & Oncology (ESTRO), MRI is recommended in diagnosis, staging, radiation treatment planning, and treatment response evaluation in locally advanced cervical cancer (LACC) [129, 130]. The better soft-tissue contrast and resolution provided can be of help in the delineation of the GTV and organs at risk, and particularly in the description of possible parametrial and vaginal invasion [131–133].

3.7.1 How Can I Use the Different MRI Sequences for EBRT Target Volume Delineation?

The MRI sequences of choice are T1w- and T2w-MRI that provide complementary information for segmentation guidance. It has to be noted that T1w-imaging often fails to adequately distinguish tumour edges, as its signal is equivalent to that of healthy tissue. On the other hand, T2w-images show the tumour as a more or less uniform area of medium or high signal, in contrast to healthy tissue (low signal) and parametrial tissue (high signal) [134]. T1w-MRI with fat suppression and contrast-enhanced sequences can help in the visualization of the tumour (Fig. 3.7a,b).

Useful physiological and functional information can be obtained from DCE and DWI [135, 136]. Nevertheless, the obtained information should be interpreted with caution, especially regarding the involvement of the parametrial tissue and stroma, as the experiences reported in the literature are controversial about this issue. An intact hypointense stromal rim on T2w-imaging is the criterion for excluding parametrial invasion, although in tumours large enough to obliterate the stromal cervical ring this is often difficult to be defined. In addition, the use of DWI for accurate parametrial invasion definition is limited by its low spatial resolution and poor anatomical detail [137, 138].

Compared with CT, the volumes segmented using MRI are generally smaller with important dosimetric implications, lower inter- and intra-observer variability and an acceptable overlap with histological examinations of the surgical specimen [139–144]. In a recent study, Song et al. [145] evaluated the different GTVs obtained using various MRI sequences. The results showed that GTV-ADC is the smallest obtained, GTV on T1w-imaging and on T1 with fat suppression are the largest while GTV-T2w-imaging is in between. The authors conclude that generating a GTV on MRI merging the information obtained by T2w-imaging and DWI might be the most appropriate choice for a correct target definition [145].

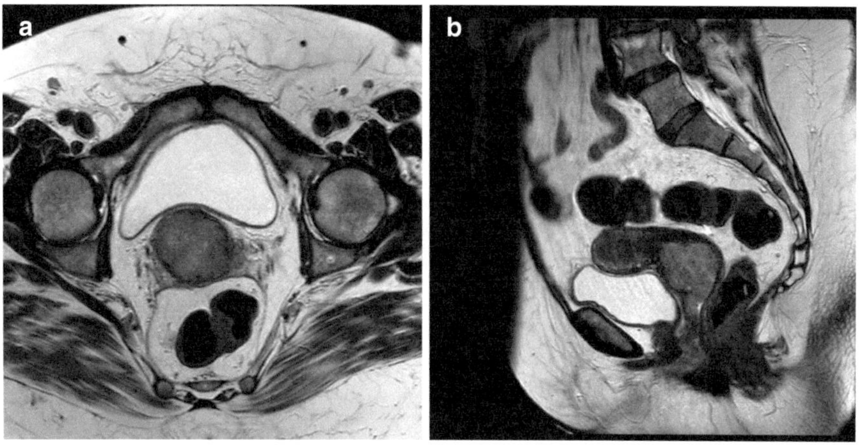

Fig. 3.7 Axial (**a**, left) and sagittal (**b**, right) T2w images of voluminous expansive-infiltrative cervical cancer. This lesion appears hyperintense in T2w sequences, spreads in both parameters and entirely occupies the vaginal canal

3.7.2 Can MRI Give Information Also during Treatment?

LACC undergoes significant regression during radiation treatment [146, 147]. Van de Bunt et al. [148] have performed weekly MRI scans on 20 patients with LACC and have shown an average reduction of tumour volume of 59.6% at the fourth week of treatment, resulting in significant changes in the position and motion of the tumour and its relationship with surrounding organs. Performing a re-evaluation scan during therapy could be therefore advantageous for replanning based on new MRI-based contours, to assess the response to the ongoing treatments, avoiding possible unnecessary exposure of healthy organs (e.g. small bowel) to high radiation doses [148, 149]. Besides morphological imaging, also functional MRI can give information in predicting the response to chemoradiation (CRT) [150].

DCE values indicating low tumour perfusion usually correlate with persistent disease, while values of high perfusion indicate a disease that should have a good response to treatment [151]. This imaging behaviour could be of help in selecting patients who are candidate for dose escalation on areas of radio-resistance, aiming to maximise the effects of external beam radiotherapy (EBRT), before performing BRT [149, 152].

3.7.3 How Can MRI Be Implemented in Brachytherapy Planning Workflow?

This aspect of imaging is in lengthy discussed in "Image-Guided Adaptive Brachytherapy" of this book. In short, MRI is the current imaging modality of choice for image-guided brachytherapy (IGBT). The GEC ESTRO working group recommends the execution of an MRI scan at the time of diagnosis and before the insertion of BT applicators for an accurate target volume delineation [153]. This indication is part of the international report for prescribing, recording and reporting brachytherapy in cervical cancer (ICRU 89) [154]. The gold standard for IGBT is to get a post-EBRT MRI scan, a pre-implantation MRI scan and then a MRI scan at the time of each applicator insertion, allowing to obtain information about the tumour regression pattern and to adapt the dose as needed [130].

The post EBRT MRI gives information about any residual disease. When the residual disease is very large or vaginal involvement is described, either an intracavitary tandem with interstitial needles or hybrid applicators can be chosen, which have been shown to improve dosimetric distribution and clinical outcomes [155, 156].

When logistically possible, real-time intraoperative MRI-guided insertion of interstitial applicators is a safe technique that helps in reducing irradiation of the organs at risk surrounding the disease [157]. A post-implantation CT scan can be acquired and co-registered to the MRI scan, to better visualize the placement of the applicators, although this method presents many uncertainties due to the image registration process and patient movements [114, 158].

3.8 Rectal Cancer

Magnetic resonance imaging represents to date the most accurate imaging modality for diagnosis, staging, evaluation of response and as support for RT treatment planning in locally advanced rectal cancer (LARC).

3.8.1 How Can MRI Be Included into LARC RT Treatment Planning?

The use of standardized diagnostic MRI protocols for rectal distension and bladder filling is important to maximize imaging reproducibility, paving the way to more reliable manual or automatic co-registration procedures with planning CT scan acquisition protocols [159, 160]. MRI-based contouring allows indeed better visualization of the GTV, the sigmoid and anorectal regions and successfully reduces intra- and inter-observer variability [161]. Tan et al. [162] compared the MRI and CT-based GTV delineation, showing that GTV-CT coverage was inadequate when anal or sigmoidal invasion was present, hampering treatment efficacy. The GTVs segmented on MRI are smaller and more accurate, reducing tumour length, width and distance from the anal verge. This results in a reduction in organs at risk toxicity and enhances the delineation quality of the target volume, safely allowing dose escalation protocols [161–163].

The LARC MRI protocol should include multiplanar conventional and high-resolution oblique T2w-, T1w-imaging and multiparametric MRI sequences including DWI and contrast-enhanced MRI. It is essential to acquire T2w- and high-resolution oblique T2w-images, perpendicular to the tumoural axis in sagittal view, should be obtained in one or more planes depending on the size and shape of the tumour (Fig. 3.8a,b). These images provide the optimal anatomic information for an improved assessment of the depth of invasion and of tumoural relationships,

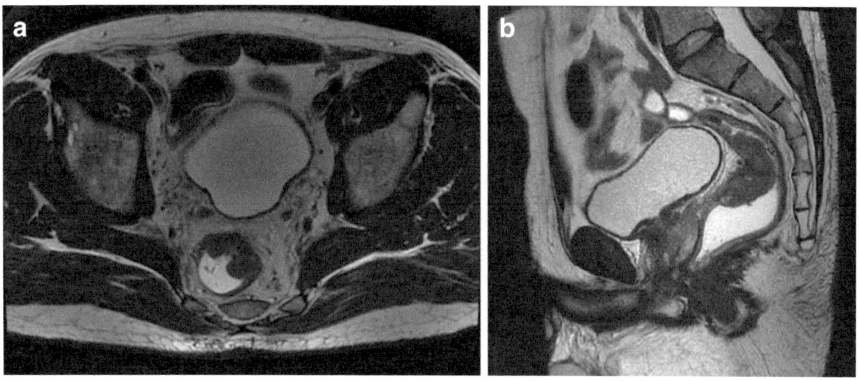

Fig. 3.8 Evidence in axial (**a**, left) and sagittal (**b**, right) T2w scans of a gross adenocarcinoma lesion at the level of the left anterolateral wall of the mid-high rectum occupying half of the lumen

such as the relation to the sphincter complex and levator ani muscle in patients affected by low rectal tumours [164–166]. DWI-MRI improves the accuracy of detecting rectal cancer and involved pelvic nodes and may be of help in response assessment [166–169].

Contrast-enhanced MRI sequences may improve the detection of malignant lymph nodes, extramural vascular invasion and facilitate the characterization of T4 tumours. DCE sequences can give information about the circumferential resection margin resection (CRM) status, while mpMRI plays a very important role in restaging [166, 170].

The evaluation of response to radio(chemo)therapy is based on assessment of local tumour status, mesorectal fascia, extramural vascular invasion and lymph node status, and is crucial for planning the appropriate treatment strategy. It is performed according to the MRI tumour regression grade (TRG) system, based on the proportion of presumed residual tumour and fibrotic change as shown on T2w-imaging. In particular, Grade 1 indicates a complete radiologic response with a linear/crescentic 1–2 mm scar in the mucosa or submucosa on MRI. However, MRI cannot give information about microscopic residual tumour or mucin lakes.

3.8.2 What Are the Recommendations for Rectal Cancer Segmentation?

The target volume includes macroscopic tumour, mesorectum and pelvic lymph nodes. At the tumour level, the entire circumference of the rectum is included due to the inability to discriminate the tumour from normal rectal tissue, while the mesorectal fascia is generally clearly visible on T2w-imaging. Primary rectal tumours are generally moderately hyperintensive on T2w-sequences, intermediate between the signal intensity of the muscularis propria and mucosa, and show enhancement after contrast agent injection. LARC lesions show restricted diffusion in DWI sequences and the depth of invasion through the rectal wall and surrounding structures are well visualized with MRI. Extracellular mucin is hyperintense on T2w-MRI and may suggest the presence of mucinous tumours. Despite the suspected histological type, it is always recommended to follow the international guidelines for target volume delineation in rectal cancer [171].

3.8.3 Can MRI Be Useful in Defining Treatment Response and Guiding Escalation Dose Protocols?

In recent years, many studies have looked for biomarkers for the training of predictive models of response to LARC neoadjuvant therapies. A successful prediction of response can lead to the personalization of oncological treatments, with the opportunity to intensify the dose of radiotherapy (i.e. boost) and use new systemic therapy approaches. Van den Begin et al. [172] have shown that tumour regression occurs more rapidly in the first 3 weeks of treatment, which was confirmed by Lambregts et al. [173] who stated that patients who have the best response to treatment had shown a significant tumour reduction in the same first 3 weeks of treatment. More recently, Fiorino et al. [174] developed a tumour early regression index based on the MRI images acquired during the second week of treatment. This index was able to predict the complete pathological response to neoadjuvant treatments and the duration of distant metastasis-free survival, with response rates to neoadjuvant CRT therapy being strictly dose-dependent [175].

The delineation of tumour volume to be boosted, especially when high doses are prescribed, cannot be based solely on the imaging acquired during the simulation phase, but must take into account any tumour regression that may have occurred during treatment. The use of MRI as an early re-evaluation imaging tool and MRI-based volume segmentation for boost guidance could help in selecting patients who could benefit from escalation dose protocols by increasing accuracy and sparing organs at risk from unnecessary irradiation [149]. Functional MRI, in particular DWI, may be used as a biomarker to select patients for dose-adaptation protocols [150, 175–177].

3.9 Anal Cancer

3.9.1 What Are the Potential Uses of MRI in Treatment Planning in Anal Cancer?

During RT planning, CT, MRI, and PET-CT images should be co-registered to the simulation CT to correctly identify the target volumes [178].

3.9.2 What Are the MRI Sequences that Can Help with Contouring?

The GTV is contoured based on clinical examination and on the tumour visible on anatomical and functional imaging. For this, apart from FDG-PET-CT, T2w- and DWI-sequences (volume of a signal restriction) are acquired in order to delineate the infiltrative component of the disease at the level of the anal canal and surrounding soft tissues (Fig. 3.9a, b). It has been shown that there is no significant inter-observer variability in GTV segmentation, when using either PET-CT or MRI. The use of these imaging modalities becomes crucial when adopting dose escalation strategies (i.e. dose painting) [179].

3.9.3 Can MRI Be Useful in Brachytherapy Planning?

Multiparametric MRI is the gold standard in IGBT of anal cancer, especially when BT is used as a boost after external beam radiotherapy and the definition of the target volumes could be complicated [180]. The advantage of this approach is mainly

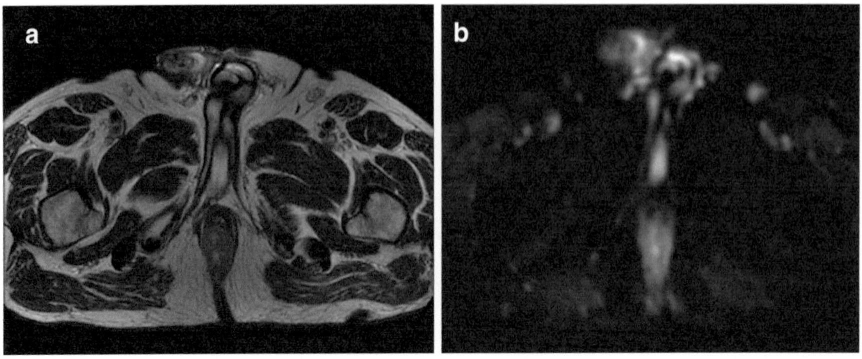

Fig. 3.9 Axial scan of anal cancer originating from the lower third of the anal canal, irregularly hyperintense in T2w sequences (**a**, left) and characterized by restricted proton diffusion in DWI sequences (**b**, right)

represented by the possibility to deliver high doses to the primary tumour volume, while accurately sparing the surrounding organs at risk, thanks to the rapid fall-off of the dose distribution. Although ultrasound is widely used, MRI remains crucial in this framework, providing better spatial resolution and allowing reliable target delineation.

3.9.4 Can MRI Be Helpful in Follow-Up?

Response is usually assessed 6–8 weeks after completion of treatment. MRI can successfully be used together with clinical response assessment through digital rectal examination. Reduction in tumour size as well as hypointensity on T2w-imaging, generally indicative of fibrosis, are findings in favour of a tumour's response to treatment [180].

3.9.5 How Can the MRI Be Used in the Future?

Recent studies have shown that not all categories of patients affected by anal cancer can benefit from RT dose escalation protocols [181]. This should be taken into account for the reduction of toxicity associated with the treatment and the possible increase of local control rates. In this context, the use of information from DWI and DCE studies can guide the clinician in the therapeutic choice. Jones et al. [182] hypothesized the execution of mpMRI during radiochemotherapy to identify imaging biomarkers in order to monitor treatment response and guide its assessment in an exploratory phase 2 study, but the available evidences need to be validated by further studies. This imaging-related information, together with information on tumour staging and HPV stage, may serve in the near future as biomarker of response to multimodal cancer therapies, addressing the high tumour heterogeneity.

The primary aim is to intensify the RT dose in patients with unfavourable biological profile and de-escalate in the ones for whom a response to lower doses is foreseen, with the aim of reducing toxicity and increasing disease control.

References

1. Nyholm T, Jonsson J. Counterpoint: opportunities and challenges of a magnetic resonance imaging-only radiotherapy work flow. Semin Radiat Oncol. 2014;24:175–80.
2. Just M, Rösler HP, Higer HP, Kutzner J, Thelen M. MRI-assisted radiation therapy planning of brain tumors--clinical experiences in 17 patients. Magn Reson Imaging. 1991;9:173–7.
3. Remedios D, France B, Alexander M. Making the best value of clinical radiology: iRefer guidelines, 8th edition. Clin Radiol. 2017;72:705–7.
4. Dirix P, Haustermans K, Vandecaveye V. The value of magnetic resonance imaging for radiotherapy planning. Semin Radiat Oncol. 2014;24:151–9.
5. Owrangi AM, Greer PB, Glide-Hurst CK. MRI-only treatment planning: benefits and challenges. Phys Med Biol. 2018;63:05TR01.
6. Fraass BA, McShan DL, Diaz RF, Ten Haken RK, Aisen A, Gebarski S, Glazer G, Lichter AS. Integration of magnetic resonance imaging into radiation therapy treatment planning: I. technical considerations. Int J Radiat Oncol Biol Phys. 1987;13:1897–908.
7. Devic S. MRI simulation for radiotherapy treatment planning. Med Phys. 2012;39:6701–11.
8. Jolicoeur M, Racine M-L, Trop I, Hathout L, Nguyen D, Derashodian T, David S. Localization of the surgical bed using supine magnetic resonance and computed tomography scan fusion for planification of breast interstitial brachytherapy. Radiother Oncol. 2011;100:480–4.
9. Steenbakkers RJHM, Deurloo KEI, Nowak PJCM, Lebesque JV, van Herk M, Rasch CRN. Reduction of dose delivered to the rectum and bulb of the penis using MRI delineation for radiotherapy of the prostate. Int J Radiat Oncol Biol Phys. 2003;57:1269–79.
10. Pötter R, Dimopoulos J, Georg P, et al. Clinical impact of MRI assisted dose volume adaptation and dose escalation in brachytherapy of locally advanced cervix cancer. Radiother Oncol. 2007;83:148–55.
11. Clinical Applications of MRI in Radiotherapy Planning | SpringerLink. https://link.springer.com/chapter/10.1007/978-3-030-14442-5_4. Accessed 25 Mar 2020.
12. Mabray MC, Barajas RF, Cha S. Modern brain tumor imaging. Brain Tumor Res Treat. 2015;3:8–23.
13. Kono K, Inoue Y, Nakayama K, Shakudo M, Morino M, Ohata K, Wakasa K, Yamada R. The role of diffusion-weighted imaging in patients with brain tumors. AJNR Am J Neuroradiol. 2001;22:1081–8.
14. Stadnik TW, Chaskis C, Michotte A, Shabana WM, van Rompaey K, Luypaert R, Budinsky L, Jellus V, Osteaux M. Diffusion-weighted MR imaging of intracerebral masses: comparison with conventional MR imaging and histologic findings. AJNR Am J Neuroradiol. 2001;22:969–76.
15. Hilario A, Sepulveda JM, Perez-Nuñez A, Salvador E, Millan JM, Hernandez-Lain A, Rodriguez-Gonzalez V, Lagares A, Ramos A. A prognostic model based on preoperative MRI predicts overall survival in patients with diffuse gliomas. AJNR Am J Neuroradiol. 2014;35:1096–102.
16. Bulakbasi N, Guvenc I, Onguru O, Erdogan E, Tayfun C, Ucoz T. The added value of the apparent diffusion coefficient calculation to magnetic resonance imaging in the differentiation and grading of malignant brain tumors. J Comput Assist Tomogr. 2004;28:735–46.
17. Haacke EM, Xu Y, Cheng Y-CN, Reichenbach JR. Susceptibility weighted imaging (SWI). Magn Reson Med. 2004;52:612–8.
18. Haacke EM, Mittal S, Wu Z, Neelavalli J, Cheng Y-CN. Susceptibility-weighted imaging: technical aspects and clinical applications, part 1. AJNR Am J Neuroradiol. 2009;30:19–30.

19. Elhawary H, Liu H, Patel P, Norton I, Rigolo L, Papademetris X, Hata N, Golby AJ. Intraoperative real-time querying of white matter tracts during frameless stereotactic neuronavigation. Neurosurgery. 2011;68:506–16; discussion 516.
20. Knopp EA, Cha S, Johnson G, Mazumdar A, Golfinos JG, Zagzag D, Miller DC, Kelly PJ, Kricheff II. Glial neoplasms: dynamic contrast-enhanced T2*-weighted MR imaging. Radiology. 1999;211:791–8.
21. Cha S. Update on brain tumor imaging: from anatomy to physiology. AJNR Am J Neuroradiol. 2006;27:475–87.
22. Horská A, Barker PB. Imaging of brain tumors: MR spectroscopy and metabolic imaging. Neuroimaging Clin N Am. 2010;20:293–310.
23. Lee MH, Smyser CD, Shimony JS. Resting-state fMRI: a review of methods and clinical applications. AJNR Am J Neuroradiol. 2013;34:1866–72.
24. White NS, McDonald CR, Farid N, Kuperman JM, Kesari S, Dale AM. Improved conspicuity and delineation of high-grade primary and metastatic brain tumors using "restriction spectrum imaging": quantitative comparison with high B-value DWI and ADC. AJNR Am J Neuroradiol. 2013;34:958–964, S1.
25. Niyazi M, Brada M, Chalmers AJ, et al. ESTRO-ACROP guideline "target delineation of glioblastomas". Radiother Oncol. 2016;118:35–42.
26. Sanai N, Chang S, Berger MS. Low-grade gliomas in adults. J Neurosurg. 2011;115:948–65.
27. Pignatti F, van den Bent M, Curran D, et al. Prognostic factors for survival in adult patients with cerebral low-grade glioma. J Clin Oncol. 2002;20:2076–84.
28. Fairchild A, Weber DC, Bar-Deroma R, Gulyban A, Fenton PA, Stupp R, Baumert BG. Quality assurance in the EORTC 22033-26033/CE5 phase III randomized trial for low grade glioma: the digital individual case review. Radiother Oncol. 2012;103:287–92.
29. Flickinger JC, Lunsford LD, Kondziolka D. Dose prescription and dose-volume effects in radiosurgery. Neurosurg Clin N Am. 1992;3:51–9.
30. Straathof CS, de Bruin HG, Dippel DW, Vecht CJ. The diagnostic accuracy of magnetic resonance imaging and cerebrospinal fluid cytology in leptomeningeal metastasis. J Neurol. 1999;246:810–4.
31. Nagai A, Shibamoto Y, Mori Y, Hashizume C, Hagiwara M, Kobayashi T. Increases in the number of brain metastases detected at frame-fixed, thin-slice MRI for gamma knife surgery planning. Neuro-Oncology. 2010;12:1187–92.
32. Gondi V, Pugh SL, Tome WA, et al. Preservation of memory with conformal avoidance of the hippocampal neural stem-cell compartment during whole-brain radiotherapy for brain metastases (RTOG 0933): a phase II multi-institutional trial. J Clin Oncol. 2014;32:3810–6.
33. Maclean J, Fersht N, Short S. Controversies in radiotherapy for meningioma. Clin Oncol (R Coll Radiol). 2014;26:51–64.
34. Rogers CL, Won M, Vogelbaum MA, et al. High-risk meningioma: initial outcomes from NRG oncology/RTOG 0539. Int J Radiat Oncol Biol Phys. 2020;106:790–9.
35. Weber DC, Ares C, Villa S, et al. Adjuvant postoperative high-dose radiotherapy for atypical and malignant meningioma: a phase-II parallel non-randomized and observation study (EORTC 22042-26042). Radiother Oncol. 2018;128:260–5.
36. Klinke T, Daboul A, Maron J, Gredes T, Puls R, Jaghsi A, Biffar R. Artifacts in magnetic resonance imaging and computed tomography caused by dental materials. PLoS One. 2012; https://doi.org/10.1371/journal.pone.0031766.
37. Khoo VS, Dearnaley DP, Finnigan DJ, Padhani A, Tanner SF, Leach MO. Magnetic resonance imaging (MRI): considerations and applications in radiotherapy treatment planning. Radiother Oncol. 1997;42:1–15.
38. Emami B, Sethi A, Petruzzelli GJ. Influence of MRI on target volume delineation and IMRT planning in nasopharyngeal carcinoma. Int J Radiat Oncol Biol Phys. 2003;57:481–8.
39. Prestwich RJD, Sykes J, Carey B, Sen M, Dyker KE, Scarsbrook AF. Improving target definition for head and neck radiotherapy: a place for magnetic resonance imaging and 18-fluoride fluorodeoxyglucose positron emission tomography? Clin Oncol (R Coll Radiol). 2012;24:577–89.

40. Abdel Khalek Abdel Razek A, King A. MRI and CT of nasopharyngeal carcinoma. AJR Am J Roentgenol. 2012;198:11–8.
41. Wippold FJ. Head and neck imaging: the role of CT and MRI. J Magn Reson Imaging. 2007;25:453–65.
42. Mathur A, Jain N, Kesavadas C, Thomas B, Kapilamoorthy T. Imaging of skull base pathologies: role of advanced magnetic resonance imaging techniques. Neuroradiol J. 2015;28:426–37.
43. Chung N-N, Ting L-L, Hsu W-C, Lui LT, Wang P-M. Impact of magnetic resonance imaging versus CT on nasopharyngeal carcinoma: primary tumor target delineation for radiotherapy. Head Neck. 2004;26:241–6.
44. Zima AJ, Wesolowski JR, Ibrahim M, Lassig AAD, Lassig J, Mukherji SK. Magnetic resonance imaging of oropharyngeal cancer. Top Magn Reson Imaging. 2007;18:237–42.
45. Abraham J. Imaging for head and neck cancer. Surg Oncol Clin N Am. 2015;24:455–71.
46. Ahmed M, Schmidt M, Sohaib A, et al. The value of magnetic resonance imaging in target volume delineation of base of tongue tumours--a study using flexible surface coils. Radiother Oncol. 2010;94:161–7.
47. Law CP, Chandra RV, Hoang JK, Phal PM. Imaging the oral cavity: key concepts for the radiologist. Br J Radiol. 2011;84:944–57.
48. Kirsch C. Oral cavity cancer. Top Magn Reson Imaging. 2007;18:269–80.
49. Lewis-Jones H, Colley S, Gibson D. Imaging in head and neck cancer: United Kingdom National Multidisciplinary Guidelines. J Laryngol Otol. 2016;130:S28–31.
50. Joshi VM, Wadhwa V, Mukherji SK. Imaging in laryngeal cancers. Indian J Radiol Imaging. 2012;22:209–26.
51. Chen AY, Hudgins PA. Pitfalls in the staging squamous cell carcinoma of the hypopharynx. Neuroimaging Clin N Am. 2013;23:67–79.
52. Kawaguchi M, Kato H, Tomita H, Mizuta K, Aoki M, Hara A, Matsuo M. Imaging characteristics of malignant Sinonasal tumors. J Clin Med. 2017; https://doi.org/10.3390/jcm6120116.
53. Freling NJ. Imaging of the salivary glands. CT and MRI. Radiologe. 1994;34:264–72.
54. Swartz JD, Rothman MI, Marlowe FI, Berger AS. MR imaging of parotid mass lesions: attempts at histopathologic differentiation. J Comput Assist Tomogr. 1989;13:789–96.
55. Afzelius P, Nielsen M-Y, Ewertsen C, Bloch KP. Imaging of the major salivary glands. Clin Physiol Funct Imaging. 2016;36:1–10.
56. Yousem DM, Kraut MA, Chalian AA. Major salivary gland imaging. Radiology. 2000;216:19–29.
57. Cardoso M, Min M, Jameson M, Tang S, Rumley C, Fowler A, Estall V, Pogson E, Holloway L, Forstner D. Evaluating diffusion-weighted magnetic resonance imaging for target volume delineation in head and neck radiotherapy. J Med Imaging Radiat Oncol. 2019;63:399–407.
58. Law BKH, King AD, Bhatia KS, Ahuja AT, Kam MKM, Ma BB, Ai QY, Mo FKF, Yuan J, Yeung DKW. Diffusion-weighted imaging of nasopharyngeal carcinoma: can pretreatment DWI predict local failure based on long-term outcome? AJNR Am J Neuroradiol. 2016;37:1706–12.
59. Samołyk-Kogaczewska N, Sierko E, Zuzda K, Gugnacki P, Szumowski P, Mojsak M, Burzyńska-Śliwowska J, Wojtukiewicz MZ, Szczecina K, Jurgilewicz DH. PET/MRI-guided GTV delineation during radiotherapy planning in patients with squamous cell carcinoma of the tongue. Strahlenther Onkol. 2019;195:780–91.
60. Choi SH, Seong J. Strategic application of radiotherapy for hepatocellular carcinoma. Clin Mol Hepatol. 2018;24:114–34.
61. Mahadevan A, Blanck O, Lanciano R, Peddada A, Sundararaman S, D'Ambrosio D, Sharma S, Perry D, Kolker J, Davis J. Stereotactic body radiotherapy (SBRT) for liver metastasis – clinical outcomes from the international multi-institutional RSSearch® patient registry. Radiat Oncol. 2018; https://doi.org/10.1186/s13014-018-0969-2.
62. Nair VJ, Pantarotto JR. Treatment of metastatic liver tumors using stereotactic ablative radiotherapy. World J Radiol. 2014;6:18–25.

63. Yang DS, Yoon WS, Lee JA, Lee NK, Lee S, Kim CY, Yim HJ, Lee SH, Chung HH, Cha SH. The effectiveness of gadolinium MRI to improve target delineation for radiotherapy in hepatocellular carcinoma: a comparative study of rigid image registration techniques. Phys Med. 2014;30:676–81.
64. Heusch P, Antoch G. Morphologic and functional imaging of non-colorectal liver metastases. Viszeralmedizin. 2015;31:387–92.
65. Voroney J-P, Brock KK, Eccles C, Haider M, Dawson LA. Prospective comparison of computed tomography and magnetic resonance imaging for liver cancer delineation using deformable image registration. Int J Radiat Oncol Biol Phys. 2006;66:780–91.
66. Pech M, Mohnike K, Wieners G, Bialek E, Dudeck O, Seidensticker M, Peters N, Wust P, Gademann G, Ricke J. Radiotherapy of liver metastases. Comparison of target volumes and dose-volume histograms employing CT- or MRI-based treatment planning. Strahlenther Onkol. 2008;184:256–61.
67. Nair VJ, Szanto J, Vandervoort E, Henderson E, Avruch L, Malone S, Jason RP. Feasibility, detectability and clinical experience with platinum fiducial seeds for MRI/CT fusion and real-time tumor tracking during CyberKnife® stereotactic ablative radiotherapy†. J Radiosurg SBRT. 2015;3:315–23.
68. Namasivayam S, Martin DR, Saini S. Imaging of liver metastases: MRI. Cancer Imaging. 2007;7:2–9.
69. Danet I-M, Semelka RC, Leonardou P, Braga L, Vaidean G, Woosley JT, Kanematsu M. Spectrum of MRI appearances of untreated metastases of the liver. AJR Am J Roentgenol. 2003;181:809–17.
70. Sica GT, Ji H, Ros PR. Computed tomography and magnetic resonance imaging of hepatic metastases. Clin Liver Dis. 2002;6:165–179, vii.
71. Kanematsu M, Goshima S, Watanabe H, Kondo H, Kawada H, Noda Y, Moriyama N. Diffusion/perfusion MR imaging of the liver: practice, challenges, and future. Magn Reson Med Sci. 2012;11:151–61.
72. Vilgrain V, Esvan M, Ronot M, Caumont-Prim A, Aubé C, Chatellier G. A meta-analysis of diffusion-weighted and gadoxetic acid-enhanced MR imaging for the detection of liver metastases. Eur Radiol. 2016;26:4595–615.
73. Lencioni R, Cioni D, Della Pina C, Crocetti L, Bartolozzi C. Imaging diagnosis. Semin Liver Dis. 2005;25:162–70.
74. Hamm B, Thoeni RF, Gould RG, Bernardino ME, Lüning M, Saini S, Mahfouz AE, Taupitz M, Wolf KJ. Focal liver lesions: characterization with nonenhanced and dynamic contrast material-enhanced MR imaging. Radiology. 1994;190:417–23.
75. Goodwin MD, Dobson JE, Sirlin CB, Lim BG, Stella DL. Diagnostic challenges and pitfalls in MR imaging with hepatocyte-specific contrast agents. Radiographics. 2011;31:1547–68.
76. Zech CJ, Herrmann KA, Reiser MF, Schoenberg SO. MR imaging in patients with suspected liver metastases: value of liver-specific contrast agent Gd-EOB-DTPA. Magn Reson Med Sci. 2007;6:43–52.
77. Marrero JA, Hussain HK, Nghiem HV, Umar R, Fontana RJ, Lok AS. Improving the prediction of hepatocellular carcinoma in cirrhotic patients with an arterially-enhancing liver mass. Liver Transpl. 2005;11:281–9.
78. Caravatta L, Macchia G, Mattiucci GC, et al. Inter-observer variability of clinical target volume delineation in radiotherapy treatment of pancreatic cancer: a multi-institutional contouring experience. Radiat Oncol. 2014;9:198.
79. Fokas E, Spezi E, Patel N, Hurt C, Nixon L, Chu K-Y, Staffurth J, Abrams R, Mukherjee S. Comparison of investigator-delineated gross tumour volumes and quality assurance in pancreatic cancer: analysis of the on-trial cases for the SCALOP trial. Radiother Oncol. 2016;120:212–6.
80. Gurney-Champion OJ, Versteijne E, van der Horst A, et al. Addition of MRI for CT-based pancreatic tumor delineation: a feasibility study. Acta Oncol. 2017;56:923–30.
81. Hall WA, Heerkens HD, Paulson ES, et al. Pancreatic gross tumor volume contouring on computed tomography (CT) compared with magnetic resonance imaging (MRI): results of an international contouring conference. Pract Radiat Oncol. 2018;8:107–15.

82. Caravatta L, Cellini F, Simoni N, et al. Magnetic resonance imaging (MRI) compared with computed tomography (CT) for interobserver agreement of gross tumor volume delineation in pancreatic cancer: a multi-institutional contouring study on behalf of the AIRO group for gastrointestinal cancers. Acta Oncol. 2019;58:439–47.
83. O'Neill E, Hammond N, Miller FH. MR imaging of the pancreas. Radiol Clin N Am. 2014;52:757–77.
84. Koay EJ, Hall W, Park PC, Erickson B, Herman JM. The role of imaging in the clinical practice of radiation oncology for pancreatic cancer. Abdom Radiol (NY). 2018;43:393–403.
85. Heerkens HD, Hall WA, Li XA, et al. Recommendations for MRI-based contouring of gross tumor volume and organs at risk for radiation therapy of pancreatic cancer. Pract Radiat Oncol. 2017;7:126–36.
86. Dalah E, Moraru I, Paulson E, Erickson B, Li XA. Variability of target and normal structure delineation using multimodality imaging for radiation therapy of pancreatic cancer. Int J Radiat Oncol Biol Phys. 2014;89:633–40.
87. Couñago F, Sancho G, Catalá V, Hernández D, Recio M, Montemuiño S, Hernández JA, Maldonado A, del Cerro E. Magnetic resonance imaging for prostate cancer before radical and salvage radiotherapy: what radiation oncologists need to know. World J Clin Oncol. 2017;8:305–19.
88. Fiorino C, Reni M, Bolognesi A, Cattaneo GM, Calandrino R. Intra- and inter-observer variability in contouring prostate and seminal vesicles: implications for conformal treatment planning. Radiother Oncol. 1998;47:285–92.
89. Milosevic M, Voruganti S, Blend R, Alasti H, Warde P, McLean M, Catton P, Catton C, Gospodarowicz M. Magnetic resonance imaging (MRI) for localization of the prostatic apex: comparison to computed tomography (CT) and urethrography. Radiother Oncol. 1998;47:277–84.
90. Moghanaki D, Turkbey B, Vapiwala N, Ehdaie B, Frank SJ, McLaughlin PW, Harisinghani M. Advances in prostate cancer magnetic resonance imaging and positron emission tomography-computed tomography for staging and radiotherapy treatment planning. Semin Radiat Oncol. 2017;27:21–33.
91. Rasch C, Barillot I, Remeijer P, Touw A, van Herk M, Lebesque JV. Definition of the prostate in CT and MRI: a multi-observer study. Int J Radiat Oncol Biol Phys. 1999;43:57–66.
92. Villeirs GM, Van Vaerenbergh K, Vakaet L, Bral S, Claus F, De Neve WJ, Verstraete KL, De Meerleer GO. Interobserver delineation variation using CT versus combined CT + MRI in intensity-modulated radiotherapy for prostate cancer. Strahlenther Onkol. 2005;181:424–30.
93. Hentschel B, Oehler W, Strauss D, Ulrich A, Malich A. Definition of the CTV prostate in CT and MRI by using CT-MRI image fusion in IMRT planning for prostate cancer. Strahlenther Onkol. 2011;187:183–90.
94. Panje C, Panje T, Putora PM, Kim S-K, Haile S, Aebersold DM, Plasswilm L. Guidance of treatment decisions in risk-adapted primary radiotherapy for prostate cancer using multiparametric magnetic resonance imaging: a single center experience. Radiat Oncol. 2015;10:47.
95. Hanvey S, Sadozye AH, McJury M, Glegg M, Foster J. The influence of MRI scan position on image registration accuracy, target delineation and calculated dose in prostatic radiotherapy. Br J Radiol. 2012;85:e1256–62.
96. Boehmer D, Maingon P, Poortmans P, Baron M-H, Miralbell R, Remouchamps V, Scrase C, Bossi A, Bolla M, EORTC Radiation Oncology Group. Guidelines for primary radiotherapy of patients with prostate cancer. Radiother Oncol. 2006;79:259–69.
97. Salembier C, Villeirs G, De Bari B, et al. ESTRO ACROP consensus guideline on CT- and MRI-based target volume delineation for primary radiation therapy of localized prostate cancer. Radiother Oncol. 2018;127:49–61.
98. Parker CC, Damyanovich A, Haycocks T, Haider M, Bayley A, Catton CN. Magnetic resonance imaging in the radiation treatment planning of localized prostate cancer using intraprostatic fiducial markers for computed tomography co-registration. Radiother Oncol. 2003;66:217–24.

99. Synopsis of the PI-RADS v2 Guidelines for Multiparametric Prostate Magnetic Resonance Imaging and Recommendations for Use. - PubMed - NCBI. https://www.ncbi.nlm.nih.gov/pubmed/26361169. Accessed 17 Feb 2020.
100. Catalá V, Vilanova JC, Gaya JM, Algaba F, Martí T. Multiparametric magnetic resonance imaging and prostate cancer: what's new? Radiologia. 2017;59:196–208.
101. Pucar D, Hricak H, Shukla-Dave A, Kuroiwa K, Drobnjak M, Eastham J, Scardino PT, Zelefsky MJ. Clinically significant prostate cancer local recurrence after radiation therapy occurs at the site of primary tumor: magnetic resonance imaging and step-section pathology evidence. Int J Radiat Oncol Biol Phys. 2007;69:62–9.
102. Cellini N, Morganti AG, Mattiucci GC, Valentini V, Leone M, Luzi S, Manfredi R, Dinapoli N, Digesu' C, Smaniotto D. Analysis of intraprostatic failures in patients treated with hormonal therapy and radiotherapy: implications for conformal therapy planning. Int J Radiat Oncol Biol Phys. 2002;53:595–9.
103. van der Heide UA, Korporaal JG, Groenendaal G, Franken S, van Vulpen M. Functional MRI for tumor delineation in prostate radiation therapy. Imaging Med. 2011;3:219.
104. Groenendaal G, van den Berg CAT, Korporaal JG, Philippens MEP, Luijten PR, van Vulpen M, van der Heide UA. Simultaneous MRI diffusion and perfusion imaging for tumor delineation in prostate cancer patients. Radiother Oncol. 2010;95:185–90.
105. Langer DL, van der Kwast TH, Evans AJ, Trachtenberg J, Wilson BC, Haider MA. Prostate cancer detection with multi-parametric MRI: logistic regression analysis of quantitative T2, diffusion-weighted imaging, and dynamic contrast-enhanced MRI. J Magn Reson Imaging. 2009;30:327–34.
106. Lips IM, van der Heide UA, Haustermans K, van Lin EN, Pos F, Franken SP, Kotte AN, van Gils CH, van Vulpen M. Single blind randomized phase III trial to investigate the benefit of a focal lesion ablative microboost in prostate cancer (FLAME-trial): study protocol for a randomized controlled trial. Trials. 2011;12:255.
107. Murray JR, Tree AC, Alexander E, et al. Standard and hypofractionated dose escalation to intraprostatic tumour nodules in localised prostate cancer: efficacy and toxicity in the DELINEATE trial. Int J Radiat Oncol Biol Phys. 2019; https://doi.org/10.1016/j.ijrobp.2019.11.402.
108. Malone S, Croke J, Roustan-Delatour N, et al. Postoperative radiotherapy for prostate cancer: a comparison of four consensus guidelines and dosimetric evaluation of 3D-CRT versus tomotherapy IMRT. Int J Radiat Oncol Biol Phys. 2012;84:725–32.
109. Lee E, Park W, Ahn SH, et al. Interobserver variation in target volume for salvage radiotherapy in recurrent prostate cancer patients after radical prostatectomy using CT versus combined CT and MRI: a multicenter study (KROG 13-11). Radiat Oncol J. 2018;36:11–6.
110. Rans K, Berghen C, Joniau S, De Meerleer G. Salvage radiotherapy for prostate cancer. Clin Oncol (R Coll Radiol). 2020;32:156–62.
111. Kitajima K, Hartman RP, Froemming AT, Hagen CE, Takahashi N, Kawashima A. Detection of local recurrence of prostate cancer after radical prostatectomy using Endorectal coil MRI at 3 T: addition of DWI and dynamic contrast enhancement to T2-weighted MRI. AJR Am J Roentgenol. 2015;205:807–16.
112. Picardi C, Perret I, Miralbell R, Zilli T. Hypofractionated radiotherapy for prostate cancer in the postoperative setting: what is the evidence so far? Cancer Treat Rev. 2018;62:91–6.
113. Gonzalez-Motta A, Roach M. Stereotactic body radiation therapy (SBRT) for high-risk prostate cancer: where are we now? Pract Radiat Oncol. 2018;8:185–202.
114. Tharmalingam H, Alonzi R, Hoskin PJ. The role of magnetic resonance imaging in brachytherapy. Clin Oncol (R Coll Radiol). 2018;30:728–36.
115. Schick U, Popowski Y, Nouet P, Bieri S, Rouzaud M, Khan H, Weber DC, Miralbell R. High-dose-rate brachytherapy boost to the dominant intra-prostatic tumor region: hemi-irradiation of prostate cancer. Prostate. 2011;71:1309–16.
116. Ménard C, Susil RC, Choyke P, et al. MRI-guided HDR prostate brachytherapy in standard 1.5T scanner. Int J Radiat Oncol Biol Phys. 2004;59:1414–23.

117. Hsu CC, Hsu H, Pickett B, et al. Feasibility of MR imaging/MR spectroscopy-planned focal partial salvage permanent prostate implant (PPI) for localized recurrence after initial PPI for prostate cancer. Int J Radiat Oncol Biol Phys. 2013;85:370–7.
118. Mason J, Al-Qaisieh B, Bownes P, Wilson D, Buckley DL, Thwaites D, Carey B, Henry A. Multi-parametric MRI-guided focal tumor boost using HDR prostate brachytherapy: a feasibility study. Brachytherapy. 2014;13:137–45.
119. Hoskin PJ, Colombo A, Henry A, Niehoff P, Paulsen Hellebust T, Siebert F-A, Kovacs G. GEC/ESTRO recommendations on high dose rate afterloading brachytherapy for localised prostate cancer: an update. Radiother Oncol. 2013;107:325–32.
120. Haack S, Nielsen SK, Lindegaard JC, Gelineck J, Tanderup K. Applicator reconstruction in MRI 3D image-based dose planning of brachytherapy for cervical cancer. Radiother Oncol. 2009;91:187–93.
121. Hu Y, Esthappan J, Mutic S, Richardson S, Gay HA, Schwarz JK, Grigsby PW. Improve definition of titanium tandems in MR-guided high dose rate brachytherapy for cervical cancer using proton density weighted MRI. Radiat Oncol. 2013;8:16.
122. de Leeuw H, Seevinck PR, Bakker CJG. Center-out radial sampling with off-resonant reconstruction for efficient and accurate localization of punctate and elongated paramagnetic structures. Magn Reson Med. 2013;69:1611–22.
123. Frank SJ, Stafford RJ, Bankson JA, Li C, Swanson DA, Kudchadker RJ, Martirosyan KS. A novel MRI marker for prostate brachytherapy. Int J Radiat Oncol Biol Phys. 2008;71:5–8.
124. Lindenberg L, Ahlman M, Turkbey B, Mena E, Choyke P. Evaluation of prostate cancer with PET/MRI. J Nucl Med. 2016;57:111S–6S.
125. Souvatzoglou M, Eiber M, Takei T, et al. Comparison of integrated whole-body [11C]choline PET/MR with PET/CT in patients with prostate cancer. Eur J Nucl Med Mol Imaging. 2013;40:1486–99.
126. Bagheri MH, Ahlman MA, Lindenberg L, et al. Advances in medical imaging for the diagnosis and management of common genitourinary cancers. Urol Oncol. 2017;35:473–91.
127. Low RN, Fuller DB, Muradyan N. Dynamic gadolinium-enhanced perfusion MRI of prostate cancer: assessment of response to hypofractionated robotic stereotactic body radiation therapy. AJR Am J Roentgenol. 2011;197:907–15.
128. Murray J, Tree AC. Prostate cancer - advantages and disadvantages of MR-guided RT. Clin Transl Radiat Oncol. 2019;18:68–73.
129. Pötter R, Haie-Meder C, Van Limbergen E, et al. Recommendations from gynaecological (GYN) GEC ESTRO working group (II): concepts and terms in 3D image-based treatment planning in cervix cancer brachytherapy-3D dose volume parameters and aspects of 3D image-based anatomy, radiation physics, radiobiology. Radiother Oncol. 2006;78:67–77.
130. Dimopoulos JCA, Petrow P, Tanderup K, Petric P, Berger D, Kirisits C, Pedersen EM, van Limbergen E, Haie-Meder C, Pötter R. Recommendations from Gynaecological (GYN) GEC-ESTRO working group (IV): basic principles and parameters for MR imaging within the frame of image based adaptive cervix cancer brachytherapy. Radiother Oncol. 2012;103:113–22.
131. Jung D-C, Kim M-K, Kang S, Seo S-S, Cho JY, Park N-H, Song Y-S, Park S-Y, Kang S-B, Kim JW. Identification of a patient group at low risk for parametrial invasion in early-stage cervical cancer. Gynecol Oncol. 2010;119:426–30.
132. Hatano K, Sekiya Y, Araki H, Sakai M, Togawa T, Narita Y, Akiyama Y, Kimura S, Ito H. Evaluation of the therapeutic effect of radiotherapy on cervical cancer using magnetic resonance imaging. Int J Radiat Oncol Biol Phys. 1999;45:639–44.
133. Lim K, Small W, Portelance L, et al. Consensus guidelines for delineation of clinical target volume for intensity-modulated pelvic radiotherapy for the definitive treatment of cervix cancer. Int J Radiat Oncol Biol Phys. 2011;79:348–55.
134. Hricak H, Lacey CG, Sandles LG, Chang YC, Winkler ML, Stern JL. Invasive cervical carcinoma: comparison of MR imaging and surgical findings. Radiology. 1988;166:623–31.

135. Torheim T, Groendahl AR, Andersen EKF, Lyng H, Malinen E, Kvaal K, Futsaether CM. Cluster analysis of dynamic contrast enhanced MRI reveals tumor subregions related to locoregional relapse for cervical cancer patients. Acta Oncol. 2016;55:1294–8.
136. McVeigh PZ, Syed AM, Milosevic M, Fyles A, Haider MA. Diffusion-weighted MRI in cervical cancer. Eur Radiol. 2008;18:1058–64.
137. Iwata S, Joja I, Okuno K, Miyagi Y, Sakaguchi Y, Kudo T, Hiraki Y. Cervical carcinoma with full-thickness stromal invasion: efficacy of dynamic MR imaging in the assessment of parametrial involvement. Radiat Med. 2002;20:247–55.
138. Kuang F, Ren J, Zhong Q, Liyuan F, Huan Y, Chen Z. The value of apparent diffusion coefficient in the assessment of cervical cancer. Eur Radiol. 2013;23:1050–8.
139. Viswanathan AN, Dimopoulos J, Kirisits C, Berger D, Pötter R. Computed tomography versus magnetic resonance imaging-based contouring in cervical cancer brachytherapy: results of a prospective trial and preliminary guidelines for standardized contours. Int J Radiat Oncol Biol Phys. 2007;68:491–8.
140. Lim K, Erickson B, Jürgenliemk-Schulz IM, et al. Variability in clinical target volume delineation for intensity modulated radiation therapy in 3 challenging cervix cancer scenarios. Pract Radiat Oncol. 2015;5:e557–65.
141. Haack S, Pedersen EM, Jespersen SN, Kallehauge JF, Lindegaard JC, Tanderup K. Apparent diffusion coefficients in GEC ESTRO target volumes for image guided adaptive brachytherapy of locally advanced cervical cancer. Acta Oncol. 2010;49:978–83.
142. van de Schoot AJAJ, de Boer P, Buist MR, Stoker J, Bleeker MCG, Stalpers LJA, Rasch CRN, Bel A. Quantification of delineation errors of the gross tumor volume on magnetic resonance imaging in uterine cervical cancer using pathology data and deformation correction. Acta Oncol. 2015;54:224–31.
143. Zhang Y, Hu J, Li J, et al. Comparison of imaging-based gross tumor volume and pathological volume determined by whole-mount serial sections in primary cervical cancer. Onco Targets Ther. 2013;6:917–23.
144. Exner M, Kühn A, Stumpp P, Höckel M, Horn L-C, Kahn T, Brandmaier P. Value of diffusion-weighted MRI in diagnosis of uterine cervical cancer: a prospective study evaluating the benefits of DWI compared to conventional MR sequences in a 3T environment. Acta Radiol. 2016;57:869–77.
145. Song Y, Erickson B, Chen X, Li G, Wu G, Paulson E, Knechtges P, Li XA. Appropriate magnetic resonance imaging techniques for gross tumor volume delineation in external beam radiation therapy of locally advanced cervical cancer. Oncotarget. 2018;9:10100–9.
146. Beadle BM, Jhingran A, Salehpour M, Sam M, Iyer RB, Eifel PJ. Cervix regression and motion during the course of external beam chemoradiation for cervical cancer. Int J Radiat Oncol Biol Phys. 2009;73:235–41.
147. van de Bunt L, Jürgenliemk-Schulz IM, de Kort GAP, Roesink JM, Tersteeg RJHA, van der Heide UA. Motion and deformation of the target volumes during IMRT for cervical cancer: what margins do we need? Radiother Oncol. 2008;88:233–40.
148. van de Bunt L, van der Heide UA, Ketelaars M, de Kort GAP, Jürgenliemk-Schulz IM. Conventional, conformal, and intensity-modulated radiation therapy treatment planning of external beam radiotherapy for cervical cancer: the impact of tumor regression. Int J Radiat Oncol Biol Phys. 2006;64:189–96.
149. White IM, Scurr E, Wetscherek A, Brown G, Sohaib A, Nill S, Oelfke U, Dearnaley D, Lalondrelle S, Bhide S. Realizing the potential of magnetic resonance image guided radiotherapy in gynaecological and rectal cancer. Br J Radiol. 2019;92:20180670.
150. Bowen SR, Yuh WTC, Hippe DS, et al. Tumor radiomic heterogeneity: multiparametric functional imaging to characterize variability and predict response following cervical cancer radiation therapy. J Magn Reson Imaging. 2018;47:1388–96.
151. Mayr NA, Wang JZ, Zhang D, et al. Longitudinal changes in tumor perfusion pattern during the radiation therapy course and its clinical impact in cervical cancer. Int J Radiat Oncol Biol Phys. 2010;77:502–8.

152. Tanderup K, Fokdal LU, Sturdza A, et al. Effect of tumor dose, volume and overall treatment time on local control after radiochemotherapy including MRI guided brachytherapy of locally advanced cervical cancer. Radiother Oncol. 2016;120:441–6.
153. Haie-Meder C, Pötter R, Van Limbergen E, et al. Recommendations from gynaecological (GYN) GEC-ESTRO working group (I): concepts and terms in 3D image based 3D treatment planning in cervix cancer brachytherapy with emphasis on MRI assessment of GTV and CTV. Radiother Oncol. 2005;74:235–45.
154. International Commission on Radiation Units and Measurements (ICRU). https://icru.org/content/reports/prescribing-recording-and-reporting-brachytherapy-for-cancer-of-the-cervix-report-no-89. Accessed 1 Mar 2020.
155. Viswanathan AN, Cormack R, Rawal B, Lee H. Increasing brachytherapy dose predicts survival for interstitial and tandem-based radiation for stage IIIB cervical cancer. Int J Gynecol Cancer. 2009;19:1402–6.
156. Fokdal L, Sturdza A, Mazeron R, et al. Image guided adaptive brachytherapy with combined intracavitary and interstitial technique improves the therapeutic ratio in locally advanced cervical cancer: analysis from the retroEMBRACE study. Radiother Oncol. 2016;120:434–40.
157. Viswanathan AN, Szymonifka J, Tempany-Afdhal CM, O'Farrell DA, Cormack RA. A prospective trial of real-time magnetic resonance-guided catheter placement in interstitial gynecologic brachytherapy. Brachytherapy. 2013;12:240–7.
158. Kapur T, Egger J, Damato A, Schmidt EJ, Viswanathan AN. 3T MR-guided brachytherapy for gynecologic malignancies. Magn Reson Imaging. 2012;30:1279–90.
159. Schmidt MA, Payne GS. Radiotherapy planning using MRI. Phys Med Biol. 2015;60:R323–61.
160. Dean CJ, Sykes JR, Cooper RA, Hatfield P, Carey B, Swift S, Bacon SE, Thwaites D, Sebag-Montefiore D, Morgan AM. An evaluation of four CT-MRI co-registration techniques for radiotherapy treatment planning of prone rectal cancer patients. Br J Radiol. 2012;85:61–8.
161. O'Neill BDP, Salerno G, Thomas K, Tait DM, Brown G. MR vs CT imaging: low rectal cancer tumour delineation for three-dimensional conformal radiotherapy. Br J Radiol. 2009;82:509–13.
162. Tan J, Lim Joon D, Fitt G, Wada M, Lim Joon M, Mercuri A, Marr M, Chao M, Khoo V. The utility of multimodality imaging with CT and MRI in defining rectal tumour volumes for radiotherapy treatment planning: a pilot study. J Med Imaging Radiat Oncol. 2010;54:562–8.
163. Seierstad T, Hole KH, Saelen E, Ree AH, Flatmark K, Malinen E. MR-guided simultaneous integrated boost in preoperative radiotherapy of locally advanced rectal cancer following neoadjuvant chemotherapy. Radiother Oncol. 2009;93:279–84.
164. Furey E, Jhaveri KS. Magnetic resonance imaging in rectal cancer. Magn Reson Imaging Clin N Am. 2014;22(165–190):v–vi.
165. Suzuki C, Torkzad MR, Tanaka S, Palmer G, Lindholm J, Holm T, Blomqvist L. The importance of rectal cancer MRI protocols on interpretation accuracy. World J Surg Oncol. 2008;6:89.
166. Jhaveri KS, Hosseini-Nik H. MRI of rectal cancer: an overview and update on recent advances. AJR Am J Roentgenol. 2015;205:W42–55.
167. Mir N, Sohaib SA, Collins D, Koh DM. Fusion of high b-value diffusion-weighted and T2-weighted MR images improves identification of lymph nodes in the pelvis. J Med Imaging Radiat Oncol. 2010;54:358–64.
168. Cong G-N, Qin M-W, You H, et al. Diffusion weighted imaging combined with magnetic resonance conventional sequences for the diagnosis of rectal cancer. Zhongguo Yi Xue Ke Xue Yuan Xue Bao. 2009;31:200–5.
169. Kuang F, Yan Z, Wang J, Rao Z. The value of diffusion-weighted MRI to evaluate the response to radiochemotherapy for cervical cancer. Magn Reson Imaging. 2014;32:342–9.
170. Alberda WJ, Dassen HPN, Dwarkasing RS, Willemssen FEJA, van der Pool AEM, de Wilt JHW, Burger JWA, Verhoef C. Prediction of tumor stage and lymph node involvement with dynamic contrast-enhanced MRI after chemoradiotherapy for locally advanced rectal cancer. Int J Color Dis. 2013;28:573–80.
171. Valentini V, Gambacorta MA, Barbaro B, et al. International consensus guidelines on clinical target volume delineation in rectal cancer. Radiother Oncol. 2016;120:195–201.

172. Van den Begin R, Kleijnen J-P, Engels B, Philippens M, van Asselen B, Raaymakers B, Reerink O, De Ridder M, Intven M. Tumor volume regression during preoperative chemoradiotherapy for rectal cancer: a prospective observational study with weekly MRI. Acta Oncol. 2018;57:723–7.
173. Lambregts DMJ, Yassien AB, Lahaye MJ, Betgen A, Maas M, Beets GL, van der Heide UA, van Triest B, Beets-Tan RGH. Monitoring early changes in rectal tumor morphology and volume during 5 weeks of preoperative chemoradiotherapy - an evaluation with sequential MRIs. Radiother Oncol. 2018;126:431–6.
174. Fiorino C, Passoni P, Palmisano A, et al. Accurate outcome prediction after neo-adjuvant radio-chemotherapy for rectal cancer based on a TCP-based early regression index. Clin Transl Radiat Oncol. 2019;19:12–6.
175. Burbach JPM, den Harder AM, Intven M, van Vulpen M, Verkooijen HM, Reerink O. Impact of radiotherapy boost on pathological complete response in patients with locally advanced rectal cancer: a systematic review and meta-analysis. Radiother Oncol. 2014;113:1–9.
176. Torkzad MR, Påhlman L, Glimelius B. Magnetic resonance imaging (MRI) in rectal cancer: a comprehensive review. Insights Imaging. 2010;1:245–67.
177. Sun Y-S, Zhang X-P, Tang L, Ji J-F, Gu J, Cai Y, Zhang X-Y. Locally advanced rectal carcinoma treated with preoperative chemotherapy and radiation therapy: preliminary analysis of diffusion-weighted MR imaging for early detection of tumor histopathologic downstaging. Radiology. 2010;254:170–8.
178. Glynne-Jones R, Tan D, Hughes R, Hoskin P. Squamous-cell carcinoma of the anus: progress in radiotherapy treatment. Nat Rev Clin Oncol. 2016;13:447–59.
179. Rusten E, Rekstad BL, Undseth C, Al-Haidari G, Hanekamp B, Hernes E, Hellebust TP, Malinen E, Guren MG. Target volume delineation of anal cancer based on magnetic resonance imaging or positron emission tomography. Radiat Oncol. 2017;12:147.
180. Glynne-Jones R, Nilsson PJ, Aschele C, Goh V, Peiffert D, Cervantes A, Arnold D, European Society for Medical Oncology (ESMO), European Society of Surgical Oncology (ESSO), European Society of Radiotherapy and Oncology (ESTRO). Anal cancer: ESMO-ESSO-ESTRO clinical practice guidelines for diagnosis, treatment and follow-up. Eur J Surg Oncol. 2014;40:1165–76.
181. Peiffert D, Tournier-Rangeard L, Gérard J-P, et al. Induction chemotherapy and dose intensification of the radiation boost in locally advanced anal canal carcinoma: final analysis of the randomized UNICANCER ACCORD 03 trial. J Clin Oncol. 2012;30:1941–8.
182. Jones M, Hruby G, Stanwell P, Gallagher S, Wong K, Arm J, Martin J. Multiparametric MRI as an outcome predictor for anal canal cancer managed with chemoradiotherapy. BMC Cancer. 2015;15:281.

Part II

Image-Guided Radiation Therapy Techniques

In-Room Systems for Patient Positioning and Motion Control

4

Patrick Wohlfahrt and Sonja Schellhammer

4.1 Introduction

The aim of radiotherapy to optimise tumour control while reducing side effects on healthy tissue is being pursued by applying dose distributions with increasingly steep gradients between the tumour and healthy organs at risk. With the introduction of advanced treatment techniques, such as three-dimensional conformal (3DCRT), stereotactic (SRT) and intensity-modulated radiation therapy (IMRT) as well as volumetric modulated arc therapy (VMAT), the precise and accurate dose delivery increasingly relies on an exact knowledge of the patient's position and anatomy during the course of treatment.

However, the patient anatomy with respect to the treatment reference point (isocentre) can strongly vary between treatment fractions (inter-fractionally) and within a treatment fraction (intra-fractionally). Inter-fractional variations can be introduced by imperfect patient setup, weight loss or gain, tumour shrinkage, oedema, post-operative tissue remodelling and inflammatory swelling. Anatomical changes due to respiration, cardiac motion, peristalsis, muscle relaxation, bowel, rectum and bladder filling as well as spontaneous motion such as swallowing during irradiation can cause intra-fractional uncertainties.

P. Wohlfahrt (✉)
Department of Radiation Oncology, Massachusetts General Hospital and Harvard Medical School, Boston, MA, USA

S. Schellhammer
OncoRay—National Center for Radiation Research in Oncology, Faculty of Medicine and University Hospital Carl Gustav Carus, Technische Universität Dresden, Helmholtz-Zentrum Dresden—Rossendorf, Dresden, Germany

Department of Radiotherapy and Radiation Oncology, Faculty of Medicine and University Hospital Carl Gustav Carus, Technische Universität Dresden, Dresden, Germany
e-mail: sonja.schellhammer@oncoray.de

E. G. C. Troost (ed.), *Image-Guided High-Precision Radiotherapy*,
https://doi.org/10.1007/978-3-031-08601-4_4

In order to ensure that a patient's tumour receives the prescribed dose in spite of these variations, a safety margin around the clinical target volume is commonly irradiated in addition to the tumour itself. As an example, this margin currently ranges between 6 and 18 mm for prostate-cancer patients positioned by aligning tattooed skin markers with the laser system in the treatment room [1]. This increases the irradiated volume by a factor of approx. two to seven. Hence, the normal tissue complication probability rises or the tumour volume needs to be underdosed.

Image-guided radiotherapy aims at reducing these safety margins by imaging essential parts of the patient anatomy in treatment position [2, 3]. Most commonly, anatomical images are acquired immediately before treatment fractions to adapt the patient position or treatment plan if necessary. Furthermore, there are techniques to monitor tissue motions and deformations in real time during irradiation [4]. By doing so, dynamic beam delivery with an enhanced dose conformality is rendered possible. Since the various modalities offer different advantages and drawbacks, most radiotherapy departments use combinations of several modalities individually tailored to the different treatment sites [5, 6].

This chapter outlines the most important modalities currently used for position verification and motion control of the patient and tumour in treatment position. Section 4.2 focuses on X-ray imaging systems, including electronic portal imaging, cone-beam CT, in-room diagnostic CT, and helical tomotherapy. Surrogate tracking systems based on optical, electromagnetic, and mechanical measurements are described in Sect. 4.3. The application of ultrasound imaging is presented in Sect. 4.4 and "Ultrasonography in Image-Guided Radiotherapy: Current Status and Future Challenges". The use of MRI for online image guidance is discussed in "Magnetic Resonance-guided Adaptive Radiotherapy: Technical Concepts" and "MR-integrated Linear Accelerators: First Clinical Results".

4.2 X-Ray Imaging Systems

The application of ionising radiation for position verification was already proposed in the early days of radiation oncology [7]. To meet the steadily increasing requirements in precision and accuracy of dose delivery, X-ray image acquisition and reconstruction were continuously improved and convenient technical solutions were implemented to enable a widespread translation into routine clinical practice [8–10].

Depending on the treatment site, complexity and intended accuracy in patient positioning as well as on the equipment available within the treatment room, two- or three-dimensional X-ray imaging is preferred. Two-dimensional X-ray imaging systems (i.e., electronic portal imaging and planar X-ray acquisition) are widely clinically applied. They are most appropriate if a patient misalignment can be sufficiently corrected by determining the geometrical difference of bony structures or of implanted fiducial markers to the position of these surrogates in the treatment plan. To properly account for internal anatomical changes induced by weight gain or loss, cavity fillings and organ motion, three-dimensional imaging using cone-beam (CBCT) or in-room CT is the current state-of-the-art method for adjusting patient positions [2, 5].

Imaging systems can use either the megavoltage (MV) X-ray spectrum provided by the linear accelerator or dedicated kilovoltage (kV) X-ray imaging systems mounted on the treatment device, connected to the treatment couch, or installed in the treatment room. Since the X-ray attenuation of megaelectronvolt (MeV) photons extracted from the linear accelerator is dominated by incoherent scattering, only tissues with a large difference in electron density can be easily distinguished, e.g. air, soft tissue and bone. In contrast to this very limited tissue contrast, X-ray spectra with common energies up to 80–140 kiloelectronvolt (keV) substantially improve the discriminability of several types of soft tissues as well as of bones, because the attenuation of low-energy photons is strongly influenced by the photoelectric effect in addition to incoherent scattering. Due to technical restrictions of on-board two- and three-dimensional X-ray imaging systems, the overall image quality is not comparable with in-room diagnostic CT systems. Furthermore, the CT acquisition time of on-board systems, i.e. cone-beam CT, is much longer, which restrains the applicability for treatment sites affected by organ motion, if no time-resolved image reconstruction is considered.

In the following paragraphs, the most common X-ray imaging systems and their respective benefits and limitations are discussed. Two-dimensional X-ray acquisitions will be addressed in the first two subsections. Sects. 4.3.3–4.3.5 are dedicated to volumetric X-ray imaging for position verification.

Overview

(+) pre-installed by manufacturers, easily applicable and individually adjustable, quantitative planar and volumetric imaging of internal anatomy, dose verification and dose tracking possible during the course of treatment.

(−) ionising radiation (therefore mostly used to adapt for inter-fractional variations), implanted fiducial markers are necessary to improve image contrast for some clinical indications, e.g. *soft-tissue tumours.*

4.2.1 Electronic Portal Imaging

MV photon treatment beams generated by the linear accelerator can be directly applied for adjusting the patient position in each fraction, verifying the treatment field before starting radiation delivery, as well as monitoring dose delivery during irradiation [11, 12]. After being shaped to the targeted region with jaws, a block and/or a multileaf collimator, the photon beam traverses the patient anatomy. The attenuation of the beam by the patient is commonly measured by an amorphous silicon active matrix flat-panel imager, a so-called electronic portal imaging detector (EPID). The cumulative dose for acquiring a single planar MV image ranges from 10 to 50 mGy in most cases [13]. Since the treatment field itself can be used for patient setup, the delivered dose can already be taken into account in the treatment plan. Furthermore, the imaging and treatment isocentre is identical and therefore no additional isocentre check is required for quality assurance (QA).

The planar projection of the patient anatomy in treatment position detected by a MV EPID can be compared with a reference MV X-ray image, a kV X-ray image acquired during patient simulation, or with a digitally reconstructed radiograph (DRR) in beam direction (Fig. 4.1). A DRR is derived from the CT scan used for treatment planning. Based on bony landmarks or fiducial markers implanted in proximity of or within the tumour region (e.g. for patients with pancreatic or prostate cancer), geometrical shifts correcting for a potential misalignment with respect to the position in the treatment plan can be determined and applied to the treatment couch. This approach is clinically appropriate for static treatment sites, where the bony anatomy or the location of fiducial markers can be assumed as a reliable

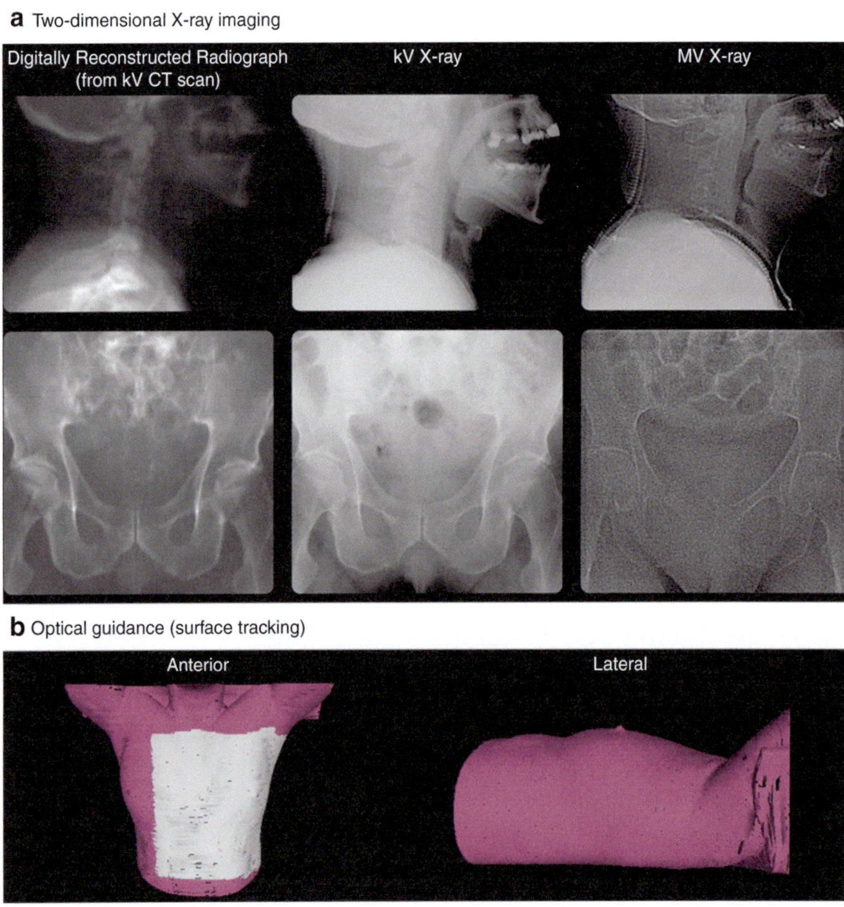

Fig. 4.1 (**a**) Exemplary two-dimensional X-ray images of the head-and-neck (top) and pelvis region (bottom). (**b**) Surface detection images (pink) of an exemplary breast-cancer patient. The white area represents the body region used for patient positioning

surrogate for the actual tumour localisation. In contrast to kV radiographs, MV X-ray images are not noticeably affected by high-density metallic implants, such as dental fillings or hip prostheses.

A geometric accuracy of 1–2 mm can be achieved in patient positioning using MV EPID. This technique is provided by all past and present vendors of linear accelerators, such as Elekta Instrument AB (Stockholm, Sweden), Siemens Healthineers (Erlangen, Germany) and Varian, a Siemens Healthineers Company (Palo Alto, CA), and can be applied to all treatment sites for setup verification [2]. However, planar MV X-ray imaging only provides a very limited tissue contrast at a relatively high imaging dose.

4.2.2 Planar kV X-Ray Imaging

As an alternative to the relatively high-dose and low-contrast planar MV imaging, the acquisition of two-dimensional kV X-ray images was proposed for setup verification (Fig. 4.1). In addition to a better differentiation of soft tissues, kV X-ray projections of the patient anatomy only require a small imaging dose of below 1 up to 3 mGy per image to be efficiently measured by an amorphous silicon flat-panel detector [13]. The imaging isocentre of the additionally implemented kV X-ray imaging system needs to be accurately aligned with the treatment isocentre to guarantee a reliable use of the radiograph for detecting and correcting potential patient misalignments. To this end, an isocentre consistency check is performed in a regular QA procedure.

The kV X-ray image is compared with a DRR derived from the CT scan used for treatment planning. A rigid registration of the two planar projections with respect to the bony anatomy, implanted fiducial markers or well-definable soft tissues yields the geometrical shift for patient setup adjustment. As opposed to MV X-ray only, three-dimensional setup information can be gathered by combining two X-ray images simultaneously acquired from different angles (mostly orthogonally). Hence, correction vectors for translations and rotations can be determined and applied to the treatment couch to further improve the accuracy in patient positioning. It is technically possible to use 2 kV or MV X-ray images, or even a combination of kV and MV X-ray acquisitions. The kV X-ray imaging system can also be applied for real-time tumour tracking in fluoroscopic mode [5].

A geometric accuracy of 1–2 mm can be achieved in patient positioning for various treatment sites using orthogonal X-ray imaging. Nowadays, several kV X-ray imaging systems are commercially available. Vendors of linear accelerators offer systems, which are directly mounted on the treatment machine orthogonally to the treatment head with their opposing EPID, e.g. the Synergy X-ray volume imaging (XVI) by Elekta Instrument AB and the On-Board Imager (OBI) from Varian, a Siemens Healthineers Company. Hence, these linear accelerators technically share the same isocentre for imaging and treatment. Other technical solutions consist of 2 kV X-ray tubes and opposing flat-panel detectors mounted to the ceiling and floor of the treatment room, respectively, such as the ExacTrac X-ray system manufactured by Brainlab AG (Munich, Germany) and the CyberKnife stereoscopic X-ray system by Accuracy, Inc. (Sunnyvale, CA). With the latter two stereoscopic X-ray solutions, a geometric accuracy of even less than 1 mm can be achieved [2, 14]. However, both MV and kV planar imaging do not provide volumetric information on the patient anatomy.

4.2.3 Cone-Beam Computed Tomography

In contrast to planar X-ray imaging, volumetric X-ray cone-beam CT provides more detailed information on inter-fractional differences in the location of internal organs and bony structures by rotating both the X-ray source and the detector around the patient. This guarantees an even more accurate three- or four-dimensional verification of the patient setup with a geometric accuracy below 1 mm and allows for an assessment of anatomical changes or monitoring of the tumour response during the course of fractionated radiation treatment [2].

Various technical solutions were developed by the vendors of linear accelerators using their MV and kV X-ray imaging systems mounted on the treatment machine (Sects. 4.3.1 and 4.3.2). While a sufficient tissue contrast for image guidance can be obtained by MV cone-beam CT, anatomical structures can be much better identified on kV cone-beam CT datasets (Fig. 4.2). To enhance the tissue contrast in MV cone-beam CT, the proportion of photons in the keV energy range of the MV photon beam can be increased by inserting a target consisting of carbon instead of tungsten and removing the flatting filter in beam direction as implemented in the In-Line kView Imaging system from Siemens Healthineers. Compared to a typical imaging dose ranging from 1 to 35 mGy for a kV cone-beam CT scan, the acquisition of MV cone-beam CT datasets is associated with much higher doses ranging from 30 to 100 mGy [15]. In the presence of high-density materials, such as metal implants in hip prostheses or multiple dental fillings, the image quality of kV cone-beam CT can be severely degraded and a MV cone-beam CT might be preferred.

To quantify the potential misalignment in patient positioning, the cone-beam CT scan is rigidly registered with the CT scan used for treatment planning and the target volume is defined as region of interest during the registration process. Due to the availability of volumetric information, correction vectors for translations and rotations can be determined and applied to the treatment couch. In addition to the bony anatomy and implanted fiducial markers, the tumour itself and internal organs can be considered for setup verification. By doing so, patients may be taken off the treatment couch in the occurrence of clinically relevant displacements of the target volume as well as of large changes in bladder, bowel or rectum fillings. These findings may give rise to a new CT scan for treatment planning or to specific instructions (e.g., intake of fluids, urination or defecation) to establish more consistent conditions with respect to the original CT scan.

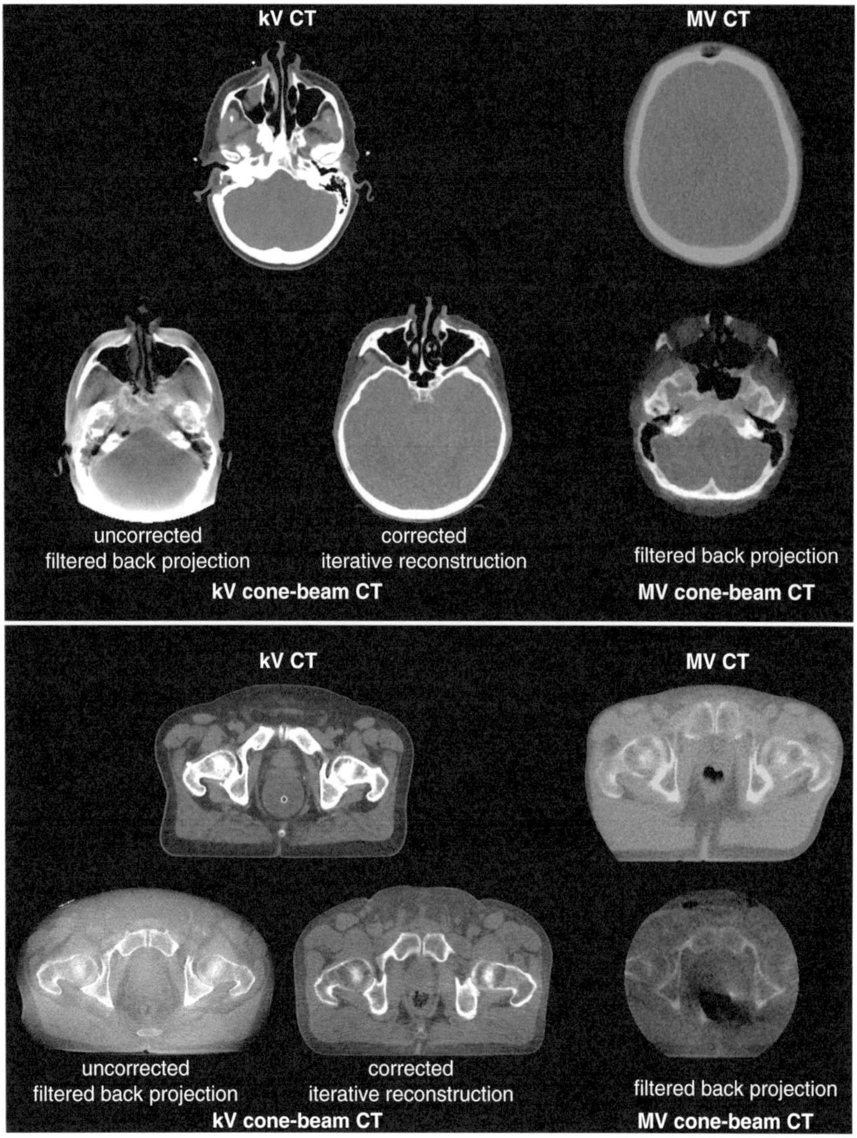

Fig. 4.2 Exemplary axial slices of three-dimensional fan-beam (upper row) and cone-beam CT scans (lower row) of the head (top) and pelvis region (bottom). The MV CT images, the uncorrected and corrected kV cone-beam CT images as well as the MV cone-beam CT images were kindly provided by Sebastian Zschaeck (Charité Universitätsmedizin, Berlin, Germany), Arthur Lalonde (Massachusetts General Hospital, Boston, MA) Julia Kirschke (Helios Klinikum, Berlin, Germany) and Nina Niebuhr (Universitätsklinikum Heidelberg, Heidelberg, Germany), respectively

The acquisition of a cone-beam CT, i.e. generating a sufficient number of X-ray projections covering an angle of 200° to 360°, takes roughly 1–2 min. Since this is a relatively slow process compared with diagnostic CT, a cone-beam CT scan represents an average view of the patient morphology and motion-induced anatomical changes are blurred. This effect can be addressed by correlating the respiratory motion with cone-beam CT acquisition. This allows for a retrospective time-resolved (4D) image reconstruction by assigning X-ray projections to specific breathing phases. Since only a portion of all projections can be used for phase-based cone-beam CT reconstruction, the poor angular sampling leads to severe streak artefacts and consequently a clearly inferior image quality with respect to static cone-beam CT. This can be partly compensated by reducing the rotation time of the linear accelerator, which results in longer acquisition times (usually 2–4 min) and thus smaller angular gaps between X-ray projections [16, 17].

Due to the technical design of such systems, a severe impact of X-ray scattering and beam hardening, especially for larger diameters and at large cone angles as in the upper abdomen or pelvic region, signal lags as well as restrictions in detector efficiency and field of view are prevalent. These technical issues in combination with patient and organ motion during the acquisition can result in a degradation of the image quality in terms of tissue contrast for tumour detection and consistency in CT numbers for dose calculation. The field of view can be increased by off-centring the detector to fully cover each half of the body in two 180° rotations separately, and then combining the projections in image reconstruction [15]. The influence of X-ray scattering on streak artefacts and CT number stability can be substantially improved by iterative reconstruction algorithms and advanced methods for scatter estimation [18–20], which might potentially lead to a more precise and accurate representation and differentiation of soft tissues in future.

Another kV cone-beam CT system consisting of a ring structure with two arms carrying the X-ray source and flat-panel detector was introduced as ImagingRing by medPhoton GmbH (Salzburg, Austria). This system can be mounted on the treatment couch or on the ceiling with a rail system and enables rotations of more than 400 degrees for full-arc acquisitions of a large field of view [21].

4.2.4 Helical Tomotherapy System

Helical tomotherapy systems deliver IMRT treatment fields divided in slices by continuously rotating a 6 MV fan-beam photon linear accelerator at a constant velocity with a binary multileaf collimator for intensity adjustment around the patient while simultaneously moving the treatment couch. The technical principle is comparable to a diagnostic X-ray CT scanner. For imaging purposes, the multileaf collimator is fully opened and the nominal electron energy is reduced to 3.5 MeV. The treatment beam in combination with the opposing detector, commonly consisting of an ion-chamber array filled with Xenon gas, can be used to acquire fan-beam MV CT scans of the patient in treatment position (Fig. 4.2). Typical imaging doses are in the range of 10–30 mGy (depending on the selected pitch) and thus comparable to kV cone-beam CT acquisitions. Since the imaging and treatment isocentre are identical, no additional isocentre QA check is required [2, 15].

The MV fan-beam CT scan is rigidly registered to the diagnostic CT scan acquired for treatment planning. A translational and rotational correction matrix is determined to adjust the patient setup with respect to the position in the planned scenario. The accuracy in image registration depends on image acquisition settings, such as pitch, slice thickness and scan length. It can also differ between body regions. In general, the image quality of MV fan-beam CT scans is less affected by X-ray scatter and beam hardening compared with kV and MV X-ray cone-beam CT. Furthermore, image artefacts caused by metallic implants hamper the image quality of kV X-ray cone-beam CT but are not present in MV fan-beam CT. However, the image noise and soft tissue contrast of volumetric MV X-ray imaging is substantially inferior to kV X-rays, but mostly still sufficient to identify clinically relevant soft tissues in addition to the bony anatomy for patient setup adjustment. The MV fan-beam CT scan can be directly used for dose calculations and the assessment of anatomical changes or tumour response during the course of treatment. In the current technical design, an axial CT slice with a field of view of 40 cm can be acquired and reconstructed within 5 s [2, 15].

A submillimetre geometric accuracy can be achieved in patient setup verification for various treatment sites with the MV fan-beam X-ray imaging system. Two helical tomotherapy solutions, TomoTherapy and Radixact, are currently commercially available from Accuracy.

4.2.5 In-Room Computed Tomography System on Rails

By the integration of a conventional CT scanner in the treatment room, the same diagnostic image quality as used for treatment planning can be deployed for patients immobilised in treatment position (Fig. 4.2). An in-room CT scanner is installed on a rail system, which is in line with the treatment couch axis and enables the movement of the CT scanner while the patient is kept still in treatment position. After isocentric positioning of the patient with respect to the room laser system, the treatment couch is rotated (usually by 180°) to align the couch orientation with the rail system. For patient treatment, the couch rotation is reversed. Since this workflow can be time-consuming sometimes, a final verification of the treatment position with two-dimensional X-ray might be appropriate. The alignment of the two coordinate systems as well as the treatment and imaging isocentre is verified in a regular QA procedure. A typical CT dose ranges from 0.5 to 10 mGy, depending on the diagnostic quality geared to the respective application – with an increasing imaging dose from (1) exclusively setup verification to (2) recalculation of dose distributions to (3) a full adaptation of the treatment plan including target delineation or quantitative tumour response assessment [2, 14, 15].

To adjust a potential misalignment of the patient with respect to the position in the treatment plan, the two CT scans, i.e. the in-room prior to treatment as well as the treatment-planning CT scan, are rigidly registered and the determined correction vectors are directly applied to the treatment couch. Due to the diagnostic image quality, bony structures and soft tissues can be easily considered for setup verification. Common in-room CT systems can be equipped with bore sizes up to 85 cm to support even bulky immobilisation devices. In-room CT scans can be reconstructed with a field of view of 50 cm (up to 60–70 cm with new CT scanner generations), which can be extended up to 80–85 cm based on extrapolated X-ray projections. Recent innovations in diagnostic CT acquisition (e.g. dual-energy CT) and image reconstruction (e.g. iterative reconstruction, beam hardening correction and metal artefact reduction) have further improved the tissue contrast, increased the CT number stability and reduced the overall imaging dose for radiotherapy solutions [22, 23].

Patient positioning for all treatment sites can be performed with a submillimetre geometric accuracy by exploiting the full diagnostic capabilities of in-room kV CT scanners on rails. Such CT systems are provided by the common vendors of CT scanners, such as Canon Medical Systems Corporation (Otawara, Japan), GE Healthcare, Inc. (Chicago, IL, USA), Philips Healthcare (Amsterdam, Netherlands) and Siemens Healthineers.

4.3 Surrogate Tracking

X-ray imaging systems, as described in the previous section, enable the direct imaging of the internal patient anatomy. Since they add ionising radiation dose to the patient, they are mainly applied to monitor inter-fractional variations. However, intra-fractional variations such as respiration and digestion can also significantly alter the delivered dose distribution. Therefore, a number of surrogate measures have been developed supplementing X-ray imaging systems.

Cameras operating in the visible or the infrared spectrum are used for position verification of superficial tumours such as breast cancer or soft tissue sarcoma (Sects. 4.3.1 and 4.3.2). Furthermore, they can generate a breathing signal, which can be applied to synchronise irradiation with the patient breathing pattern. Such a breathing signal can also be generated by spirometry (Sect. 4.3.3) and mechanical gauges (Sect. 4.3.4). Finally, electromagnetic transponders implanted in the tumour can facilitate the tracking of the tumour position (Sect. 4.3.5).

In general, the correlation of these surrogate signals with the patient anatomy, i.e. the position and shape of the tumour and healthy tissue, is limited [24, 25]. Therefore, they are not used as alternative to, but rather in combination with X-ray imaging systems.

Overview

(+) easy installation and use, real-time information during irradiation, no ionising radiation.

(−) no volumetric images, limited correlation between surrogate position and internal patient anatomy.

4.3.1 Optical Guidance

Optical guidance can be performed by cameras monitoring the patient's surface (Fig. 4.1). Light sources project a grid pattern on the patient's surface, which is detected by one to three high-definition cameras and converted into a three-dimensional map in real time. To determine the translation and rotation necessary for correcting the patient position, this virtual surface is mapped onto the external body contour derived from the treatment planning CT scan by rigid or deformable registration. Furthermore, breath-synchronised irradiation and patient motion monitoring can be facilitated by integrated systems that pause irradiation automatically whenever the monitored surface leaves a defined volume [26, 27].

Due to computational costs, there is a trade-off between the spatial resolution, the temporal resolution, and the imaged volume. Most commonly, a high resolution is prioritised, for example, in cranial applications, whereas a large volume and high temporal resolution are chosen for breath-synchronised irradiation. The geometric accuracy of optical guidance typically ranges from 1 to 2 mm if room lighting is optimal and the patient is unclothed [3].

The advantages of this system lie in its straightforward implementation, its real-time capability, and the absence of radiation dose. However, it provides no information on the internal patient anatomy. Furthermore, the correlation between surface and target motion can be unreliable for many body regions, especially for deep-seated tumours. Optical image guidance is therefore best suited for superficial tumours, whose position correlates reliably with the patient surface, such as skin tumours, superficial soft-tissue sarcoma, and whole breast irradiation [28]. The real-time imaging capabilities of optical image guidance systems are most commonly used for breath-gated irradiation of the breast in combination with deep-inspiration breath-hold.

The most common commercial optical surface tracking systems in radiotherapy are AlignRT (VisionRT, London, UK), Catalyst (C-Rad, Uppsala, Sweden) and Identify (Varian, a Siemens Healthineers Company).

4.3.2 Infrared Markers

As an alternative to the visible range of the electromagnetic spectrum, infrared light can be used to monitor the patient's surface. This is facilitated by either passive infrared reflectors or active infrared emitters attached to the patient, the treatment couch or patient positioning equipment. Before and during irradiation, stereoscopic cameras installed in the ceiling of the treatment room record the marker position in three dimensions at a frame rate of up to 100 frames per second. This enables both position verification and online motion monitoring. In integrated systems, beam-on can be triggered automatically during patient breath-hold [29].

Such systems are relatively easy to implement, provide real-time information of the reflector position, and do not add radiation dose to the patient. Hence, they are a commonly used option for motion monitoring during irradiation. However, the reflector position provides limited information of the patient's anatomy and serves only as a surrogate for the tumour position. Furthermore, the repeated marker positioning on the patient skin adds to the treatment time and causes reproducibility uncertainty.

Infrared systems are therefore mostly used in combination with other position verification systems and to generate a breathing signal for gated treatment delivery. Comparative studies have shown residual setup errors for treatments of the breast and internal organs in the order of 3–4 mm [30, 31].

Common infrared monitoring systems are the Real-time Position Management system (Varian, a Siemens Healthineers Company), ExacTrac (Brainlab AG) and SMART DX (BTS Bioengineering, Garbagnate Milanese, Italy).

4.3.3 Spirometry

Spirometers can be used as a means to control the air volume inhaled by the patient. They are attached to the patient via a mouthpiece and a valve acting to restrict the inhaled air volume to a pre-defined level. This technique, referred to as active breathing control (ABC), enforces a reproducible lung volume, and has been applied for Hodgkin's disease, breast and lung tumours [32, 33]. Integration with the linear accelerator ensures an automatic synchronisation of the irradiation with the patient breathing pattern. A common ABC system is the Active Breathing Coordinator (Elekta Instrument AB).

This technique is free from ionising radiation and relatively easy to implement. However, the correlation of the inhaled air volume with the position and shape of the tumour and healthy organs is not always reliable due to variations of the thoracic and abdominal breathing motion [34]. Furthermore, patients need to be trained to properly breathe under ABC, which requires a good compliance and communication.

4.3.4 Mechanical Gauges

Mechanical gauges used to monitor the patient respiration are non-invasive and very easy to implement. One such method relies on expanding belts. Here, a belt is placed around the abdomen of the patient, which expands and contracts in conjunction with the patient surface. A pressure sensor converts the pressure changes to a digital gating signal. This signal can be used to synchronise irradiation with the breathing cycle. Common pressure belt systems are ANZAI (Anzai Medical Co., Tokyo, Japan) and Bellows (Philips Healthcare) [35, 36].

Another mechanical system is a sensor consisting of two arms placed on the abdomen and the chest of the patient. Respiration-induced motion of these arms is translated mechanically to a needle indicating the current respiration height on a scale. The patient receives breathing instructions via speakers in the treatment room and watches the needle through a mirror to control the respiration level in real time. This system does not require electricity, but patient compliance and flawless communication between the radiotherapist and the patient. It is commercially available as Abches (APEX Medical Inc., Tokyo, Japan) [37, 38].

4.3.5 Electromagnetic Transponders

Electromagnetic transponders are mainly used for inter- and intra-fractional motion control of the prostate. They can be placed inside the tumour volume through a minimally invasive intervention. When the patient is positioned on the treatment couch, the transponders are excited by an external coil array at a resonance frequency unique to each transponder. During de-excitation, a radiofrequency signal is emitted by the transponders and recorded by receiver coils. This allows for a real-time monitoring of the position and motion of the target, both before and during irradiation, with an accuracy better than 2 mm [39, 40].

One of the main limitations of these markers is the need of a surgical intervention. Furthermore, the markers can produce artefacts in MR images, require a non-conducting couch top, and can only be used up to a depth of about 20 cm due to signal degradation. The most common system is Calypso (Varian, a Siemens Healthineers Company).

4.4 Ultrasound

Since ultrasound is covered in "Ultrasonography in Image-Guided Radiotherapy: Current Status and Future Challenges", only a brief overview for completeness of the topic is given here. Ultrasound imaging is based on acoustic waves (typically 2–8 MHz) being sent into the patient tissue by a piezoelectric transducer placed on the patient's surface. Part of these waves are reflected at interfaces between tissues of different acoustic impedance and in inhomogeneous tissues. The transducer then records the resulting echo alongside its amplitude and time of flight (echo time). Assuming a constant speed of sound (typically 1540 m/s), the time of flight is converted to depth in tissue and the echo amplitude is plotted as a function of depth.

An array of successively activated transducer elements allows to generate two-dimensional images of the patient anatomy, most commonly with the echo amplitude encoded as brightness (B-mode) [41]. This technique can be extended to three dimensions, for example, by moving the transducer array along the patient skin and tracking the transducer with a position sensor, or by use of a two-dimensional transducer array. Due to a high repetition rate, four-dimensional imaging (i.e. continuous real-time 3D imaging) can be performed.

Ultrasound can be used for inter-fractional patient positioning by matching an ultrasound image acquired in treatment position to either the planning CT scan (inter-modality matching) or another ultrasound image acquired directly before or after the planning CT scan (intra-modality matching). For both methods, the position of the transducer in the reference frame of the linear accelerator can be determined optically (by cameras and markers), electromagnetically (by electromagnetic emitters and detectors) or mechanically (by an ultrasound probe holder affixed to the accelerator).

The axial resolution of this technique commonly amounts to about 0.5 mm, depending on the depth of the tissue to be monitored and the corresponding required ultrasound frequency. The lateral and longitudinal resolution typically range between 2 and 5 mm, depending on the transducer element dimension and the depth in tissue [42]. The positional accuracy of this technique, as determined by comparison to a kV X-ray with fiducial markers, is in the order of a few millimetres. The relatively high sensitivity to differences in acoustic impedance allows for a high contrast between tissues.

This method can provide markerless, high-contrast volumetric images in real time while being cost-effective, well-tolerated and free from ionising irradiation. On the other hand, a number of limitations hinder its application in most clinical practices [43, 44]:

- Pressure applied to the transducer can deform the patient's anatomy.
- The inter-modality matching and registration of the ultrasound and reference frame of the linear accelerator introduce geometric uncertainties.
- A significant inter- and intra-user variability has been demonstrated for the acquired images.
- The field of view is limited and electron density information is lacking.
- Image artefacts due to inhomogeneities in the speed of sound, multiple reflections and strong differences in echogeneity are common.
- Ultrasound waves hardly propagate through bone and air.

For these reasons, the field of application for ultrasound imaging in radiotherapy is mainly limited to position verification of the prostate, either by transperineal or transabdominal ultrasound [45]. Current research is directed at decreasing the user-dependence, for example, by robotic probe holders and adhesive phased crystal probes.

The most common commercial ultrasound systems used in radiotherapy are the B-Mode Acquisition and Targeting (BAT) system (NOMOS Corp., Cranberry Township, USA), the SonArray system (Varian, a Siemens Healthineers Company), and the Clarity System (Elekta Instrument AB).

Overview

(+) markerless (non-invasive), high soft-tissue contrast, real-time information during irradiation, no ionising radiation.

(−) no image information behind bones and air, small field of view, prone to artefacts and geometrical uncertainties, lack of electron density information.

References

1. Yartsev S, Bauman G. Target margins in radiotherapy of prostate cancer. Br J Radiol. 2016;89:20160312.
2. De Los SJ, Popple R, Agazaryan N, et al. Image guided radiation therapy (IGRT) technologies for radiation therapy localization and delivery. Int J Radiat Oncol Biol Phys. 2013;87:33–45.
3. Goyal S, Kataria T. Image guidance in radiation therapy: techniques and applications. Radiol Res Pract. 2014;2014:1–10.
4. Bertholet J, Knopf A, Eiben B, et al. Real-time intrafraction motion monitoring in external beam radiotherapy. Phys Med Biol. 2019;64:15TR01.
5. Zou W, Dong L, Kevin Teo B-K. Current state of image guidance in radiation oncology: implications for PTV margin expansion and adaptive therapy. Semin Radiat Oncol. 2018;28:238–47.
6. International Atomic Energy Agency. Introduction of image guided radiotherapy into clinical practice. Vienna: International Atomic Energy Agency; 2019.
7. Verellen D, De Ridder M, Storme G. A (short) history of image-guided radiotherapy. Radiother Oncol. 2008;86:4–13.
8. Dawson LA, Sharpe MB. Image-guided radiotherapy: rationale, benefits, and limitations. Lancet Oncol. 2006;7:848–58.
9. Verellen D, De Ridder M, Linthout N, Tournel K, Soete G, Storme G. Innovations in image-guided radiotherapy. Nat Rev Cancer. 2007;7:949–60.
10. Jaffray DA. Image-guided radiotherapy: from current concept to future perspectives. Nat Rev Clin Oncol. 2012;9:688–99.
11. Boyer AL, Antonuk L, Fenster A, Van Herk M, Meertens H, Munro P, Reinstein LE, Wong J. A review of electronic portal imaging devices (EPIDs). Med Phys. 1992;19:1–16.
12. van Elmpt W, McDermott L, Nijsten S, Wendling M, Lambin P, Mijnheer B. A literature review of electronic portal imaging for radiotherapy dosimetry. Radiother Oncol. 2008;88:289–309.
13. Murphy MJ, Balter J, Balter S, et al. The Management of Imaging Dose during Image-Guided Radiotherapy: report of the AAPM task group 75. Med Phys. 2007;34:4041–63.
14. Yin F-F, Wong J. The role of in-room kV X-ray imaging for patient setup and target localization. Alexandria VA: AAPM; 2009.
15. Bissonnette J-P, Balter PA, Dong L, Langen KM, Lovelock DM, Miften M, Moseley DJ, Pouliot J, Sonke J-J, Yoo S. Quality Assurance for Image-Guided Radiation Therapy Utilizing CT-based technologies: a report of the AAPM TG-179. Med Phys. 2012;39:1946–63.
16. Bryce-Atkinson A, Marchant T, Rodgers J, Budgell G, McWilliam A, Faivre-Finn C, Whitfield G, van Herk M. Quantitative evaluation of 4D cone beam CT scans with reduced scan time in lung cancer patients. Radiother Oncol. 2019;136:64–70.
17. Liang J, Lack D, Zhou J, Liu Q, Grills I, Yan D. Intrafraction 4D-cone beam CT acquired during volumetric arc radiotherapy delivery: KV parameter optimization and 4D motion accuracy for lung stereotactic body radiotherapy (SBRT) patients. J Appl Clin Med Phys. 2019;20:10–24.
18. Yan H, Wang X, Shi F, Bai T, Folkerts M, Cervino L, Jiang SB, Jia X. Towards the clinical implementation of iterative low-dose cone-beam CT reconstruction in image-guided radiation therapy: cone/ring artifact correction and multiple GPU implementation. Med Phys. 2014;41:111912.
19. Cai B, Laugeman E, Mazur TR, Park JC, Henke LE, Kim H, Hugo GD, Mutic S, Li H. Characterization of a prototype rapid Kilovoltage X-ray image guidance system designed for a ring shape radiation therapy unit. Med Phys. 2019;46:1355–70.
20. Maier J, Eulig E, Vöth T, Knaup M, Kuntz J, Sawall S, Kachelrieß M. Real-time scatter estimation for medical CT using the deep scatter estimation: method and robustness analysis with respect to different anatomies, dose levels, tube voltages, and data truncation. Med Phys. 2019;46:238–49.

21. Rit S, Clackdoyle R, Keuschnigg P, Steininger P. Filtered-Backprojection reconstruction for a cone-beam computed tomography scanner with independent source and detector rotations. Med Phys. 2016;43:2344–52.
22. van Elmpt W, Landry G, Das M, Verhaegen F. Dual energy CT in radiotherapy: current applications and future outlook. Radiother Oncol. 2016;119:137–44.
23. Wohlfahrt P, Richter C. Status and innovations in pre-treatment CT imaging for proton therapy. Br J Radiol. 2020;93:20190590.
24. Gierga DP, Brewer J, Sharp GC, Betke M, Willett CG, Chen GTY. The correlation between internal and external markers for abdominal tumors: implications for respiratory gating. Int J Radiat Oncol Biol Phys. 2005;61:1551–8.
25. Korreman SS, Juhler-Nøttrup T, Boyer AL. Respiratory gated beam delivery cannot facilitate margin reduction, unless combined with respiratory correlated image guidance. Radiother Oncol. 2008;86:61–8.
26. Bert C, Metheany KG, Doppke KP, Taghian AG, Powell SN, Chen GTY. Clinical experience with a 3D surface patient setup system for alignment of partial-breast irradiation patients. Int J Radiat Oncol Biol Phys. 2006;64:1265–74.
27. Hamming VC, Visser C, Batin E, McDermott LN, Busz DM, Both S, Langendijk JA, Sijtsema NM. Evaluation of a 3D surface imaging system for deep inspiration breath-hold patient positioning and intra-fraction monitoring. Radiat Oncol. 2019;14:125.
28. Hoisak JDP, Pawlicki T. The role of optical surface imaging systems in radiation therapy. Semin Radiat Oncol. 2018;28:185–93.
29. Baroni G, Garibaldi C, Scabini M, Riboldi M, Catalano G, Tosi G, Orecchia R, Pedotti A. Dosimetric effects within target and organs at risk of interfractional patient mispositioning in left breast cancer radiotherapy. Int J Radiat Oncol Biol Phys. 2004;59:861–71.
30. Li R, Mok E, Han B, Koong A, Xing L. Evaluation of the geometric accuracy of surrogate-based gated VMAT using Intrafraction Kilovoltage X-ray images. Med Phys. 2012;39:2686–93.
31. Fassi A, Ivaldi GB, de Fatis PT, Liotta M, Meaglia I, Porcu P, Regolo L, Riboldi M, Baroni G. Target position reproducibility in left-breast irradiation with deep inspiration breath-hold using multiple optical surface control points. J Appl Clin Med Phys. 2018;19:35–43.
32. Wong JW, Sharpe MB, Jaffray DA, Kini VR, Robertson JM, Stromberg JS, Martinez AA. The use of active breathing control (ABC) to reduce margin for breathing motion. Int J Radiat Oncol Biol Phys. 1999;44:911–9.
33. McNair HA, Brock J, Symonds-Tayler JRN, Ashley S, Eagle S, Evans PM, Kavanagh A, Panakis N, Brada M. Feasibility of the use of the active breathing co Ordinator™ (ABC) in patients receiving radical radiotherapy for non-small cell lung cancer (NSCLC). Radiother Oncol. 2009;93:424–9.
34. Fassi A, Ivaldi GB, Meaglia I, Porcu P, Fatis PT, Liotta M, Riboldi M, Baroni G. Reproducibility of the external surface position in left-breast DIBH radiotherapy with spirometer-based monitoring: methodological mistake. J Appl Clin Med Phys. 2014;15:401.
35. Li XA, Stepaniak C, Gore E. Technical and dosimetric aspects of respiratory gating using a pressure-sensor motion monitoring system. Med Phys. 2005;33:145–54.
36. Liu J, Lin T, Fan J, Chen L, Price R, Ma C-MC. Evaluation of the combined use of two different respiratory monitoring systems for 4D CT simulation and gated treatment. J Appl Clin Med Phys. 2018;19:666–75.
37. Bengua G, Ishikawa M, Sutherland K, et al. Evaluation of the effectiveness of the stereotactic body frame in reducing respiratory intrafractional organ motion using the real-time tumor-tracking radiotherapy system. Int J Radiat Oncol. 2010;77:630–6.
38. Yeh T-C, Chi M-S, Chi K-H, Hsu C-H. Evaluation of Abches and volumetric modulated arc therapy under deep inspiration breath-hold technique for patients with left-sided breast cancer. Medicine (Baltimore). 2019;98:e17340.
39. Willoughby TR, Kupelian PA, Pouliot J, et al. Target localization and real-time tracking using the calypso 4D localization system in patients with localized prostate cancer. Int J Radiat Oncol Biol Phys. 2006;65:528–34.

40. Foster RD, Solberg TD, Li HS, Kerkhoff A, Enke CA, Willoughby TR, Kupelian PA. Comparison of transabdominal ultrasound and electromagnetic transponders for prostate localization. J Appl Clin Med Phys. 2010;11:57–67.
41. Wild JJ. The use of ultrasonic pulses for the measurement of biologic tissues and the detection of tissue density changes. Surgery. 1950;27:183–8.
42. Fontanarosa D, van der Meer S, Bamber J, Harris E, O'Shea T, Verhaegen F. Review of ultrasound image guidance in external beam radiotherapy: I. treatment planning and inter-fraction motion management. Phys Med Biol. 2015;60:R77–R114.
43. Fuss M, Salter BJ, Cavanaugh SX, Fuss C, Sadeghi A, Fuller CD, Ameduri A, Hevezi JM, Herman TS, Thomas CR. Daily ultrasound-based image-guided targeting for radiotherapy of upper abdominal malignancies. Int J Radiat Oncol Biol Phys. 2004;59:1245–56.
44. Western C, Hristov D, Schlosser J. Ultrasound imaging in radiation therapy: from Interfractional to Intrafractional guidance. Cureus. 2015;7:23–4.
45. Camps SM, Fontanarosa D, de With PHN, Verhaegen F, Vanneste BGL. The use of ultrasound imaging in the external beam radiotherapy workflow of prostate cancer patients. Biomed Res Int. 2018;2018:1–16.

IMRT/VMAT-SABR

5

Pablo Carrasco de Fez and Núria Jornet

5.1 The Technology-Driven Evolution of Radiotherapy

Technological changes are deeply changing society, in general, and medicine, in particular. Radiotherapy (RT) is a very technical branch of medicine. Consequently, technological changes are having great impact on radiotherapy. New technologies and new techniques, such as Intensity Modulated Radiation Therapy (IMRT) and Volumetric Modulated Arc Therapy (VMAT), have allowed increasing the radiation dose delivered to the tumour while reducing the absorbed dose delivered to healthy tissues nearby, by significantly improving our ability to adapt dose delivery to the target (i.e., conformality). An increase in absorbed dose to the tumour is, to a large extent, related with an increase in tumour control probability. Any reduction of absorbed dose to healthy tissues is related to a decrease in the probability of treatment toxicity. As a result, technological changes have helped to increase the success of radiation treatments, understood as the proportion of cancer cases that can be cured with an acceptable level of toxicity. However, the more we shape the dose distribution to the target volume the higher the risk is of missing a part of it. Therefore, this success would have not been possible without the addition of imaging systems to radiation treatment units. We can now 'see' more precisely where we are pointing at with the radiation beams. Modern imaging systems allow delivering of radiotherapy with an accuracy below 1 mm.

The aforementioned improved accuracy in treatment delivery has also allowed performing ablative treatments. In this kind of treatments, high radiation doses are delivered in one or a few fractions. For ablative treatments, such as Stereotactic Ablative Body Radiotherapy (SABR), it is of paramount importance to minimize the irradiation of healthy tissues. In this scenario, the absorbed dose falloff with

P. Carrasco de Fez (✉) · N. Jornet
Servei de Radiofísica i Radioprotecció, Hospital de la Santa Creu i Sant Pau, Barcelona, Spain
e-mail: PCarrasco@santpau.cat; NJornet@santpau.cat

E. G. C. Troost (ed.), *Image-Guided High-Precision Radiotherapy*,
https://doi.org/10.1007/978-3-031-08601-4_5

distance has to be very steep and safety margins that are related to setup uncertainties have to be minimized. It is also crucial to direct the radiation very accurately and precisely towards the target.

All in all, modern radiotherapy is a world of interlaced new delivery techniques and imaging systems. The increasing complexity of this world also requires intensive quality assurance programs in a multidisciplinary approach. The present chapter will describe the main aspects of each technique as they are implemented in the clinical practice at present time, but before going through modern techniques it is convenient to recall the radiotherapy workflow from prescription to delivery.

5.2 The Radiation Therapy Workflow

Radiation treatments are aimed at delivering the prescribed absorbed dose to a 'target'. This absorbed dose must be high enough to produce the desired therapeutic effect. The endpoint for curative treatments is most frequently tumour control. However, for palliative treatments it is commonly relief of symptoms, such as pain, neurological deficits, or bleeding. At the same time, the absorbed dose to healthy tissues that are close to the 'target' has to be minimized in order to avoid treatment toxicity. To achieve these goals, three main requirements can be identified. First, imaging systems to acquire 3D information about the patient geometry and the extent of the disease are required. Secondly, a systematic way of defining what the 'target' is, is needed. And thirdly, some software to design the treatment plan and to calculate the absorbed dose distribution in the patient (known as treatment planning system, or TPS) is required. Although these requirements might seem independent of one another, the first one and the third one are not: computed tomography (CT) scans are used as the primary imaging modality to calculate absorbed dose in a patient, because CT images themselves give information on the absorption of energy within the patient's tissues. Consequently, CT scans not only provide morphological information about the patient, but also give information on how radiation interacts with the patient.

As a result, CT is required for radiation treatment planning. However, CT has low soft-tissue contrast and lacks functional information. For this reason, other imaging modalities are used to complement CT information when needed. For instance, MRI overcomes the soft-tissue limitation of CT when soft-tissue contrast is required, and it also offers complementary functional information (see "Use of Anatomical and Functional MRI in Radiation Treatment Planning"). At present time, however, the preferred source of imaging for functional information is PET (see "Use of [^{18}F]FDG PET/CT for Target Volume Definition in Radiotherapy" and "Specific PET Tracers for Solid Tumors and for Definition of the Biological Target Volume"). Radiation oncologists combine the information provided by these three main imaging modalities and define what the 'target' is for each patient.

The International Commission on Radiation Units and Measurements (ICRU) standardized in reports 50 and 62 [1, 2] how the 'target' must be defined. These documents specify that the radiation oncologist has to define several volumes integrating the information given by different imaging systems and the knowledge about the tumour biology and tumour progression patterns. The main volumes defined by ICRU are:

- The gross tumour volume (GTV): it is the gross demonstrable extent and location of the malignant growth. It consists of primary tumour and possibly metastatic lymphadenopathy or other metastases.
- The clinical target volume (CTV): it is a volume that contains the demonstrable GTV and/or subclinical malignant disease that must be eliminated. This volume must be treated adequately in order to achieve the aim of radical therapy. The CTV is a clinical-anatomical concept and can be described as including structures with clinically suspected but unproved involvement (called *subclinical disease*), in addition to known tumour.
- The planning target volume (PTV): it is a geometrical concept used for treatment planning, and it is defined to select appropriate beam sizes and beam arrangements, to ensure that the prescribed dose is actually delivered to the CTV. It is designed as an expanded volume derived from the CTV that takes into account that the patient geometry on a daily basis can differ from the set of images used for treatment planning. Computation of dose distribution is done for a set of images acquired at a specific point of time (a 'snapshot'). However, when the treatment is delivered, there are variations in positions, sizes, shapes, and orientations of the tissues and the beams with respect to this snapshot. By treating the PTV (the CTV plus some suitable margins), correct irradiation of the CTV is guaranteed throughout the treatment. CTV-PTV margins are therefore related to the degree of reproducibility that can be achieved for a given treatment and patient. The next subsection will tackle this issue.

5.2.1 Immobilization: Dealing with Patient Position Reproducibility in Radiotherapy

As radiation treatments are delivered fractionated and therefore repeated on different days, it is of outmost importance to guarantee reproducibility of patient position and anatomy between radiation treatment planning and each fraction delivery, as well as during the treatment fraction, i.e. inter- and intra-fractional reproducibility. Any change would compromise target coverage and increase radiation doses to organs at risk.

Immobilization and positioning devices are the first step to guarantee reproducibility of patient geometry during the radiotherapy process (Fig. 5.1). The need for reproducibility also applies from the moment when the different imaging modalities (CT, MRI, PET) are used to acquire images for treatment planning until the last treatment session. The kind of positioning/immobilization device that is used depends on the treatment site. For head and neck tumours, head supports and individualized thermoplastic masks covering the head to the shoulders are used. These masks are made of a plastic material of polymeric composition that may incorporate

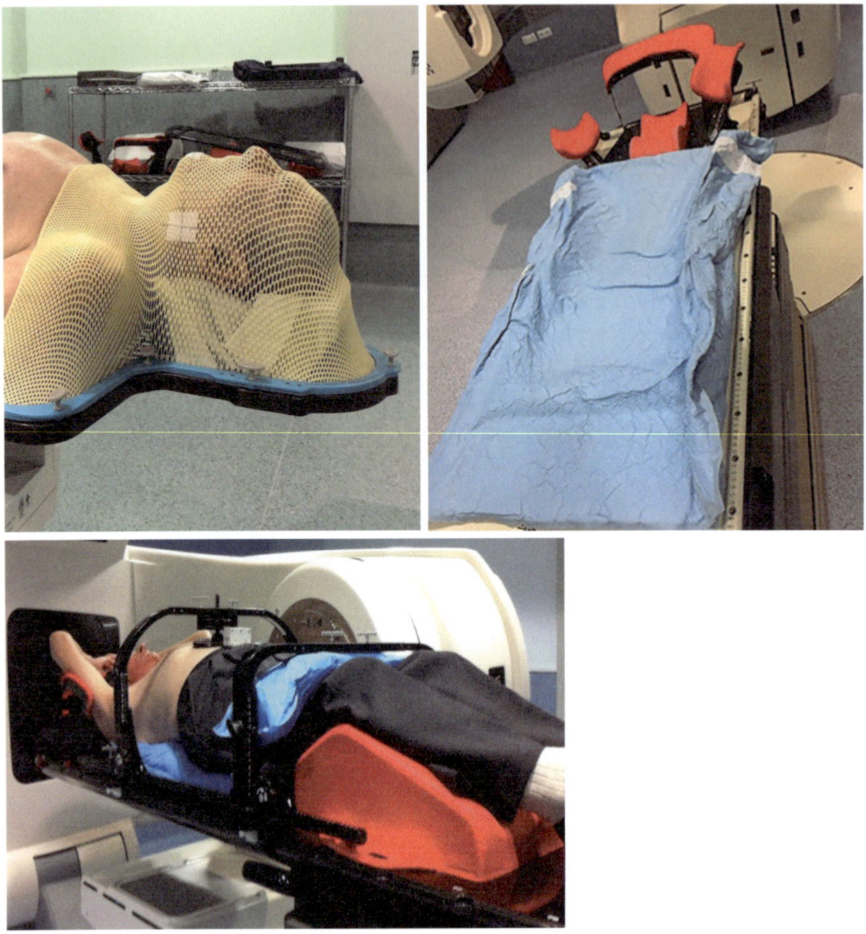

Fig. 5.1 The top left panel shows a thermoplastic mask used for head and neck treatments. The top right panel shows a head and arm support and a vacuum mattress. This mattress consists of a bag filled with little porexpan spheres, which is sucked vacuum when the patient is lying on it. Thus, the mattress turns rigid and keeps the patient's shape. The left bottom panel shows a patient lying on the treatment couch with several positioning and immobilization devices: a knees fixation, an abdominal compression plate, an arm and head support, and a vacuum mattress

Kevlar fibre. When heated this material in a water bath it can be deformed, but once cooled down it turns rigid. The deformation and cooling down processes are done with the mask covering the patient's head and neck, and fixed to the treatment table. The mask thus acquires the shape of the head and neck region and restricts movements inside it. Literature shows that movements within head and neck masks can be limited to 3 mm [3]. Masks are produced with small holes perforated in the material they are made of. The holes enable patients to breath.

There are more sophisticated systems to guarantee the reproducibility of patient positioning, such as those based on surface scanning (Catalyst, Align RT). These systems project structured light and by means of two cameras reconstruct the patient's actual surface, which is compared with the reference surface at the day of image acquisition. In these systems, the user predefines the tolerances that should apply to the positioning of the patient. The tighter the tolerance, the more accurate the positioning is, but the longer it takes.

Nevertheless, for prostate or gynaecological treatments, thermoplastic masks or surface scanning systems offer little improvement, as the position of the prostate or the uterus is weakly correlated with the patient surface. In these cases, providing the patient with some dietary and drinking instructions to guarantee a reproducible filling of rectum and bladder and placing a simple positioning device, such as a knee support increases reproducibility. The reason for this is that the main movement is not a movement of the patient but a movement of the prostate or uterus itself inside the patient. Due to variable bladder and rectum filling, the prostate and uterus change their position with respect to the pelvic bones. Their relative position can even change during the treatment in a short-time scale. There are techniques that allow interrupting the beam if the change in position exceeds certain thresholds and resuming the irradiation when the problem is solved. For prostate cancer, the optimal strategy is to implant some small radio-opaque markers, usually made of gold or of PEEK with a steel core, inside the prostate (3 or more; also see "Artificial Intelligence in Radiation Oncology: A Rapidly Evolving Picture"). Consequently, for daily positioning, the radio-opaque markers, as seen on daily radiological images acquired with the imaging systems of the linear accelerator, i.e., orthogonal X-ray imaging or cone beam-computed tomography (CBCT), are made to match their projected positions on the planning CT. Another possibility is to acquire a (CB)CT scan prior to the treatment fraction and to match the prostate position of that particular day with its position on the planning CT. There are other approaches that do not use radiological images, such as the Calypso® 4D localization system (today provided by Varian Medical Systems) [4]. The Calypso system uses some small radiofrequency transponders (cylinders of 8 mm long and 2 mm diameter) that are implanted in the prostate and thus act as antennas for a detector that tracks the prostate position.

There are other treatment sites where the motion control strategy can be more complicated, because the target position and shape is affected by respiratory motion. This is the case for tumours of the lung, breast, oesophagus, mediastinum, liver, or pancreas [5–7]. For these cases, some specific strategies have been developed and will be discussed in Sect. 5.5.

5.2.2 Image Acquisition

The choice of the positioning and immobilization device depends on the treatment site and on the required degree of accuracy. After immobilizing the patient, a coordinate system origin must be defined. This coordinate system will be common both for image acquisition and for treatment delivery. The origin of this coordinate system is indicated by alignment lasers. These lasers are attached to the walls of the CT scan rooms that are dedicated to treatment planning image acquisition and to the walls of the treatment units. After positioning the patient correctly on the imaging unit, the projections of the lasers are transferred onto the patient's skin using tattoos or long-lasting ink or marked on the thermoplastic mask. These tattoos/marks will also be used for patient repositioning every day on the treatment unit. For image acquisition, very small metallic markers (below 1 mm) are placed attached onto these marks or tattoos to make them visible on the CT images that are to be acquired. Image acquisition for treatment planning is then performed. If MRI is used for treatment planning, other markers are used because metallic markers are not visible on MRI. The acquired imaging information must not be restricted to the volume to be treated, since radiation fields often enter from distant regions. Furthermore, complete organ information is also required to evaluate possible toxicities of the treatment. As a result, when acquiring information for a lung tumour, for example, the entire thorax from the neck down to the abdomen has to be scanned; and the field of view has to be wide enough to include the complete patient contour.

5.2.3 Contouring, Margin Calculation and Dose Prescription

Once the planning CT has been acquired, the radiation oncologist will delineate the volume(s) to be treated. To do so, spatial or functional information from other image modalities may be needed. Therefore, all image modalities must have a common coordinate system in the TPS in order to match them with the planning CT that will be used for dose calculation. The process that leads all image modalities to be referred to the reference coordinate system of the CT scan used for treatment planning is called *registration*. Once images are registered, the radiation oncologist delineates the contour of the area with demonstrable malignancy (GTV) on each slice of the planning CT scan, aided by the other image modalities and the clinical information. Then, the CTV has to be created taking into account the GTV and all areas with risk of subclinical malignancy. To delineate the CTV international guidelines must be followed. These guidelines specify how to proceed for each treatment site, pathology and tumour stage.

As previously mentioned, the PTV is a geometrical concept that accounts for uncertainties (delineation and also positioning). These uncertainties have to be estimated and accounted for. The different kinds of uncertainty, that will be detailed later in this section, have different relevance in the mathematical formulae that provides the value of the margins that should be added to the CTV to define the PTV [8, 9]. The magnitude of the CTV to PTV margin also depends on the management of patient positioning by means of image guidance during the treatment. In the following paragraphs, some detail is given about these concepts.

Positioning uncertainties can occur systematically and randomly. Systematic uncertainties are due to differences between image acquisition for treatment planning and treatment execution. Consequently, these uncertainties impact on the entire course of treatment. They can stem from technical and mechanical differences in some systems, for example, a positioning laser misalignment. They can be rooted in some difference in the patient itself, for instance, weight loss between image acquisition for treatment planning and treatment delivery. But they can also stem from the patient's different psychological status at the time of acquiring the treatment planning CT and at treatment sessions. Patients tend to be more nervous during image acquisition for treatment planning than on routine daily treatment delivery, because image acquisition is one of the first contacts with the radiation oncology department. This translates in a different muscular tone and a slightly different geometry. Systematic uncertainties introduce a particular systematic error for each patient, which will be constant all through the treatment.

Random uncertainties, conversely, are unpredictable and change every single day. They are introduced by patient positioning, by patient movements or are due to physiological processes such as respiration, circulation, the degree of bladder filling, and the presence of gas pockets in the rectum or peristalsis. About daily patient setup, it must be considered that patients are not rigid solids. The process of alignment of skin tattoos or markers against positioning lasers cannot be therefore carried out with infinite accuracy. As a consequence, daily setup errors are always present.

Systematic uncertainties are the largest source of error and have also the largest impact on treatments [8, 9]. Without a procedure to correct for systematic errors margins from CTV to PTV should be increased. This would involve the irradiation of more healthy tissue or organs at risk. One of the approaches used to remove the systematic error is to monitor the patient position by imaging using the treatment unit x-ray or CBCT capacities before the fraction delivery during a number of fractions (usually from 3 to 5). The shifts that have to be applied to the patient for correct positioning during the first treatment sessions are recorded and are used as a statistical sample and their average is calculated. For subsequent treatment sessions the average shift is applied, and systematic errors are almost removed. After this correction, weekly monitoring can be followed to keep track of any anatomical changes produced during the treatment. With this approach, only random errors and residual systematic errors, which are of small magnitude, have to be included in the formula for margin calculation, leading to smaller margins. The values to be included in the formula for margin calculation in this case can be obtained from a series of patients for each treatment site. The evaluation of these margins has to be performed at each department as its value depends on the procedures for patient positioning.

Random errors can also be corrected, but only with daily imaging. This alternative reduces further the margins but translates into extra radiation dose to the patient due to imaging that may be non-negligible if x-ray-based equipment is used. At present time there are recommendations on this issue [10]. However, random errors are of less importance and have less impact on normo-fractionated treatments (i.e.

2 Gy per fraction) made up of many treatment fractions (i.e. typically 30–35 in curatively intended treatments). Depending on the accuracy requirements of a specific treatment, either only the systematic errors or both, systematic and random errors, are corrected for.

Beyond state-of-the-art, LINACs equipped with low- or high-field MRI do not have the problem of the additional absorbed dose to the patient due to imaging. MR-LINACs offer additional advantages over those LINACs equipped with X-ray-based imaging because of their exceptional soft-tissue contrast (see "Magnetic Resonance-guided Adaptive Radiotherapy: Technical Concepts"). These LINACs can therefore facilitate daily imaging, random error correction and consequent margin reduction without additional radiation dose to the patient.

In addition to 'target' volumes (GTV, CTV and PTV), the contours of all organs at risk (OARs) in the vicinity of the PTV have to be delineated on each CT slice. OAR contouring is commonly done by radiation therapists. Radiation oncologists supervise and approve these contours later. TPSs reconstruct all volumes (GTV, CTV, PTV and OARs) from contours delineated on individual CT slices.

Once completed the contouring process, the radiation oncologist prescribes the radiation treatment. Treatment prescription includes: treatment site, the values of total dose and dose per fraction that have to be delivered to each PTV, the total number of fractions, the fractions per day, and the dose-volume constraints for OARs that should be respected in order to prevent toxicity. These dose-volume constraints are commonly expressed as maximum doses to the OARs or the maximum percentage volumes of each OAR that can receive certain dose levels. Several dose-volume constraints are usually specified for each OAR.

5.2.4 Treatment Planning

Treatment planning is the process that follows contouring in the RT workflow. During treatment planning, the treatment technique and beam energies are selected, and the number of beams, field sizes and gantry, collimator and couch angles are determined, in order to adequately irradiate the PTV. Treatment planning is carried out by different professionals depending on the country. In some countries, medical physicists are responsible for designing the treatment plan. However, in other countries radiation technologists are in charge of making treatment plans and medical physicists supervise and approve them afterwards. The final responsibility of the treatment plan, though, lies with the radiation oncologist, that at the end of the process approves the whole treatment.

Treatment planning is an iterative process. At the end of each iteration, the user ends up by calculating the absorbed dose distribution in the patient and comparing the resulting dose-volume parameters with the pre-set dose-volume constraints. Then, the next iteration is started to further improve the treatment plan whenever possible. There are two approaches to carry out each iteration in treatment planning: *forward planning* and *inverse planning*. In the 'forward' approach the user 'guesses' what arrangement of beams and beam options and parameters would lead to good absorbed distribution and then choose these options. Then, the absorbed dose distribution and the dose-volume parameters are calculated. The 'inverse' approach goes the other way round. The planner chooses some values for the dose-volume parameters and the TPS through an automatic iterative process will find the optimal beam arrangements to achieve the dose-volume parameters proposed by the planner. Then, the absorbed dose distribution and the final dose-volume parameters are calculated. These concepts will be tackled with greater detail in the next sections, which deal with the various planning and delivery techniques.

5.2.5 Treatment Delivery

Once the treatment plan is approved by the radiation oncologist, the treatment is ready for delivery. The patient will be positioned in the treatment unit reproducing the position on the day where the planning CT was taken. Positioning and patient anatomy will be checked by in-room imaging. Adjustments in positioning will be made if necessary. Then, the treatment will be delivered according to the radiation beam arrangements as defined by the treatment plan.

A schema summarizing the patient workflow from the first consultation in the radiation therapy department to treatment delivery is shown in Fig. 5.2. This complex process involves different professionals (radiation oncologists, medical physicists, radiation technologists, nurses) that have to work as a team in order to deliver safe and up to quality standards radiotherapy.

5.3 Radiotherapy Techniques

Once the radiation oncologists have prescribed the treatment and defined the target volumes and organs at risk on the planning images, there are several available radiotherapy techniques. Choosing one or the other will depend on available equipment and personnel, on the demands for dose conformation to the PTV and the constraints to the OARs and on the delivery accuracy demands, amongst other factors. On this section, all these techniques will be described.

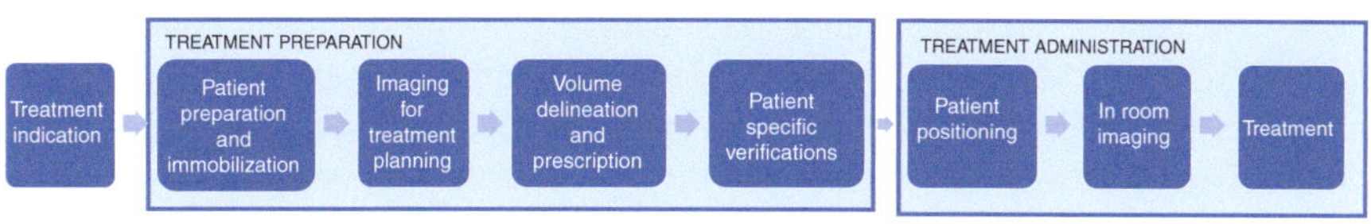

Fig. 5.2 Schematic overview of the various steps that make up the radiation therapy workflow. These steps can be categorized into two main groups: treatment preparation and treatment administration

5.3.1 Conventional Radiotherapy: Three-Dimensional Conformal RT

When a specific radiation dose value is prescribed to a PTV, the whole PTV is intended to receive a homogeneous absorbed dose. The dose at any point within the PTV should be equal to the prescribed dose plus or minus some tight tolerance values (−5% to +7% following ICRU recommendations [1, 2]). Keeping this in mind, medical linear accelerators (LINACs) have traditionally been designed, such that photon radiation beams that emerge from them are mostly of uniform fluence. This means that for a given photon beam it has the same number of photons per unit area all across the beam. When a PTV is irradiated by a uniform beam, and the beam axis is perpendicular to the body entrance surface, the absorbed dose distribution inside the PTV is flat in a plane parallel to the entrance surface. However, the absorbed dose decreases in depth because for each parallel plane the photons that interacted in a previous plane were removed from the beam. If an additional radiation beam coming from the opposite side of the PTV is added, the aforementioned absorbed dose decrease in depth can be somewhat compensated by the photons coming from the opposed field.

In general, an isotropous arrangement of several photon beams directed to the PTV with equal space between them leads to homogeneous irradiation of the PTV. In order to minimize the irradiation of healthy tissues within the body, each beam is shaped to fit the outline of the PTV from the point of view of the beam (*Beam's Eye View*, or BEV). This conformation is achieved by means of the multileaf collimator (MLC). Additionally, to avoid damage of healthy OARs close to the target, beam entries (beam portals) are chosen such that they do not traverse OARs. When this is not possible, the number of beams that crosses a given OAR and the intensities of those beams are adjusted so that the absorbed dose at that OAR is below the threshold that would cause toxicity (tolerance dose). This treatment strategy is known as *3D Conformal Radiotherapy* (3DCRT).

For 3DCRT only a further consideration has to be taken into account: there are three situations that could result in a non-homogeneous absorbed dose within the PTV. First, when the incidence of a radiation beam and the body surface are not perpendicular. Second, when there are heterogeneities within the body, such as bones or air cavities, which can attenuate a part of the beam more (or less) than the rest of it. Third, when the radiation beam arrangement that would lead to OAR doses below tolerance values has not equally spaced beams. In these cases, that are most common, to guarantee dose homogeneity within the target volume non-uniform radiation beams are required. For 3DCRT techniques, the traditional beam modifiers are *wedge filters*. Wedge filters are metal filters with the shape of a wedge that are placed between the LINAC and the patient. Due to the varying thickness of the wedges, these filters attenuate the beam more on one side (thick side of wedge) than on the opposite side (thin part of wedge), leading to a beam with a dose gradient in one direction but uniform in the perpendicular direction. The same effect can also be obtained by moving one of the LINAC collimators while a beam is on, which is called *dynamic wedge*. 3DCRT is a forward planning technique; and it was the technique of choice till two decades ago. 3DCRT is still used for some treatment indications, such as tangential fields for breast early stage cancer or for irradiation of symptomatic bone metastasis.

5.3.2 From Convex to Concave: The Need for Modulations

The result of 3DCRT is that the intersection of all radiation beams defines a convex volume that encompasses the PTV. Within this convex volume, a high and uniform dose is delivered. This poses a major problem: what happens when an OAR is partially surrounded by the target, and it is included within this convex volume? The answer is that this OAR will be irradiated up to a dose that in some cases could lead to severe or even fatal toxicity. To avoid excessive toxicity in an OAR, the radiation oncologist is sometimes forced to lower the prescribed dose to the PTV so that the constraints to the involved OARs are fulfilled, and thus below the dose that would most likely lead to tumour control and patient cure. To avoid such a situation, a technique resulting in concave dose distributions or, in general, in dose distributions of any shape is required. This necessity is the reason why intensity-modulated radiation therapy, IMRT, was developed. The urgent need of IMRT caused its very fast widespread in the beginning of this century. Figure 5.3 compares dose distributions planned by means of 3DCRT against those planned with IMRT or VMAT.

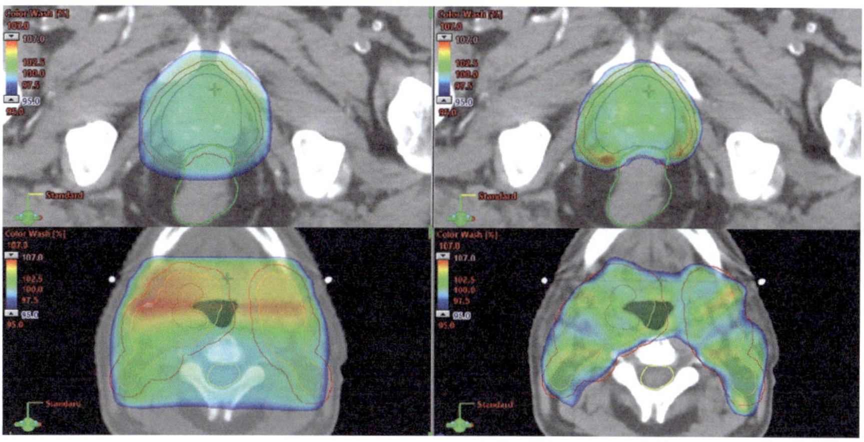

Fig. 5.3 Calculated dose distributions for a prostate treatment plan (upper panels) and for a head and neck treatment plan (lower panels). 3DCRT distributions are shown on the left panels and VMAT/IMRT dose distributions are shown on the right panels. The dose level of 95% of the prescribed dose is shown in colour overlying the CT scan image. The three concentric contours shown on each image correspond to GTV, CTV and PTV, going from the inner contour to the outer contour. The main organs at risk at the level of these CT slices are also shown as contours. For the prostate plan, the rectum is shown in green. For the head and neck plan, the spinal cord is shown in yellow. The right panels clearly show that the concavity generated in the dose distribution by IMRT spares better the rectum (upper panel) and the spinal cord (lower panel) than the corresponding 3DCRT distributions on the left panels

5.3.3 Modulated Techniques: IMRT and VMAT

The advent of computerized multileaf collimator (MLC) systems triggered the development of IMRT [11]. MLCs were initially designed to give shape to the radiation beam. They are composed of leaves that are made of high-density metal materials, such as tungsten. They are a few millimetres wide but several centimetres long, and thick in the direction of the photons that come from the LINAC source. As a result, they block out more than 99% of the photons that impinge on them. Each individual leaf is computer-controlled and, if the leaves move while the beam is irradiating, a beam with non-uniform fluence is produced. This technique is called *sliding windows*. Another way of generating non-uniform fluences for a treatment field consists of adding up several subfields with different MLC shapes, and delivering sequentially each subfield. This technique is named *step-and-shoot*. Potentially, one could deliver any arbitrary desired fluence by predefining how the leaves should move during the irradiation, for *sliding windows*, or with a sufficient number of subfields, for *step-and-shoot*. In reality, mechanical restrictions concerning the maximum possible leaf speed and acceleration limit the possibility of delivering any arbitrary fluence for the *sliding windows* technique, and the number of subfields cannot be infinite for the *step-and-shoot* technique. As a result, fluences that would be optimal for a specific case can differ from those that can actually be accurately delivered. Furthermore, dose calculation accuracy can be jeopardized for very complex deliveries. These limitations make a quality control program for individual patient treatment plans necessary. Patient-specific pre-treatment verifications test whether dose distributions that were calculated can be delivered within some maximum tolerance deviations detailed in various international guidelines [12].

In IMRT, several photon beams are planned with fixed LINAC gantry angles, e.g. 7 gantry angles in head and neck tumours. For each gantry angle, the fluence of the beam is modulated. Literature shows that more than nine modulated beams offer little improvement in the final dose distribution [13]. Modulation can be performed in a forward manner (*forward planning*). In this strategy, one has to 'guess' how fluences should be in order to get the desired final dose distribution. Conventional forward planning mostly depends on geometric relationship between the tumour and nearby sensitive structures. Usually, institutions using this approach create what are called 'class solutions', which can, with minor changes, be applied for typical treatment sites and typical PTV shapes [11]. However, at present time most IMRT treatments are designed in an inverse manner (*inverse planning*). In this strategy, the input for the software are the absorbed doses that should be delivered to PTVs, and the OAR dose-volume constraints to avoid toxicities. In most inverse planning IMRT optimizing software, PTV doses and OAR dose-volume constraints can be prioritized relatively to one another to guide the software towards the desired dose distribution. When the optimization process is completed, the final dose distribution is calculated. As explained in Sect. 5.2.4, then, the user must compare the resulting dose-volume parameters with the dose-volume constraints for the OARs, and the compliance of the dose calculated for the PTV with the homogeneity requirements of the ICRU criteria. In case of failure, the values that served as input for the optimizer have to be changed, and the process is restarted. Thus, the optimal final dose distribution is achieved by an iterative process.

In VMAT, the irradiation of the PTV is carried out during the movement of the LINAC gantry following an arc. This arc can be one or more complete rotation(s) (360°) or a partial arc, to minimize the irradiation of particular OARs or to avoid a collision of the gantry with the treatment couch, the patient or the immobilization devices. In this technique, the MLC leaves are continuously moving during the gantry rotation (with varying speed) defining a different pattern at each gantry angle. However, there is no movement of the leaves at each specific gantry position. Therefore, strictly speaking, in VMAT there is no real modulation of the beam. Since the treatment is delivered with such a large number of beams (up to 178), though, this compensates for the lack of modulation at each individual angle. There is a continuity restriction on the shape that the MLC can define between two contiguous gantry angles: if the MLC leaves define a given shape at one gantry angle and they had to define an arbitrary and very different shape at the following gantry angle, the required leaf speed and acceleration could exceed the maximum possible leaf speed and the acceleration limit of the leaves. As these limits are real physical limits, there is a restriction on the maximum change of the leaves between two contiguous gantry angles. This restriction is similar to that posed in IMRT by the maximum speed by which the leaves can travel. As opposed to IMRT, VMAT treatment planning is always performed in an inverse manner, and the inverse planning optimization procedure is the same. As a matter of fact, most software uses a single user interface for both techniques at present time.

The main advantage of VMAT over IMRT is efficiency. The results of dose distributions for both techniques are comparable, although treatment delivery is faster with VMAT than with IMRT. The reduction in delivery times is the key factor that sparked the very fast change from IMRT to VMAT in most departments all over the world. Some studies showed improvement in VMAT dose distributions compared to those obtained for IMRT for various treatment sites [14–21]. There are even theoretical studies that showed that VMAT might be superior to IMRT [22, 23]. However, one factor that most influences the quality of a treatment plan is the expertise of the planner [24, 25]. The question of whether the dose distribution can be further improved once the PTV goals and the OAR dose constraints are met has a simple answer: again it depends on the expertise of the individual that is performing the treatment plan calculation, and on the workload of the department. To eliminate these dependences, automatic solutions with minimum human interaction are today being developed, and starting to be commercialized and routinely used.

Dose distributions resulting from modulated techniques (IMRT and VMAT) show two main differences compared to those resulting from 3DCRT. First, the prescribed dose level more conformally encompasses the PTV shape (increased conformality). Second, low dose levels are more spread out all around the patient body for IMRT and VMAT than for 3DCRT. This last effect is sometimes called the 'dose-bath'. Since mainly high doses are expected to be related to toxicity, modulated techniques are believed to decrease toxicity compared to 3DCRT. However, low dose-baths are related to an increased probability of radiation-induced secondary malignancies [26, 27]. Consequently, they should be avoided in children and in patients with a long life expectancy, e.g. early breast cancer in young patients, because they are more radio-sensitive and have a longer life expectancy. Therefore, an individualized analysis of the technique of choice is required before the treatment planning process is initiated.

In current clinical radiotherapy practice, different doses are prescribed at different volumes that have to be irradiated depending on the tumour cells' radiosensitivity and/or the probability of tumour spread in those volumes. To achieve this goal in 3DCRT, a sequential approach has been traditionally followed. First, a treatment plan was prepared to irradiate all volumes during some days until the lowest prescribed dose was delivered to all volumes. Then, a second treatment plan ('boost') was prepared to irradiate a smaller volume corresponding to the following prescribed dose level. And so on. This strategy poses the problem that during irradiation of each boost dose level we are re-irradiating volumes that had already been irradiated. Therefore, low and medium doses increase in some regions. In modulated techniques, however, fluence modulation enables the delivery of different absorbed doses at different volumes during the delivery of a single treatment plan. Consequently, in a given number of fractions, we can deliver simultaneously a different total dose to different volumes. In short, IMRT and VMAT allow delivering what are called 'simultaneous integrated boosts' (SIB) with optimal dose distributions in tumour surrounding tissues. Figure 5.4 shows an example of SIB in a head and neck treatment.

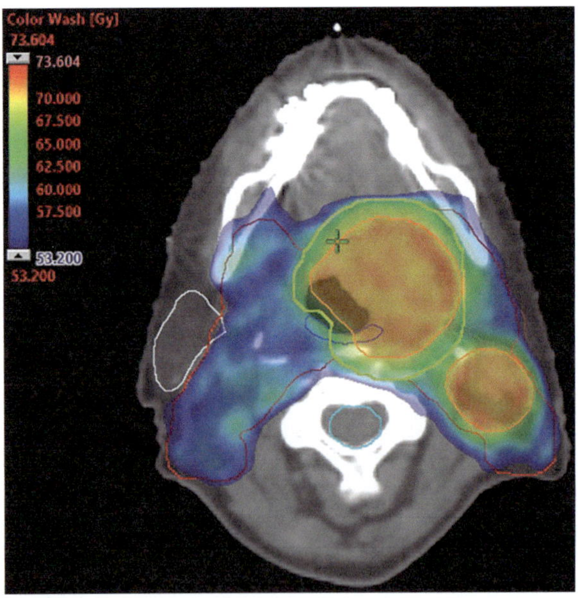

Fig. 5.4 Example of SIB in a head and neck treatment planned with VMAT. Various PTVs are irradiated simultaneously. A low-risk PTV shown in red contour was prescribed 56 Gy, a medium-risk PTV shown in pink contour was prescribed 63 Gy and two high-risk PTVs shown with orange contour were prescribed 70 Gy. Isodose levels are overlaid in colour wash. The bluish colour corresponds to 95% of the prescription dose of the low-risk PTV. The greenish colour corresponds to 95% of the medium-risk PTV, and the orange colour corresponds to the prescription dose of the high-risk PTV. The right parotid gland and the spinal canal are shown in white and cyan contours, respectively

As previously mentioned, high dose levels for IMRT and VMAT techniques fit PTVs very tightly while sparing OARs. This sparing enables dose escalation in the PTV with acceptable toxicity rates. And dose escalation means higher tumour control for some pathologies. As a result, modulated techniques could potentially achieve higher tumour control rates. Moreover, they also enable focal therapy for some treatments (still in experimental set at present time) [28]. As an example, in radiotherapy for prostate, the target is usually the whole prostate. By means of MRI or PET, the dominant intraprostatic lesion can be determined and by using modulated techniques, the dose to this focus can be increased up to four times compared to the whole prostate prescription dose, while keeping the dose at OAR the same. This strategy could potentially open the therapeutic window of radiotherapy.

5.3.3.1 The Need for Image Guidance and Motion Control in Modulated Techniques

For IMRT and VMAT, the tight conformation of the line of prescription dose to the shape of the PTV poses a challenge compared to 3DCRT: geometrical inaccuracies due to patient mal-positioning, organ motion during irradiation, and mechanical machine inaccuracies may lead to geographical target misses. Inaccuracies must therefore be minimized, controlled and accounted for, or even be removed. In addition, if we want to take maximum advantage of the conformation possibilities of modulated techniques, we should reduce CTV to PTV margins. For example, in the treatment of a head and neck tumour close to the parotid glands, large margins would make it impossible to sufficiently reduce the radiation dose in these glands to prevent xerostomia from occurring. Usually, a margin of 5–10 mm is used, depending on the anatomical region and immobilization tools in place [3]. To safely reduce safety margins, patient anatomy and positioning has to be guaranteed with a high level of reproducibility, and a strict procedure has to be followed using image guidance.

5.3.4 Stereotactic Ablative Body Radiotherapy

Delivery of conventional radiotherapy, regardless of technique, e.g. 3DCRT, IMRT or VMAT, is performed following fractionated schedules. This means that the fraction dose to the tumour is restricted to 1.8–2.0 Gy and that treatment is delivered 5 days per week. Normal cells can usually repair the damage caused by radiation better than tumour cells. Fractionated radiotherapy, therefore, allows normal tissues to recover between fractions to a greater extent than tumour cells. Fractionation thus enhances the therapeutic window for radiation therapy. However, if radiation therapy is focused only to the tumour and the PTV does not contain any significant volume of healthy tissues, fractionated radiotherapy could be of limited interest.

It is within this frame that stereotactic ablative body radiotherapy (SABR) was developed. SABR is also named 'stereotactic body radiation therapy' (SBRT) in literature. The goal of this technique is to ablate the tumour by delivering a single or a few fraction(s) of high-dose radiotherapy. Usually, the number of scheduled fractions is less than five, although some schemes allow up to eight fractions when there is risk of severe toxicity for specific OARs. Even if the prescribed dose per fraction is much higher than that of standard radiation treatments, the total prescribed dose may be approximately the same value or even lower since the treatment consists of fewer fractions. Having said that, since the physical radiation dose per fraction is between 5 and 24 Gy and therefore we don't let the cells to repair sublethal damage, the biological total dose achieved with SABR is by far higher than with conventional RT. Examples of SABR schedules for early stage lung cancer include: a single fraction of 30 Gy, 3 fractions of 15–20 Gy per fraction, 5 fractions of 10–12 Gy, or 8 fractions of 7.5 Gy per fraction [29–35]. In fact, several clinical studies on SABR for lung tumours reported on excellent local control rates of approximately 85–95% [30, 36, 37], which is much larger than the 55% 2-year disease-free survival obtained with conventional schemes [38]. Local control of lung SABR is therefore similar to that achieved by surgery, whereas the toxicity of SABR is much lower [29, 39]. Unfortunately, randomised clinical studies comparing SABR to surgery in early-stage non-small cell lung cancer have repeatedly failed due to slow and insufficient patient accrual [40].

At present time, lung SABR treatments are indicated in clinical guidelines for early-stage non-small cell lung cancer for unfit patients or those that refuse surgery, and for patients with oligometastatic disease that have a contra-indication for surgery.

As pointed out in the introduction, in SABR the dose falloff around the PTV must be very steep. The reason for this is that the absorbed dose outside the PTV ought to be low in order to not lead to ablative effect outside the target volume. Dosimetric criteria are somewhat different for SABR compared to 3DCRT. The treatment is aimed at delivering a dose equal to or greater than the prescribed dose to any point of the PTV, or at least to 95% of the points of the PTV volume [29], and with maximum dose gradient outside. For SABR, dose homogeneity inside the PTV is not the priority. The ICRU recommendation that the dose values in the PTV should be confined between 95% and 107% of the prescribed dose mentioned in Sect. 5.3.1 is not in use for SABR, since some clinicians prefer a high dose in the middle of the target and most clinical experience was obtained with this kind of inhomogeneous dose distributions [41].

SABR treatments can be planned using 3DCRT, IMRT or VMAT techniques. Dose distributions are quite similar for all techniques, although they tend to be more homogeneous inside the PTV for IMRT and VMAT than for 3DCRT. As for other radiation treatment planning, in case of close contact between a tumour and an OAR, a modulated technique (IMRT or VMAT) may be required to spare the OAR. In order to achieve maximum dose gradient around the PTV, ideally non-coplanar fields or arcs have to be planned. However, the risk of collision of the LINAC gantry with the treatment couch sometimes limits possible beam incidences. It is important to mention here that ring-based linacs, such as tomotherapy or MRI-linacs, can only deliver co-planar beams.

When treating lung lesions, PTVs are heterogeneous because they include not only the lesion but also a volume of lung tissue, both consisting of different tissue densities. As a consequence of this heterogeneity, the maximum dose gradients for lung SABR treatments with 3DCRT are achieved close to isodose values of 60–80% of the dose maximum. Consequently, prescribing the dose to the isodose that covers the PTV, i.e. 60–80% leads to maximum doses inside the PTV of approximately 120–140% of the prescription dose. The use of IMRT and VMAT, as mentioned before, increases dose homogeneity inside the PTV with maximum values rarely exceeding 120% of the prescribed dose. For these techniques, it is important to include objectives in the inverse optimization process that lead to dose gradients outside the tumour as steep as possible. A prerequisite to achieve steep dose falloffs, regardless of the planning technique, is that the PTV is smaller than 5 cm in the maximum dimension. Dose distributions that result from irradiating larger volumes, i.e. 5 cm, usually do not meet the requirements of dose falloff for SABR treatments.

SABR treatments are not only performed for lung metastases. Metastases in lymph nodes, liver, brain, pancreas, adrenal glands and bones can be treated with a similar approach. There is a main difference for these other sites compared to lung: the tissue densities are more homogeneous, resulting in dose distributions to be more homogeneous and in maximum radiation doses of approximately 110%. Obviously, also the fractionation schemes differ for each treated site. Typical SABR treatment plans for lung and brain metastases are shown in Figs. 5.5 and 5.6.

It must be kept in mind that breathing motion affects most sites where SBRT treatments are delivered (lung, liver, pancreas and other abdominal sites). In a scenario of margin reduction and ablative treatments, breathing monitoring, motion management and on-line daily imaging are required.

When the respiratory movement has to be taken into account, the most common image guidance workflow for SABR treatments is based on CBCT and fluoroscopy. CBCT is acquired with equipment mounted on the linear accelerator head and resembles a slow CT scan that integrates several breathing cycles. Tumours with large movement show a smoothed periphery on the CBCT. On the one hand, CBCT gives a true time-averaged image of the tumour position and is therefore suitable for overall image matching of moving tumours. On the other hand, fluoroscopy gives a time-resolved high-resolution image of the tumour during its trajectory for given projections. Fluoroscopy therefore allows assessing the tumour position at a particular point of the breathing cycle on a daily basis. When fluoroscopy is combined with a gating system, tumour motion can be monitored and irradiation is only allowed when the tumour is inside the PTV. The most recent linear accelerators allow acquiring 4D CBCT studies. These can therefore substitute fluoroscopy or allow for other strategies, such as image registration and gating based on a specific breathing phase.

In cases, in which the tumour is not visible in X-ray images, such as pancreas or liver, some kind of surrogate for tumour position and tumour movement is required. Implanted markers close to the tumour are commonly used for image guidance for the pancreas and for the liver. These are dealt with in "Artificial Intelligence in Radiation Oncology: A Rapidly Evolving Picture".

When dealing with breathing motion management it is important that the overall treatment time be reasonably short. Treatments performed in times longer than about 30 min result in significant intra-fraction patient motion and larger

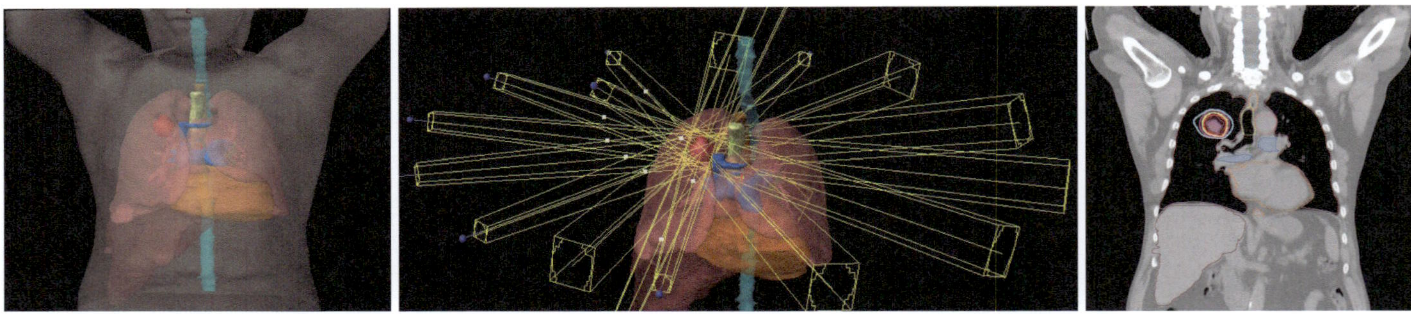

Fig. 5.5 SABR treatment of a lung metastasis performed with 3DCRT. Non-coplanar fields were used. The left panel shows the internal geometry of the patient. Lungs are shown in pink, the heart in orange, the liver in brown, the great vessels in dark blue, the aorta in pink, the spinal cord in cyan and the trachea in yellow. The PTV, which was derived from a CT scan corrected for breathing motion, i.e. 4D, is highlighted in red. The central panel shows the beam arrangement. The beam arrangement is non-coplanar, i.e. all beams are not included in a single plane perpendicular to the cranial-caudal axis of the patient, which would be the result of just turning the gantry angle from beam to beam. If radiation beams were co-planar all entrance and exit of radiation beams would be irradiating a specific 'slice' of the patient. That would increase the dose to healthy tissues on this 'slice'. Non-coplanar beams spread out low doses to other 'slices' but lead to steeper dose decrease with distance close to the tumour. Non-coplanar beams are achieved by means of couch rotation together with gantry rotation. The right panel shows a coronal reconstruction of the CT exam with the 50% (blue), 70% (magenta), 90% (yellow) and 100% (red) isodose lines. Percentages refer to the prescription dose

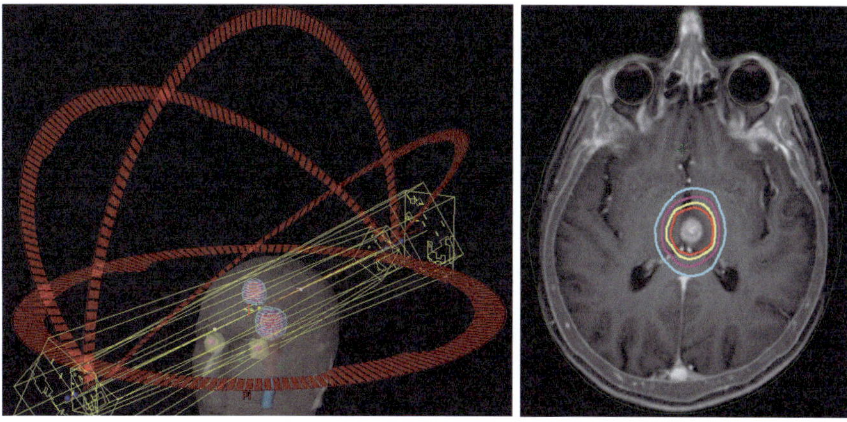

Fig. 5.6 SABR treatment of two brain metastases planned and calculated using VMAT. The left panel shows the internal geometry of the patient. The eyes are shown in yellow, the lenses in pink, the brainstem in brown and the spinal cord in cyan. PTVs are highlighted in red. The trajectories of the four planned arcs are shown in red around the patient's head. One complete arc and three partial arcs with treatment couch rotation (non-coplanar arcs) were planned. The right panel shows an axial slice of the MR scan with 50% (blue), 70% (magenta), 90% (yellow) and 100% (red) isodose lines. Percentages refer to the prescription dose. The same isodose lines are shown in the left panel as contours around both metastases

positioning uncertainties [42]. The time to be minimized includes setup, immobilization, image guidance, beam-on time and intra-fraction downtime. The staff must therefore be well-trained to perform all actions effectively and efficiently to reduce all these times. Nonetheless, there is also a technical development that helps to significantly reduce the beam-on time for SABR treatments. Modern LINACs can be purchased with beams where the so-called "flattening filter" is not used. The flattening filter is a metal filter with conical shape that is traditionally placed inside the LINAC head behind the target. Electron beams accelerated by the LINAC that impinge on the target produce photon beams that are more intense on the beam axis than at the periphery. The flattening filter is then used to obtain photon beams with a flat fluence. However, the photons that are removed by the flattening filter decrease the photon beam fluence around the central axis. If the flattening filter is removed, the dose rate of the LINAC is therefore increased. An increase in dose rate leads to a decrease in beam-on time for a given dose. For modulated beams, primary beams (before the MLC) with flat fluence are not required because the movement of the MLC leaves creates the final modulated photon fluence. Consequently, removal of the flattening filter is possible for IMRT and VMAT treatments [43]. For SABR treatments, where large doses per fraction are delivered, flattening filter-free (FFF) beams are recommended as they reduce beam on times and inhomogeneity is not an issue for such small beams.

For SABR treatments of the brain or bone metastases intra-fraction motion management is not an issue and set up uncertainties can be minimized by specific immobilization masks that offer a higher degree of fixation than ordinary immobilization masks. Patient positioning is guided only by means of CBCT. Immediately after assessing the position of the patient and properly correcting it, if needed, the treatment is delivered.

5.4 Considerations on Dose Calculations for IMRT, VMAT and SABR Treatment Planning

Treatment plans for IMRT and VMAT may result in MLC patterns where most of the beam is blocked by the MLC and only a small part of it is of use for the irradiation of the PTV. The result is that the tumour is irradiated by small *beamlets*. Small radiation fields are also used for SABR, that is meant for treatment of small tumours.

Dose calculation uncertainty can be large for all those small radiation beams for many dose calculation algorithms. This large uncertainty has two main sources.

The first source is the beam model configured in those software used to calculate absorbed dose distributions. The beam model is initially configured with measurements made on the treatment beams after installation of the treatment unit and before starting to treat patients. Standard detectors might be too large to correctly describe small fields. And some detectors are even too large to characterize any radiation fields with enough spatial resolution. As a result, dose calculations for small fields might be inaccurate [44–46]. For small dynamic beams, it is also important to have an accurate multileaf collimator (MLC) model that should be configured by means of dedicated equipment and specific dosimetry codes of practice.

The second source is inherent dose calculation algorithms themselves. There are algorithms that rely on charge-particle equilibrium inside radiation fields, but for very small fields there is no charge-particle equilibrium anywhere within the beam. This issue gains special relevance for low-density media, such as the lung, because secondary electrons travel further and they are produced in less quantity in low-density media compared to other human tissues. Some calculation algorithms perform better than others under these circumstances. For dose calculation of lung SABR treatments, the most advanced calculation algorithms should be used [21]. These algorithms are based on the Monte Carlo method or on the Boltzmann transport equation. The minimum requirement for an algorithm to be used on lung SABR calculations is that it takes into account lateral electron transport. The collapsed cone algorithm, and the anisotropic analytical algorithm (AAA) to a lesser extent, fit into this category. However, simpler algorithms such as pencil beam are unable to calculate reliable dose distributions for small lung tumours and should not be used for lung SABR treatment planning [21]. Indeed, there are even clinical studies that showed that local control for SABR depended on the dose calculation algorithm that was used [47].

Not only because of the dose calculation, but also due to the complexity of the delivery itself for IMRT, VMAT and SBRT, it is common practice to verify every treatment before starting the treatment. Pre-treatment verifications are usually performed by means of 2D detectors that can be flat or with a cylindrical surface. 2D dose measurements can be analysed in two ways. First, dose distributions measured with 2D detectors can be compared against expected 2D dose distributions that result from the treatment plan at the level of the detectors. Second, 3D dose distributions reconstructed from 2D measurements by means of specific software can be compared against the treatment plan 3D dose distribution [48].

5.5 Dealing with Organ Motion in Radiotherapy

It is commonly accepted that organ movement should be accounted for and managed when its range is larger than 5 mm [7].

Depending on the timescale there are two types of organ movements in radiotherapy: interfraction and intrafraction [5]. Interfraction movements are due to different positions of the organs at different treatment sessions. Good positioning and immobilization with clear instructions and pictures obtained during image acquisition for treatment planning is the first step to manage interfraction movement. To further minimize interfraction organ position for some treatment sites, it is convenient to provide the patient with preparation guidelines on diet and drinking as mentioned in the previous section so as the internal geometry be reproducible along the treatment. Intrafraction movements are those happening during a treatment session. They can be transitory or periodical. Transitory movements are mostly unpredictable. An example of transitory movement is prostate movement due to the transit of a gas pocket through the rectum. Another example could be rectum or bladder filling. Periodical movements have two origins: respiration and heart beating. Respiration has larger range and impact than cardiac movements and is usually accounted for. Cardiac movement is commonly neglected.

There are five main systems to monitor breathing motion [49]. The first is to monitor the flow of air that is inhaled and exhaled by the patient by means of a spirometer. The second is to monitor the pressure of the abdomen of the patient against a belt. The third is to monitor the position of the thorax or the abdomen with the aid of a marker block that is detected by a camera mounted on the wall, the ceiling or the treatment table. Some studies show the degree of correlation between internal organ movement and the external marker block movement [50, 51]. The fourth is based on the detection of the position of the patient surface itself by means of a surface scanner system mounted on the ceiling. The fifth is to detect some metallic markers implanted inside the tumour with fluoroscopy. This last method supposes extra radiation dose to the patient. To minimize this dose a hybrid system has also been developed. This system uses x-ray images and external reflectors placed on the patient's surface. At the beginning of the procedure, a correlation model is built between the internal markers' movement and the external reflectors' movement. This model is checked at regular intervals with x-rays, but most of the time the motion is monitored with the skin reflectors.

There are several strategies to account for organ movement due to respiration in radiotherapy [7]. The less demanding strategy is just to take the movement into account being the patient's respiration in free breathing. Modern multi-slice CTs allows acquiring data for each point of the patient during a whole breathing cycle.

Afterwards, they reconstruct data at predefined phases of the breathing cycle, for instance, at maximum inspiration, maximum expiration and some phases in between. It is common practice to reconstruct a total of 6–10 respiratory phases. As a result, the user has several 3D CT studies that change with time. The result is called a '4DCT' study, and they can even be visualized as a 3D study in motion. One can delineate the tumour on each phase CT study and create the envelope of the tumour for all phases. The resulting structure is called the internal target volume (ITV). If the PTV is created from the ITV, and we irradiate the whole PTV, we will be irradiating the tumour all along its trajectory. This is a simple strategy but it has a main drawback: the PTV may include a large amount of healthy tissue. A prerequisite for this strategy is that the breathing is stable. Otherwise, the tumour might lay outside the ITV on respiratory cycles that differ from that when we acquired images. Breathing monitoring should therefore also be performed during treatment to guarantee that the motion during treatment delivery be consistent with that recorded during image acquisition.

The second strategy is to limit the movement and to create an ITV with a reduced movement range. Abdominal compression by means of a compression plate or a compression belt has shown a reduction in organ motion below 7 and 8 mm [7, 52]. 4DCT is also used for image acquisition. This strategy can be applied to all patients and is well tolerated. However, the tolerable level of compression and therefore the level of movement reduction depend on the patient.

The third strategy, named 'gating', is the synchronization of radiation delivery with organ motion. Treatment is only delivered when the respiration is around at specific phase of the breathing cycle (phase gating) or around a specific position (amplitude gating). The two points of choice for gated treatments are those that are inflexion points of the movement, because the tumour position is almost steady: maximum inspiration and maximum expiration. Maximum expiration is the most stable phase because lungs are emptied very similarly every breathing cycle. The amount of air that is taken at maximum inspiration changes significantly between different respiratory cycles. It is therefore preferred maximum expiration for some abdominal treatments with gating because of the increased stability [53]. However, maximum inspiration offers an important advantage for some treatment sites such as the breast: the distance between the breast and the heart is increased. As a result the dose to the heart decreases. To carry out gating techniques successfully, respiration has to be stable and periodical. It is therefore required respiration monitoring and a training session for the patient. For this session audio and visual coaching is recommended [54, 55]. Audio coaching is performed with some instructions that tell the patient when to breathe in and when to breathe out. This way, the frequency of respiration is regularized [56]. Visual coaching is done with the aid of a screen or video goggles that show the patient a region that has not to be exceeded when inspiring. It regularizes therefore the amplitude of the breathing [56]. Ideally, simultaneous audio and video coaching would make respiration an almost sinusoidal pattern. However, not all patients are able to follow both instructions simultaneously [55]. Gating is the most demanding strategy for motion management. And it has three main drawbacks. First, not all patients can comply. Second, it requires special equipment and human resources. Third, and most importantly, it increases significantly treatment times. In a gating technique that irradiates only in a tenth of the respiratory cycle, the delivery time is ten-fold the time in a non-gated technique. And this would be with an ideal respiration perfectly periodic. Real respirations have irregularities that further increase treatment times. Any increase in treatment times is related to patient involuntary movements that degrade the delivered treatment quality. As a result, gating treatments that irradiate during 30% of the breathing cycle are most common [57], and they may incorporate some residual movement.

The problems described above have made a move towards a fourth strategy, named deep inspiration breath-hold (DIBH). DIBH is simpler and a more efficient technique than gating. Patients are trained to breathe deeply and hold their breath during some 20 s when they are told to do so. During this time, images for treatment planning are acquired. Later, during the treatment, they must repeat the procedure for any positioning imaging and also during the delivery of the treatment. DIBH almost stops any movement. It therefore minimizes motion management issues. However, to carry out optimally and efficiently a DIBH strategy, the requirements about patient training and monitoring, and about coaching equipment are similar to those mentioned for gating techniques. The treatment is usually planned with the highest available dose rate and the number of beams is adjusted so that each beam can be delivered on less than 20 s. This allows the delivery of the beam in a single breath-hold. Additionally, all the gating instrumentation is adjusted as a backup system. It automatically stops the treatment if the patient cannot hold the breath all the time required to deliver a beam or an arc in a VMAT treatment. As a result, not being able to hold the breath all the required time does not translate into wrong delivery, because the treatment is stopped and subsequently resumed when the patient comes back to the predefined breath-hold level. Unlike for gating techniques, most patients can comply with DIBH, and treatment times are not significantly larger than for non-motion-managed treatments. Consequently, it is becoming the preferred strategy for motion management in today's radiotherapy.

References

1. International Commission of Radiation Units and Measurements. ICRU Report 50. Prescribing, recording, and reporting photon beam therapy. Journal of the ICRU. Bethesda, Maryland 20814; 1994.
2. International Commission on Radiation Units and Measurements. ICRU Report 62. Prescribing, Recording and Reporting Photon Beam Therapy (Supplement to ICRU Report 50). Bethesda, Maryland 20814; 1999. 1–52 p.
3. Chen AM, Farwell DG, Luu Q, Donald PJ, Perks J, Purdy JA. Evaluation of the planning target volume in the treatment of head and neck cancer with intensity-modulated radiotherapy: what is the appropriate expansion margin in the setting of daily image guidance? Int J Radiat Oncol Biol Phys. 2011;81(4):943–9.
4. Silva C, Mateus D, Eiras M, Vieira S. Calypso® 4D localization system: a review. J Radiother Pract. 2013;13(4):473–83.
5. Langen KM, Jones DTL. Organ motion and its management. Int J Radiat Oncol Biol Phys. 2001;50(1):265–78.

6. George R, Keall PJ, Kini VR, Vedam SS, Siebers JV, Wu Q, et al. Quantifying the effect of intrafraction motion during breast IMRT planning and dose delivery. Med Phys. 2003;30(4):552–62.
7. Keall PJ, Mageras GS, Balter JM, Emery RS, Forster KM, Jiang SB, et al. The management of respiratory motion in radiation oncology report of AAPM task group 76. Med Phys. 2006;33(10):3874–900.
8. Van Herk M, Remeijer P, Rasch C, Lebesque JV. The probability of correct target dosage: dose-population histograms for deriving treatment margins in radiotherapy. Int J Radiat Oncol Biol Phys. 2000;47(4):1121–35.
9. Stroom JC, Heijmen BJM. Geometrical uncertainties, radiotherapy planning margins, and the ICRU-62 report. Radiother Oncol. 2002;64(1):75–83.
10. Ding GX, Alaei P, Curran B, Flynn R, Gossman M, Mackie TR, et al. Image guidance doses delivered during radiotherapy: quantification, management, and reduction: report of the AAPM therapy physics committee task group 180. Med Phys. 2018;45(5):e84–99.
11. Webb S. Intensity-modulated radiation therapy. Bristol: Institute of Physics Publication; 2001. 435p.
12. Ezzell GA, Burmeister JW, Dogan N, Losasso TJ, Mechalakos JG, Mihailidis D, et al. IMRT commissioning: multiple institution planning and dosimetry comparisons, a report from AAPM task group 119. Med Phys. 2009;36(11):5359–73.
13. Pirzkall A, Carol MP, Pickett B, Xia P, Roach M, Verhey LJ. The effect of beam energy and number of fields on photon-based IMRT for deep-seated targets. Int J Radiat Oncol Biol Phys. 2002;53(2):434–42.
14. Cozzi L, Dinshaw KA, Shrivastava SK, Mahantshetty U, Engineer R, Deshpande DD, et al. A treatment planning study comparing volumetric arc modulation with RapidArc and fixed field IMRT for cervix uteri radiotherapy. Radiother Oncol [Internet]. 2008;89(2):180–91. https://doi.org/10.1016/j.radonc.2008.06.013.
15. Fogliata A, Clivio A, Nicolini G, Vanetti E, Cozzi L. Intensity modulation with photons for benign intracranial tumours: a planning comparison of volumetric single arc, helical arc and fixed gantry techniques. Radiother Oncol [Internet]. 2008;89(3):254–62. https://doi.org/10.1016/j.radonc.2008.07.021.
16. Palma D, Vollans E, James K, Nakano S, Moiseenko V, Shaffer R, et al. Volumetric modulated arc therapy for delivery of prostate radiotherapy: comparison with intensity-modulated radiotherapy and three-dimensional conformal radiotherapy. Int J Radiat Oncol Biol Phys. 2008;72(4):996–1001.
17. Kjær-Kristoffersen F, Ohlhues L, Medin J, Korreman S. RapidArc volumetric modulated therapy planning for prostate cancer patients. Acta Oncol. 2009;48(2):227–32.
18. Vanetti E, Clivio A, Nicolini G, Fogliata A, Ghosh-Laskar S, Agarwal JP, et al. Volumetric modulated arc radiotherapy for carcinomas of the oro-pharynx, hypo-pharynx and larynx: a treatment planning comparison with fixed field IMRT. Radiother Oncol [Internet]. 2009;92(1):111–7. https://doi.org/10.1016/j.radonc.2008.12.008.
19. Verbakel WFAR, Cuijpers JP, Hoffmans D, Bieker M, Slotman BJ, Senan S. Volumetric intensity-modulated arc therapy vs. conventional IMRT in head-and-neck cancer: a comparative planning and dosimetric study. Int J Radiat Oncol Biol Phys. 2009;74(1):252–9.
20. Clivio A, Fogliata A, Franzetti-Pellanda A, Nicolini G, Vanetti E, Wyttenbach R, et al. Volumetric-modulated arc radiotherapy for carcinomas of the anal canal: a treatment planning comparison with fixed field IMRT. Radiother Oncol [Internet]. 2009;92(1):118–24. https://doi.org/10.1016/j.radonc.2008.12.020.
21. Fogliata A, Cozzi L. Dose calculation algorithm accuracy for small fields in non-homogeneous media: the lung SBRT case. Phys Medica [Internet]. 2017;44:157–62. https://doi.org/10.1016/j.ejmp.2016.11.104.
22. Bortfeld T. The number of beams in IMRT - theoretical investigations and implications for single-arc IMRT. Phys Med Biol. 2010;55(1):83–97.
23. Bortfeld T, Webb S. Single-arc IMRT? Phys Med Biol. 2009;54(1):N9–20.

24. Berry SL, Ma R, Boczkowski A, Jackson A, Zhang P, Hunt M. Evaluating inter-campus plan consistency using a knowledge based planning model. Radiother Oncol [Internet]. 2016;120(2):349–55. https://doi.org/10.1016/j.radonc.2016.06.010.
25. Nelms BE, Robinson G, Markham J, Velasco K, Boyd S, Narayan S, et al. Variation in external beam treatment plan quality: an inter-institutional study of planners and planning systems. Pract Radiat Oncol. 2012;2(4):296–305.
26. Hall EJ, Wuu CS. Radiation-induced second cancers: the impact of 3D-CRT and IMRT. Int J Radiat Oncol Biol Phys. 2003;56(1):83–8.
27. Schneider U, Zwahlen D, Ross D, Kaser-Hotz B. Estimation of radiation-induced cancer from three-dimensional dose distributions: concept of organ equivalent dose. Int J Radiat Oncol Biol Phys. 2005;61(5):1510–5.
28. Feutren T, Herrera FG. Prostate irradiation with focal dose escalation to the intraprostatic dominant nodule: a systematic review. In: Prostate International, vol. 6. Amsterdam: Elsevier B.V.; 2018. p. 75–87.
29. Hurkmans CW, Cuijpers JP, Lagerwaard FJ, Widder J, Van der Heide UA, Schuring D, et al. Recommendations for implementing stereotactic radiotherapy in peripheral stage IA non-small cell lung cancer: report from the quality assurance working party of the randomised phase III ROSEL study. Radiat Oncol. 2009;4:1–14.
30. Timmerman RD, Paulus R, Pass HI, Gore EM, Edelman MJ, Galvin J, et al. Stereotactic body radiation therapy for operable early-stage lung cancer findings from the NRG oncology RTOG 0618 trial. JAMA Oncol. 2018;4(9):1263–6.
31. Ricardi U, Badellino S, Filippi AR. Stereotactic radiotherapy for early stage non-small cell lung cancer. Radiat Oncol J. 2015;33(2):57–65.
32. Bradley J. Radiographic response and clinical toxicity following SBRT for stage I lung cancer. J Thorac Oncol [Internet]. 2007;2(7 Suppl. 3):S118–24. https://doi.org/10.1097/JTO.0b013e318074e50c.
33. Zhang B, Zhu F, Ma X, Tian Y, Cao D, Luo S, et al. Matched-pair comparisons of stereotactic body radiotherapy (SBRT) versus surgery for the treatment of early stage non-small cell lung cancer: a systematic review and meta-analysis. Radiother Oncol [Internet]. 2014;112(2):250–5. https://doi.org/10.1016/j.radonc.2014.08.031.
34. Yu XJ, Dai WR, Xu Y. Survival outcome after stereotactic body radiation therapy and surgery for early stage non-small cell lung cancer: a meta-analysis. J Investig Surg [internet]. 2018;31(5):440–7. https://doi.org/10.1080/08941939.2017.1341573.
35. Onishi H, Shirato H, Nagata Y, Hiraoka M, Fujino M, Gomi K, et al. Stereotactic body radiotherapy (SBRT) for operable stage i non-small-cell lung cancer: can SBRT be comparable to surgery? Int J Radiat Oncol Biol Phys. 2011;81(5):1352–8.
36. Nagata Y, Takayama K, Matsuo Y, Norihisa Y, Mizowaki T, Sakamoto T, et al. Clinical outcomes of a phase I/II study of 48 Gy of stereotactic body radiotherapy in 4 fractions for primary lung cancer using a stereotactic body frame. Int J Radiat Oncol Biol Phys. 2005;63(5):1427–31.
37. McGarry RC, Papiez L, Williams M, Whitford T, Timmerman RD. Stereotactic body radiation therapy of early-stage non-small-cell lung carcinoma: phase I study. Int J Radiat Oncol Biol Phys. 2005;63(4):1010–5.
38. Dosoretz DE, Katin MJ, Blitzer PH, Rubenstein JH, Salenius S, Rashid M, et al. Radiation therapy in the management of medically inoperable carcinoma of the lungs: results and implications for future treatment strategies. Int J Radiat Oncol Biol Phys. 1992;24(1):3–9.
39. Shirvani SM, Jiang J, Chang JY, Welsh JW, Gomez DR, Swisher S, et al. Comparative effectiveness of 5 treatment strategies for early-stage non-small cell lung cancer in the elderly. Int J Radiat Oncol Biol Phys [Internet]. 2012;84(5):1060–70. https://doi.org/10.1016/j.ijrobp.2012.07.2354.
40. Chang JY, Senan S, Paul MA, Mehran RJ, Louie AV, Balter P, et al. Stereotactic ablative radiotherapy versus lobectomy for operable stage I non-small-cell lung cancer: a pooled analysis of two randomised trials. Lancet Oncol. 2015;16(6):630–7.
41. J Int Comm Radiat Units Meas. ICRU Report 91: Prescribing, Recording and Reporting of Stereotactic Treatments with Small Photon Beams. J Int Comm Radiat Units Meas [Internet]. 2014;14(2):1–152. https://journals.sagepub.com/doi/toc/crua/14/2.

42. Purdie TG, Bissonnette JP, Franks K, Bezjak A, Payne D, Sie F, et al. Cone-beam computed tomography for on-line image guidance of lung stereotactic radiotherapy: localization, verification, and Intrafraction tumor position. Int J Radiat Oncol Biol Phys. 2007;68(1):243–52.
43. Gasic D, Ohlhues L, Brodin NP, Fog LS, Pommer T, Bangsgaard JP, et al. A treatment planning and delivery comparison of volumetric modulated arc therapy with or without flattening filter for gliomas, brain metastases, prostate, head/neck and early stage lung cancer. Acta Oncol. 2014;53(8):1005–11.
44. Lechner W, Wesolowska P, Azangwe G, Arib M, Alves VGL, Suming L, et al. A multinational audit of small field output factors calculated by treatment planning systems used in radiotherapy. Phys Imaging Radiat Oncol [internet]. 2018;5(September 2017):58–63. https://doi.org/10.1016/j.phro.2018.02.005.
45. Lechner W, Primeβnig A, Nenoff L, Wesolowska P, Izewska J, Georg D. The influence of errors in small field dosimetry on the dosimetric accuracy of treatment plans. Acta Oncol. [internet]. 2020;59(5):511–17. https://doi.org/10.1080/0284186X.2019.1685127.
46. Carrasco P, Jornet N, Duch MA, Weber L, Ginjaume M, Eudaldo T, et al. Comparison of dose calculation algorithms in phantoms with lung equivalent heterogeneities under conditions of lateral electronic disequilibrium. Med Phys. 2004;31(10):2899–911.
47. Latifi K, Oliver J, Baker R, Dilling TJ, Stevens CW, Kim J, et al. Study of 201 non-small cell lung cancer patients given stereotactic ablative radiation therapy shows local control dependence on dose calculation algorithm. Int J Radiat Oncol Biol Phys. 2014;88(5):1108–13.
48. Miften M, Olch A, Mihailidis D, Moran J, Pawlicki T, Molineu A, et al. Tolerance limits and methodologies for IMRT measurement-based verification QA: recommendations of AAPM task group no. 218. Med Phys. 2018;45(4):e53–83.
49. Korreman SS. Motion in radiotherapy: photon therapy. Phys Med Biol. 2012;57(23):R161–91.
50. Mageras GS. Fluoroscopic evaluation of diaphragmatic motion reduction with a respiratory gated radiotherapy system. J Appl Clin Med Phys. 2001;2(4):191.
51. Chi PCM, Balter P, Luo D, Mohan R, Pan T. Relation of external surface to internal tumor motion studied with cine CT. Med Phys. 2006;33(9):3116–23.
52. Heinzerling JH, Anderson JF, Papiez L, Boike T, Chien S, Zhang G, et al. Four-dimensional computed tomography scan analysis of tumor and organ motion at varying levels of abdominal compression during stereotactic treatment of lung and liver. Int J Radiat Oncol Biol Phys. 2008;70(5):1571–8.
53. Vedam SS, Keall PJ, Kini VR, Mohan R. Determining parameters for respiration-gated radiotherapy. Med Phys. 2001;28(10):2139–46.
54. George R, Chung TD, Vedam SS, Ramakrishnan V, Mohan R, Weiss E, et al. Audio-visual biofeedback for respiratory-gated radiotherapy: impact of audio instruction and audio-visual biofeedback on respiratory-gated radiotherapy. Int J Radiat Oncol Biol Phys. 2006;65(3):924–33.
55. Neicu T, Berbeco R, Wolfgang J, Jiang SB. Synchronized moving aperture radiation therapy (SMART): improvement of breathing pattern reproducibility using respiratory coaching. Phys Med Biol. 2006;51(3):617–36.
56. Kini VR, Vedam SS, Keall PJ, Patil S, Chen C, Mohan R. Patient training in respiratory-gated radiotherapy. Med Dosim [Internet]. 2003;28(1):7–11. https://linkinghub.elsevier.com/retrieve/pii/S095839470200136X
57. Pollock S, Keall R, Keall P. Breathing guidance in radiation oncology and radiology: a systematic review of patient and healthy volunteer studies. Med Phys. 2015;42(9):5490–509.

Magnetic Resonance-Guided Adaptive Radiotherapy: Technical Concepts

6

Sara Hackett, Bram van Asselen, Marielle Philippens, Simon Woodings, and Jochem Wolthaus

6.1 Image Guidance and Adaptive Radiotherapy

Adaptive radiotherapy uses imaging information acquired at the time of treatment to address anatomical deformations relative to the planning image data, which are generally computed tomography (CT) images [1]. These deformations may arise from inter-fractional changes, such as organ filling, weight loss, or relative displacements of multiple targets, or from intra-fractional changes, such as respiratory or cardiac motion. The adaptive process therefore requires both clear visualization of the target and organs at risk, and an image acquisition frequency as high as, if not higher than the frequency of the changes that the adaptation is intended to address.

Image guidance with cone-beam CT (CBCT) is widely used in radiotherapy for position verification of the tumour and surrounding tissue. The modality enables correction of positional misalignments through translations and rotations of the treatment couch (Chap. 4 and [2]). The contrast of CBCT images is based on density differences, so interfaces between structures with large differences in density such as between lung and tissue, or tissue and bone, can be clearly visualized. The primary limitation of the CBCT for image-guided radiotherapy is the lack of soft tissue contrast, which is often insufficient for identification of target structures. The long acquisition time of the scans also precludes any real-time monitoring of intrafraction motion. Finally, each CBCT scan acquired to monitor the position of the target will deliver extra radiation dose to the patient.

Unlike CBCT and CT modalities, magnetic resonance imaging (MRI) provides excellent soft-tissue contrast, (see Fig. 6.1), and has therefore become a highly valuable diagnostic tool in oncology. The images can be acquired in almost real time, whilst the patient is on the treatment table to capture the motion of the target and its

S. Hackett (✉) · B. van Asselen · M. Philippens · S. Woodings · J. Wolthaus
Department of Radiotherapy, University Medical Center Utrecht, Utrecht, The Netherlands
e-mail: S.S.Hackett@umcutrecht.nl; B.vanAsselen@umcutrecht.nl; M.Philippens@umcutrecht.nl; jwooding@umcutrecht.nl; J.Wolthaus@umcutrecht.nl

E. G. C. Troost (ed.), *Image-Guided High-Precision Radiotherapy*,
https://doi.org/10.1007/978-3-031-08601-4_6

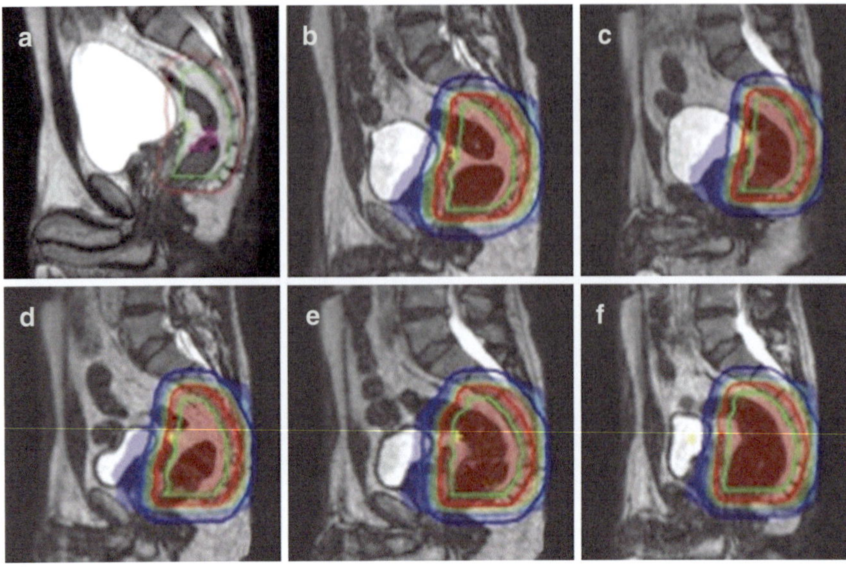

Fig. 6.1 Daily MR images (T2-weighted TSE sequence) of a rectum cancer patient undergoing neoadjuvant radiotherapy. The change in the gross tumour volume (outlined in green) and the bladder, relative to the pre-treatment dataset (**a**) is clearly visible over fractions one to five (images **b–f**, respectively)

surroundings at a high temporal resolution. Functional MR imaging modalities are also available to probe biological function and physiology [3]. Technical developments over the last decades have led to scanners with sufficiently wide bores (up to 70 cm in diameter) and sufficiently rapid image acquisition sequences for pre-treatment imaging of the tumour for radiotherapy applications. Tumour definition and delineation, which has historically hindered the accuracy with which target volumes could be identified, can be improved through the inclusion of MR data in the diagnostic and treatment planning process [4–7]. For example, quantitative MR images that reflect blood flow and vessel permeability are now frequently used for delineation of the gross tumour volume (GTV) of the prostate [8, 9]. MR therefore affords the possibility of adapting the radiotherapy to the biological as well as geometric characteristics of the anatomy.

The soft-tissue contrast and the speed at which images can be acquired are the primary reasons why MR is an ideal imaging modality for adaptive radiotherapy. Furthermore, the MR imaging process does not expose the patient to ionizing radiation, which is a concern for X-ray based modalities, so images can be acquired as frequently as necessary for the adaptive process without extra radiation dose to the patient. The excellent soft-tissue contrast facilitates adaptation of the radiation delivery to the target and organs at risk, and frequent, rapid imaging throughout the treatment delivery will enable adaptation of the dose to the mobile anatomy in real time. These features of MR imaging motivated the development of MR-guided radiotherapy (MRgRT) devices. There are currently two commercially available

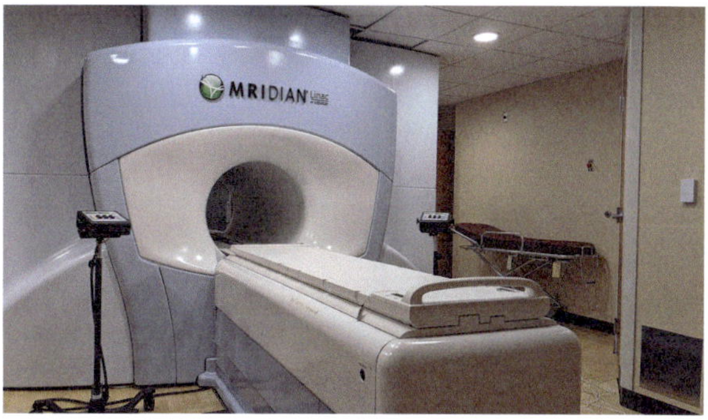

Fig. 6.2 Clinically used ViewRay MRIdian MR-linac at Washington University in St Louis, USA. (Courtesy of Dr. Olga Green)

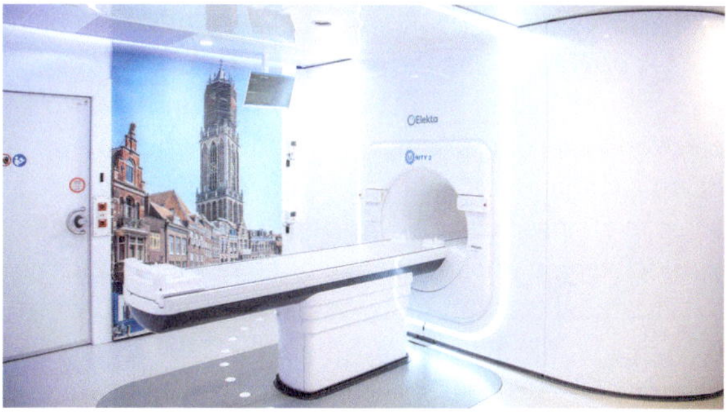

Fig. 6.3 Clinically used Elekta Unity MRI-Linac at the UMC Utrecht hospital, Utrecht, The Netherlands

radiotherapy systems with integrated MR-guidance; the ViewRay MRIdian (Fig. 6.2) and the Elekta Unity (Fig. 6.3). Two other systems are under development at the University of Alberta [10] and within the Australian MR-linac consortium [11].

6.1.1 Development of MR-Guided Radiotherapy Systems

Integration of an MR scanner and a radiation delivery system is far from straightforward, as the mechanism of MR image acquisition can interfere with the process of generating the radiation beam of the linac, and vice versa. The strong magnetic field of the MR scanner influences the trajectories of the accelerating electrons in the linac, which necessitates modifications to the linac design. It should be noted that even the beam generation systems of conventional linacs with travelling waveguides must be dynamically corrected to account for the orientation of the earth's magnetic field, which is three to four orders of magnitude weaker than the magnetic fields used in MRgRT systems. Conversely, the radio-frequency (RF) noise generated by the linac interferes with the radio-waves used for image acquisition of the MR scanner. The modifications implemented for MRgRT systems include a re-design of the Faraday cage, so that the cage wraps around the linac and the cryostat of the MR-scanner, to prevent RF interference on MR signal acquisition. The systems also use standing-wave linac designs as the waveguides of these linacs are relatively compact. The influence of the magnetic field on the beam generation system can be further minimized by either passive shielding of the system with mu-metal, or by placing the linac and other electronic components sensitive to the magnetic field within a torus of very low magnetic field around the MR magnet.

6.1.2 The ViewRay System

The ViewRay MRIdian system (ViewRay Inc., Oakwood, OH) was the first commercially available device for MRI-integrated radiotherapy [12]. Clinical treatments with this system began in 2014 at Washington University in St. Louis [13]. The system uses a 0.35 T MR scanner with a split bore of 70 cm diameter. The magnetic field is oriented along the +y-axis of the IEC 61217 coordinate system, perpendicular to the radiation beam. The MRI comprises two superconducting self-shielded electromagnets, a 75 cm wide gradient coil and a surface receiver coil with low beam attenuation. Planar and volumetric imaging are available, with a field of view of up to 50 cm. Planar MR imaging for motion monitoring is possible during radiation delivery, with a frame rate of up to four frames per second of a single slice.

The initial version of this system was equipped with three equidistant ^{60}Co-sources mounted on the gantry ring within the split of the scanner bore [12]. In the current version, the ^{60}Co-sources have been replaced by a single standing-wave linac with a 6 MV flattening-filter free (FFF) beam, which can deliver a dose rate of 5.5 Gy per minute at the isocenter [14]. The source-axis distance of the linac is 90 cm. The beam is shaped by double-focused multi-leaf collimators (MLC) and does not pass through any of the MRI components before entering the bore. The available field size ranges from 0.5×0.5 to 24.1×27.4 cm^2, and the system can deliver both IMRT and 3D-conformal treatment plans.

6.1.3 The Unity System

The Unity MRI-linac was developed at the University Medical Center in Utrecht, in collaboration with Elekta and Philips [15–17]. A first-in-man study to demonstrate the safety and the dosimetric and geometric accuracy of treatment delivery on the clinical prototype MR-linac was performed in 2017 [18]. The Unity system was clinically released in 2018 after CE-certification.

The system comprises a 1.5 T MRI scanner, with a diameter of 70 cm, and a standing-wave linac with a 7 MV FFF beam. The magnetic field is oriented along the −y-axis of the IEC 61217 coordinate system, perpendicular to the radiation beam. The MR scanner offers a wide range of volumetric image sequences and motion monitoring via 2D cine-loop imaging. The linac gantry is mounted behind the covers of the closed bore of the MR scanner so the gantry can safely be rotated at a speed of up to six rotations per minute. The radiation beam travels through a portal in the cryostat of the MR scanner, in between the superconducting coils. The portal is constructed to minimize attenuation of the radiation beam. The projected leaf width at isocentre is 7.2 mm, and field sizes range from 0.5×0.5 to 22×57 cm^2. The maximum dose rate at isocentre is approximately 4.3 Gy per minute.

6.1.4 MRgRT Systems under Development

Two MRgRT systems are under development and have not yet been clinically used. The Australian Magnetic Resonance Imaging-linac program has built a prototype system with an actively shielded 1.0 T open-bore magnet with a 50 cm gap between the coils [11]. The second system, located at the University of Alberta (Edmonton, Canada) [10], comprises a biplanar superconducting open-bore 0.6 T magnet capable of operating at high temperatures and a 6 MV linac. Both systems feature the possibility to orient the magnetic field parallel as well as perpendicular to the radiation beam by rotating the MRI magnet relative to both the patient couch and radiation beam. When the magnetic field is oriented parallel to the radiation beam, the lateral scatter of electrons away from the radiation beam will be reduced. This reduction of lateral scatter avoids concerns about high doses at density interfaces, as described later in this chapter, at the cost of hugely increasing the skin dose at the entrance of the beam [19, 20]. The systems are also designed so that the radiation beam does not pass through the cryostat.

6.2 The Effect of the Magnetic Field on the Dose Distribution

6.2.1 The Lorentz Force

MR-guided radiotherapy delivers dose to a patient in the presence of a (strong) magnetic field. The photon fluence as well as the resulting photon-electron interactions (i.e., the photoelectric effect, Compton scatter and pair production) are not affected by the magnetic field. The resulting secondary electrons are, however, affected by the Lorentz force, which will change their trajectory. The Lorentz force is given by:

$$\vec{F}_L = q\vec{v} \times \vec{B}$$

where q is the charge of the particle, $\vec{v}$ is the particle velocity and $\vec{B}$ the magnetic field. The trajectory of the secondary electrons in a medium in the presence of a magnetic field therefore depends on two factors: interactions with the surrounding medium and the Lorentz force acting on the electron. Since no energy is lost through the Lorentz force, the path length of the electron will be unchanged by the presence of the magnetic field. However, as the electron loses energy via interactions with the medium, as determined by the stopping power, the velocity will decrease, and therefore the Lorentz force experienced by the electron will decrease. As a result, the gyroradius of the electron will also decrease.

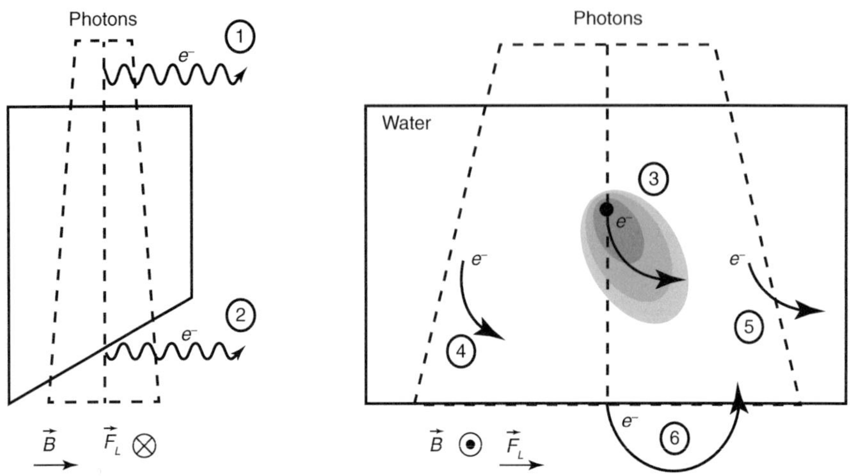

Fig. 6.4 Effects of the magnetic field on the dose distribution in and out of the primary radiation beam. (1) Contaminant electron spiralling away from entry beam. (2) Electron at distal end of beam spiralling away from surface along magnetic field lines. (3) Tilted dose kernel around point of interaction. (4) Electron swept towards central axis, resulting in sharper penumbra. (5) Electron swept away from central axis, resulting in broader penumbra. Effects (4) and (5) result in an asymmetry of the penumbra in the axis perpendicular to the magnetic field. (6) Electron return effect at interface between water and air

6.3 The Dose Distribution in a Transverse Magnetic Field

6.3.1 Beam Entry

As the radiation beam passes through air it will generate contamination electrons before reaching the patient. In a transverse magnetic field these electrons will experience a Lorentz force, which will cause them to spiral around the magnetic field lines and travel along the axis of the field away from the incident beam [21, 22]. These electrons can cause a modest increase of the skin dose outside the primary field (less than 5% of the maximum dose within the field). This process is illustrated as effect 1 in Fig. 6.4. However, as these electrons are swept away from the primary beam they will not contribute to the surface dose of the beam. The skin dose in a 0.35 T magnetic field is comparable to the case without a magnetic field. However, the skin dose increases with field strength, as the electrons in the patient are swept sideways and deposit dose closer to the point of interaction [23, 24].

6.3.2 Beam Exit

Electrons generated at the distal end of the beam usually exit the patient, but in a magnetic field the trajectories of the electrons can spiral and return to the patient surface, depositing their remaining dose on the patient skin. This well-documented phenomenon is known as the electron return effect (ERE), and is generally characterized as a dose peak at the distal end of the beam [19, 23–26]. The effect is shown in Fig. 6.4 as effect 6. However, ejected electrons can also spiral along magnetic field lines, as shown as effect 2 in Fig. 6.4. This effect, known as the electron streaming effect (ESE) [27], can lead to unexpectedly high skin doses outside the radiation field as these electrons can deposit dose at surfaces perpendicular to the magnetic field axis outside the irradiated volume.

6.3.3 Penumbra

The Lorentz force also causes a detectable shift in the dose distribution in the plane orthogonal to both the beam central axis and the magnetic field. On one side of the radiation beam the electrons will be swept towards the central axis as illustrated by effect 4 in Fig. 6.4, and on the other side the electrons will be directed away from the central axis (see effect 5 in Fig. 6.4). The penumbra and dose profile will therefore be asymmetrical [25, 28, 29].

6.3.4 Central Axis

The magnetic field exerts a lateral force on electrons, which causes a lateral shift of the kernel of dose deposition around the point of photon interaction, shown by the asymmetric kernel in Fig. 6.4 (effect 3). The dose is therefore deposited closer to point of interaction, resulting in a shift of the percentage depth dose curve towards the surface. Dose as a function of depth therefore more closely resembles the Kerma as a function of depth than the 0 T case. The percentage depth dose also shows a shorter region of dose build-up and a shallower depth of maximum dose. These changes become more pronounced with increasing magnetic field strength [30, 31].

6.4 Dose Measurements in a Magnetic Field

High-precision measurements of dose and dose distributions are required for high precision of dose delivery in MRgRT. The presence of the magnetic field not only changes the dose distributions, but also the detector response to radiation [30, 31]. Further, detectors and associated equipment (such as holders, motors and phantoms) must be MR-compatible.

Practical concerns regarding dosimetry in a magnetic field include (1) equipment that is not MR-compatible, (2) accurate localization of detectors within a bore treatment unit that has no light field, and (3) disruption of electronic equilibrium at density interfaces. Most of these problems have now been solved [32, 33]. Manufacturers now often provide MR-compatible versions of radiotherapy equipment [34–38]. Accurate positioning of detectors can be achieved by using an equipment positioning template or a displaced isocenter indicator, such as lasers, or by imaging the detector in situ [29]. These positioning methods need precise table movements in order to adjust or reproduce a detector position. Commercially available MRgRT systems can satisfy the requirements for accuracy of table positioning.

The ideal detector for MRgRT would also be visible in MR images, as this would enable dosimetry as part of the clinical adaptive MRgRT workflow. Geometrically accurate MR-imaging of detectors with metal components is not achievable, but clinical workflows can be performed with phantoms including films and with gel dosimeters. Another option is to use a dummy detector or phantom insert for imaging, and then to replace these components for dosimetric measurements, although the risk of perturbing the phantom while replacing the components must be considered.

6.5 Reference Dosimetry

The gold-standard detector for quantitative dosimetry for radiotherapy is the ionization chamber. Secondary electrons travel through the chamber, ionizing molecules along their path. The resultant charged particles are collected by electrodes and recorded by an electrometer. The magnetic field will cause the trajectories of the secondary electrons to curve and, as discussed above, the gyroradius of these trajectories will depend on the magnetic field strength, relative orientation of the radiation beam, magnetic field and the chamber, and beam energy [24, 39, 40]. The number of ionizations inside the cavity for a given secondary electron fluence will therefore change, and consequently the relationship between dose in medium and collected charge released in air is altered.

The change of trajectory of secondary electrons induced by the magnetic field means that the effective origin of these particles will differ in a magnetic field, which thereby changes the effective point of measurement of the detector [41]. In extreme cases the magnetic field can affect the physical structure of detector components, such as bending the central electrode [42], which may also influence the chamber response to radiation. Thin layers of air around detectors can also influence measurements [32, 33, 43–45]. Reference dosimetry should therefore be performed with waterproof Farmer-type ionization chambers in a water phantom.

The influence of the magnetic field on the response of the chamber to a given electron fluence depends on the magnetic field strength and the relative orientations of the photon beam, chamber and magnetic field. It is necessary to correct the chamber reading for an absolute derivation of dose [30, 44]. The dose to water, $D_{w,Q}^{\vec{B}}$, in the presence of a magnetic field $\vec{B}$ for beam quality Q is given by

$$D_{w,Q}^{\vec{B}} = k_{\vec{B},Q} M_Q^{\vec{B}} N_{D,w,Q_0} k_{Q,Q_0} = c_{\vec{B}} k_{\vec{B},M,Q} M_Q^{\vec{B}} N_{D,w,Q_0} k_{Q,Q_0}$$

where $k_{\vec{B},Q}$ accounts for the change in the chamber calibration factor, N_{D,w,Q_0} due to the magnetic field, $M_Q^{\vec{B}}$ is the raw chamber reading in the magnetic field, corrected for polarity, recombination, relative humidity, temperature and pressure, and k_{Q,Q_0} corrects for the difference in beam quality between the reference beam and the beam of the MRgRT system. The $k_{\vec{B},Q}$ factor comprises an extrinsic component,

$c_{\vec{B}}$, which accounts for the change in dose to water at the reference point due to the magnetic field, and an intrinsic component $k_{\vec{B},M,Q}$, which accounts for the change in the raw chamber reading due to the magnetic field.

For magnetic field strengths of commercially available MRgRT systems, it is possible to choose an orientation of the chamber (namely, parallel or anti-parallel to magnetic field) such that the $k_{\vec{B},Q}$ correction factor is close to unity [30, 46]. The correction factor can be determined directly for a specific chamber and orientation using a primary standard such as a calorimeter, as the response of the calorimeter to radiation is not affected by the presence of a magnetic field. However, calorimeters, particularly those modified for use in a magnetic field, are not available at most institutions [47]. The correction factor can also be obtained via cross-calibration with a dosimeter such as alanine, via Monte Carlo simulations or by using a combination of Monte Carlo simulations and measurements [30, 31, 46, 48].

Detailed Monte Carlo simulations have been performed for many detector types and $k_{\vec{B},Q}$ factors determined from these simulations, or from experimental methods, are available in the literature [43, 49–51]. It has been demonstrated from measurements of multiple chambers that, for at least two types of Farmer chamber, the $k_{\vec{B},Q}$ values are consistent for each chamber type [46, 52]. Literature values of $k_{\vec{B},Q}$ for a specific chamber model could therefore be used for individual chambers if the measurements or simulations are appropriately conducted. The correction factors will be specific to the chamber orientation relative to the magnetic field, beam quality and the strength of the magnetic field.

6.6 Relative Dosimetry

Detectors used for relative dosimetry may also be influenced by the presence of a magnetic field. The angular dependence of detectors may change in a magnetic field, and this dependence should be investigated before use [41, 46, 53]. Two- and three-dimensional detector arrays typically include density interfaces and layers of air around the detectors. The angular sensitivity of each system should be evaluated and profiles should be compared with measurements in 3D scanning water phantoms. Scanning water phantoms have been developed for MRgRT systems [37]. The new phantoms have non-standard sizes to pass within the bores and to measure the available field sizes. The phantoms use MR-compatible ultrasonic motors instead of standard electric motors.

Film remains the detector of choice for high spatial resolution measurements in an MR-linac and is suitable for dosimetry in a magnetic field [54]. Attention must be given to avoid thin layers of air between the film and any solid phantom. Film phantoms have been designed with materials of high electron density sandwiching the film. These materials effectively stop all secondary electrons, thus negating the effect of the magnetic field on the electron trajectories. The film can then be used to assess the geometric characteristics of the photon beam, such as for quality assurance of the multi-leaf collimators (MLCs) or identification of the radiation isocenter on a spoke film [55] (Fig. 6.5).

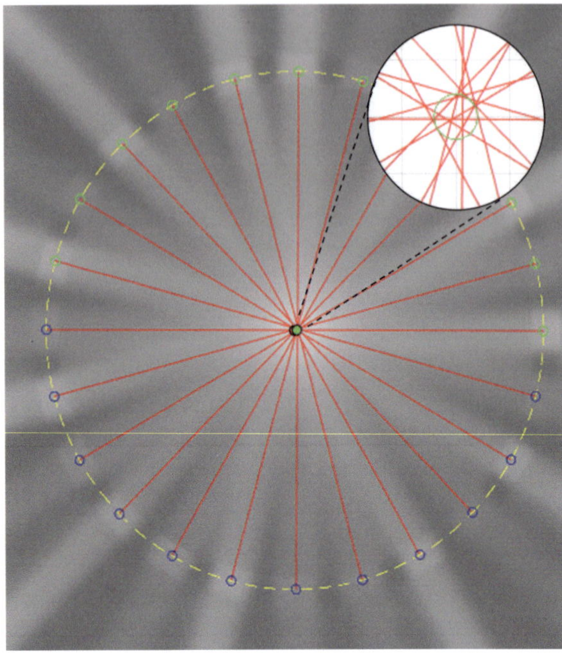

Fig. 6.5 Spoke film showing a locus of radius of gantry isocenter of 0.4 mm. The film was acquired on a Unity MR-linac using a phantom with copper rings to avoid the influence of the Lorentz force on each spoke

The Unity system incorporates an in-built megavoltage imager (MVI) [56]. This imager has a limited field of view, approximately 22 cm wide and 9 cm long. The imager itself is located in a region where the magnetic field strength is only 0.01 T [57] and therefore can be used for dosimetry without concerns of magnetic field effects, although the usual caveats for beam hardening, scatter and energy sensitivity still exist. A particular advantage of the MVI panel is that images can be recorded at all gantry angles and can therefore be used for constancy checks of dose output, dose profiles, and field edges. These measurements are not easy to perform with other detectors as a detector cannot be mounted on the head of the linac, and no commercially-available rotating platform is currently available.

An independent monitor chamber can be valuable for obtaining highly accurate measurements for reference dosimetry, or for removing the effects of fluctuations in output or dose rate on relative dosimetric measurements. The use of monitor chambers in MR-linacs has proven challenging. A transmission chamber cannot be easily used as it cannot be mounted on the head of the linac, as it would be for a conventional system. It should also be noted that, for certain combinations of detector, beam and phantom orientations, detectors in the bore may record a measurable dose from the electron streaming effect [22, 58].

It has been demonstrated that MR images can be acquired during beam delivery [38], and that the MRI radiofrequency pulses during imaging do not affect the radiation dose distribution [29].

6.7 Magnetic Resonance Imaging for MRgRT

6.7.1 Magnetic Resonance Imaging

MR images acquired on the MR-linac are used for multiple purposes over the course of the treatment, including daily localization of the tumour and organs at risk, delineation of structures for adaptive treatment planning, motion monitoring, and assessment of the treatment response. Each purpose has associated and specific imaging objectives. The geometrical accuracy of images used for delineation and motion monitoring is of course essential, as is a high contrast-to-noise ratio, whereas good visualization of biomarkers is of greater importance for images used for response assessment [59]. Before the scanner is installed in the department, MRI safety procedures must be in place to ensure safe working conditions in the vicinity of a magnetic field for both staff and patients [60].

6.7.2 Safety

An MR scanner consists of multiple hardware components that present safety concerns [61]. The most obvious is the magnet with a (strong) static magnetic field, as well as field gradients for imaging and radiofrequency coils to transmit and receive signals. In addition to the effects of the magnetic field on the patient's body, special attention must be paid to passive and active implants (e.g., prostheses and pacemakers) [62]. The static magnetic field will exert rotational (i.e., torque) and translational (i.e., attractive) forces on a ferromagnetic object in the proximity of the magnet, which can be very dangerous for both patients and staff. These forces are dependent on both the field strength and the gradient of the magnetic stray field. Careful screening is therefore warranted.

To produce an image, the gradient system has to switch at a high frequency. This frequent switching of the field may cause perineural stimulation (PNS), i.e., stimulation of nerves, and produces acoustic noise due to the Lorentz force on the gradient coils while changing currents. Effective hearing protection for the patient is therefore necessary. The acoustic noise is determined by both the magnetic field strength and the gradient strength. Finally, the transmit coils deposit radio-frequency (RF) power in the body, and deposition increases with magnetic field strength [63]. This process is monitored carefully via the acquisition protocols so as not to exceed specified limits for heating of the body. If non-ferrous implants are present, linear structures in the implants can act as a resonant antenna, which will cause further heating. The length of the implant and the field strength will determine whether it is safe to image the patient. The safety regulations are generally more stringent with increasing field strength.

6.7.3 Image Acquisition

As indicated above, geometric accuracy of MR images for radiotherapy is of great importance. The two sources of geometric distortions are non-linearity of the field gradient and susceptibility-induced inhomogeneities in the magnetic field [64, 65]. Non-linearity of the gradient violates the assumed linear relationship between spin location and the local field strength controlled by the gradient system, and manifests as a shift in pixel location. The displacements increase with distance from the iso-center and are dependent on the design of the gradient coil but not on the imaging sequence [66]. Most vendors apply correction algorithms, which can largely mitigate distortions. However, the correction can only be applied in the in-plane axes of a multi-slice image. In a 3D image with two phase-encoded directions, the unwarping can be performed in all three dimensions, making 3D acquisition preferable for MRgRT.

Susceptibility artefacts are caused by local inhomogeneities in the magnetic field arising from an inherent variation of the susceptibility of the imaged object. Susceptibility-induced distortions are dependent on the acquisition technique and parameters. Echo-planar imaging, which is used for diffusion-weighted imaging, is highly sensitive to susceptibility effects, whereas a 3D fast spin-echo sequence is relatively insensitive to susceptibility variations of the tissue [67, 68]. The sensitivity of a particular sequence to magnetic field deviations is determined by the bandwidth and the resolution of the images. This bandwidth is also referred to as water-fat shift. A small water-fat shift, i.e., a high bandwidth, means that the sequence is insensitive to magnetic field offsets. The drawback of increasing the bandwidth of a sequence is that the signal to noise ratio will decrease [65, 69].

6.7.4 Image Quality

Image acquisition with MRI is relatively slow compared with CT. For the purpose of MRgRT the image contrast and resolution therefore have to be balanced with the scan time. The scan time for the MR image used for registration, delineation and treatment planning should be less than approximately 5 min. The treatment planning system requires a 3D dataset, so this requirement directs the choice of imaging protocol. Generally, a spoiled gradient recalled (SPGR) sequence (for T1-weighted images), a 3D turbo spin-echo (TSE) sequence (for T2-weighted images) or a 3D balanced steady-state free precession (SSFP) or fast imaging with steady-state precession (TRUFI) sequence [70, 71] will be used for tumour and organs at risk delineation. These 3D-acquired images are not optimal for diagnosis and tumour staging as the contrast is weaker and the in-plane resolution is lower than would typically be demanded for radiology images. However, for daily delineation of structures, these images suffice. The choice of contrast is directed by the location of the tumour and by the field strength of the MRI scanner.

At low field strengths (0.35 T) the balanced SSFP sequence is normally used, while for the 1.5 T scanner the SPGR and T2TSE sequences are typically used. The balanced SSFP is more effective at low field because of the relatively long T2 and short T1 relaxation times. The T2 fast spin-echo sequences become more useful at high field strengths and can provide a cleaner T2 contrast.

Due to the nature of the image acquisition, MRI is prone to geometric and intensity distortions. Geometrical uncertainties of standard T2-weighted MR images at locations 18 cm from the centre of the bore are typically up to 1.3 mm [72]. The geometrical accuracy of images is crucial for the planning and delivery of radiotherapy, so such image-related uncertainties must be carefully considered. Limitations for treatment of particular tumour sites (such as breast) may apply, but novel MRI sequences dedicated to reducing geometric distortions and geometrical correction techniques will further extend the use of MRI in radiotherapy simulation, treatment planning and treatment guidance. An example of the geometric distortions of a B0-map sequence acquired on the 1.5 T scanner of the Unity is shown in Fig. 6.6.

The imaging frequency required for real-time motion management is determined by the motion of the target and the surrounding tissues. A high imaging frequency is not necessary to assess and correct for the drift of the target position over the course of a treatment fraction. For exception gating, i.e., gating of the delivery if the target moves out of the high dose region, a scan time of up to 10 s is sufficient, which is long enough for dynamic 3D imaging. However, for real-time guidance with tracking of the target, fast cine imaging with short loop latency times is needed. The time required for reconstruction and data transfer, which depends on the filling of *k*-space [73], as well as the scan time are of crucial importance. The gradient coils are designed to prevent damage from ionizing radiation to the electrical components and to reduce the attenuation of the beam by the coil by splitting the coil in two, with a gap of approximately 20 cm. This design constrains the performance of the scanner as it limits the maximum gradient amplitude and gradient slope, which therefore reduces the imaging speed and signal-to-noise ratio because of the longer echo times. However, the performance reductions are generally small. The relatively low field strength of the 0.35 T MR scanner of the ViewRay system also limits the signal-to-noise ratio, but the design of the receive coil and the distance between the receive coil and the patient also reduces the signal of the 1.5 T Unity MR scanner.

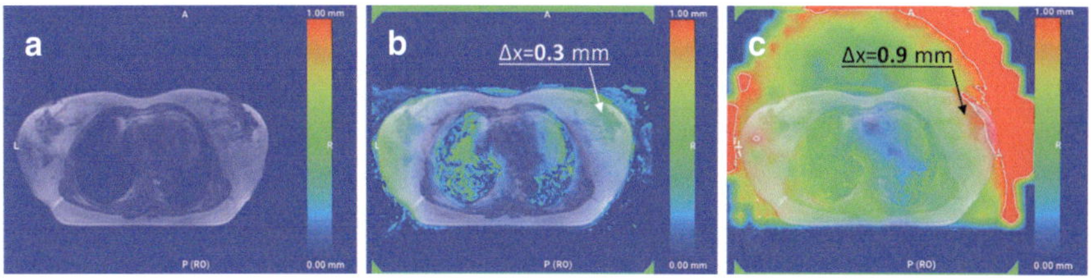

Fig. 6.6 Geometric distortions in the breast of a B0-map sequence acquired with the patient centred in the bore of the Unity 1.5 T scanner. The distortions induced by the B0-field are shown in the centre image, and the total geometric distortion (including gradient-induced distortions) is shown in the image on the right

6.8 Treatment Planning for the MR-Linac

The magnetic field of the MR-linac influences the dose distribution in the patient, as discussed above, and so the effects of the magnetic field on charged particle trajectories must be simulated in the treatment planning process. Monte Carlo codes provide the only feasible means of accurately generating and calculating treatment plans in a magnetic field. The effects of a 1.5 T magnetic field on dose distributions can be accurately simulated with the EGSNRC [74], PENELOPE [75] and GEANT4 [76] codes.

However, online adaptive planning demands both speed and accuracy of dose calculations. The graphics processing unit Monte Carlo dose (GPUMCD) code [77] parallelizes simulations over multiple GPU threads to increase computational power, and includes simplifications of the simulated physical structures and processes in order to speed up calculations [78]. The code has also been modified to incorporate magnetic field effects [79]. The GPUMCD code has been implemented in treatment planning systems for the Unity MR-linac. The code used by the ViewRay treatment planning system is based on the VMC [80] and EGSNRC code and also simulates the effects of the 0.35 T magnetic field on the dose distribution [81].

A comparison of treatment planning strategies for lymph node oligometastases planned for the Unity MR-linac showed that a complete re-optimization and calculation of a treatment plan could be achieved in under 2 min [82, 83]. A comparable average time of 2.9 min was reported for re-optimization and calculation of prostate plans for the ViewRay system [81]. The time required to achieve a clinically acceptable plan adaptation will of course depend on the factors such as the resolution of the dose grid, the required statistical uncertainty of the dose calculation and the dimensions of the calculation volume. However, it is clear that further gains in planning and calculation speed must be made for real-time plan adaptation.

6.8.1 Quality Assurance

Online adaptive radiotherapy is particularly challenging regarding quality assurance of patient-specific, or rather, fraction-specific plans. The patient must remain in the treatment position on the couch for the entire online workflow, which imposes both time and logistical constraints on any QA measures. Quality assurance steps performed by centres currently delivering MRgRT typically include one or more of the following:

- Visual inspection of new contours and electron density map.
- Independent three-dimensional calculation of the planned dose distribution [84].
- Verification of integrity of transferred data from the treatment planning system to the record-and-verify system [85].
- Verification of treatment delivery log files [86–88].
- Post-delivery measurement of treatment plans [89].

6.9 Workflows for Adaptive MRgRT

6.9.1 Offline Workflows

Treatments for commercially available MR-linac systems start with an offline patient dataset and treatment plan. The delineations and electron density information of the dataset and the initial treatment plan serve as references for plan adaptation. Challenges regarding planning on MR data, particularly the lack of information about electron densities in MR images used for online plan adaptation, are discussed in Chap. 3. Patient-specific data on electron densities of delineated structures can be obtained from a simulation CT. Many centres also acquire simulation MR datasets as part of the clinical preparation for an MR-linac treatment [18, 81, 82]. The reference plan can be calculated directly on the CT, but using the MR images as the offline reference dataset, with electron density information supplemented from the CT, can improve the registration process in online workflow due to the similar tissue contrast on the two images [90, 91].

6.9.2 Online Workflows

The online component of the treatment includes many of the standard steps for delivery of a conventional radiotherapy plan: acquisition of an (MR) image with the patient in the treatment position, image registration, delineation, treatment planning, position verification, quality assurance of the treatment plan, and treatment delivery. The workflow for online adaptive MRgRT for a specific patient can be tailored according to the nature and frequency of the intra- and inter-fraction anatomical changes. The strategy chosen for a particular treatment must balance the optimization time with the plan quality that can be achieved.

A brief summary of the online adaptive workflow is as follows: the patient is brought into the treatment room and positioned on the couch of the MR-linac. A volumetric MR scan is acquired and the offline image dataset is rigidly registered to the online MR scan. The delineated volumes must be modified to account for deformations of the online anatomy relative to the reference dataset. This process is usually initiated via deformable registration-based auto-contouring, which generates contours of the structures delineated on the reference dataset on the online MR image. These contours require reviewing and may need to be manually modified. The electron densities of the structures of the reference dataset will also be mapped to the corresponding structures of the online MR dataset; the electron density distribution of the online dataset should also be reviewed. Average times of 10 min were reported for prostate [81, 92] and abdominal stereotactic ablative body radiotherapy [83], although the time required for reviewing and editing will of course depend on the treatment site and staff experience. Improvements in auto-contouring via artificial intelligence and deep learning are thus essential to reducing the time, with which MRgRT can be delivered and to the introduction of real-time plan adaptation [93–96].

After the online dataset has been reviewed and approved, the reference plan can be adapted to the new patient dataset. There are a number of strategies available to generate an online plan. The apertures of the original plan can be adapted to the new target volume [97–99]. The shapes and/or weights of these apertures can then be optimized. It should be noted that this optimization process must also account for the non-uniform profile of the flattening-filter free beams used in commercial MRgRT systems. Alternatively, the fluence of the original plan can be re-optimized and re-segmented. The most time-consuming option is to create a new plan based on a full optimization of the fluence for the new anatomy and constraints.

The full optimization strategy is shown in the bottom workflow in Fig. 6.7, and is the only means of addressing changes in the dose to organs at risk due to anatomical deformations. The workflow shown in Fig. 6.8 for an oligometastatic lymph node illustrates both a change of the position of the target lymph node relative to the nearby organs at risk, as well as deformations in these organs at risk. Although the form of the target volume is relatively unchanged between treatments, the deformations in the organs at risk and the change in proximity between the organs at risk and the target volume necessitate a full re-optimization of the fluence, followed by segmentation and calculation of the plan dose.

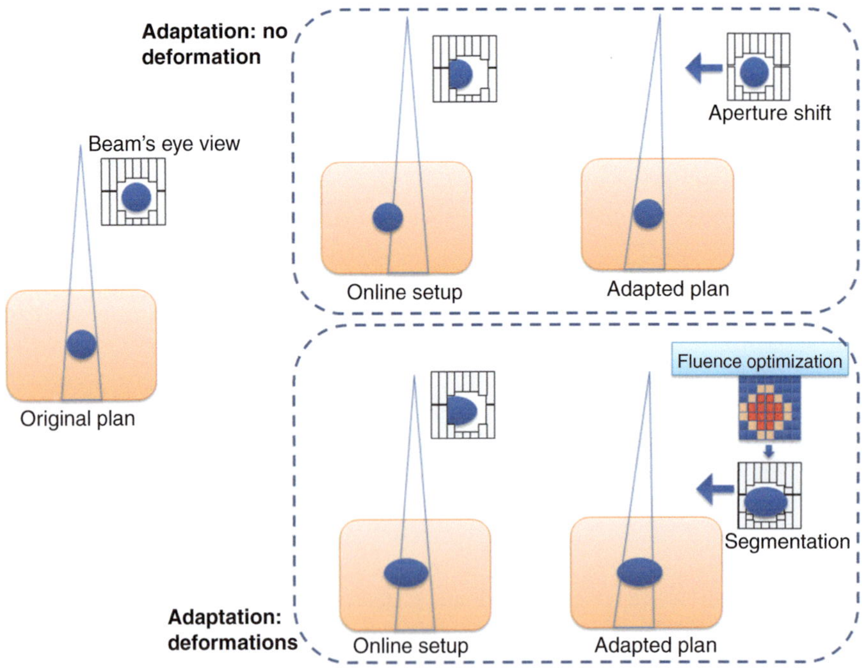

Fig. 6.7 Plan adaptation process. Top workflow: adaptation of segment to account for position of target relative to isocentre. Bottom workflow: optimization from fluence to account for deformation of target volume, followed by segmentation of the plan

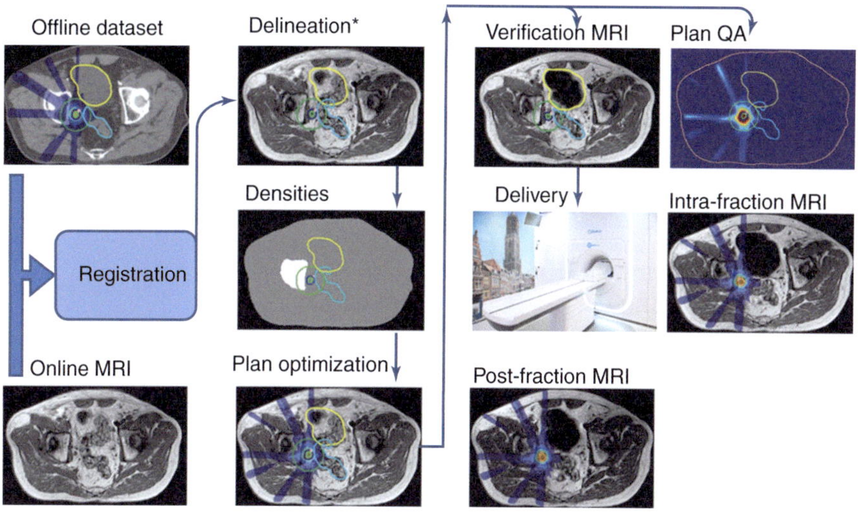

Fig. 6.8 Example workflow for MRgRT for an oligometastatic lymph node. The deformations of the organs at risk of the online MR relative to the offline dataset are particularly obvious, and the target lymph node is also closer to the bowel. In this case, without re-optimizing the fluence it is not possible to satisfy the planning constraints

It should be noted that the registered original dataset, including electron density information, can also be used for plan generation and dose calculation. The plan segments may need to be repositioned and the shapes and weights re-optimized to account for the position of the target volume relative to the isocenter and the profile of the FFF beam. This workflow, shown in the upper workflow in Fig. 6.7, is comparable to an image-guided treatment on a CBCT linac, and such an MRgRT workflow can be superior to a CBCT-guided workflow if the visibility of the target on the CBCT images is poor. However, the workflow cannot account for deformations of the target volume, such as can be seen in Fig. 6.1, or the organs at risk.

Once a treatment plan has been generated and reviewed, it is necessary to verify that the patient anatomy has not substantially changed since the online MR scan was acquired. A verification MR scan is acquired during the planning process and compared with the initial online dataset. If anatomical changes are acceptably small, plan quality approval is performed and the plan is delivered. Unacceptable anatomical changes necessitate repeating the workflow process. It should be noted that the frequency and complexity of plan adaptation increases the duration of each treatment fraction, which increases the burden for both patient and staff [100].

6.9.3 Intra-Fraction Monitoring and Adaptation

Two- and three-dimensional MR images can also be acquired during plan delivery. These images can be used to monitor intra-fraction motion and changes [101, 102], and, if necessary, for further adaptation of the treatment plan during irradiation.

Current MRgRT systems allow for exceptional gating in treatment delivery, and, if necessary, for the remaining plan to be adapted to account for a drift in the position of the target volume. Respiratory gating of treatments, so that radiation is only delivered during a specified phase of the respiratory cycle (see Chap. 4), is also possible [103]. However, both these processes lengthen the treatment process [104] and cannot address deformations of the target or organs at risk during delivery.

6.10 The Future of MRgRT

Tracking of the tumour with the radiation beam during delivery, to account for both drift of the mean position of the tumour and for respiratory motion [105, 106] is currently under development, and shows particular benefit for reducing normal tissue complication probabilities [107, 108]. Implementation of tracking is predicated on real-time MRI with adequate signal and temporal resolution. The ultimate goal of adaptive MR-guided radiotherapy is of course a system that can not only visualize anatomical changes in real time, but also continuously adapt and optimize the plan in real time based on these changes [109]. This process is hugely challenging as it not only requires rapid image acquisition but also rapid calculation of deformation vector fields, fluence optimization, beam segmentation, dose calculation and dose accumulation.

However, the benefits of combining real-time online MR imaging with high-precision real-time plan adaptation are clear. An improved definition of the target and improved accuracy of the delivered dose would enable reduction of uncertainty margins [110, 111] and thereby an increase of the therapeutic index through dose escalation [112] or a reduction in toxicity [13, 113, 114]. The margin reductions could also allow safe hypofractionation of treatments to improve both treatment outcomes and patient quality of life. Finally, the inclusion of functional MR data in the radiotherapy process can facilitate targeting the dose to biologically active regions of the tumour. This combination of immediate visualization of disease and immediate treatment would essentially make the MRgRT process one resembling interventional radiology.

References

1. Yan D, Vicini F, Wong J, Martinez A. Adaptive radiation therapy. Phys Med Biol. 1997;42:123–32.
2. Jaffray DA, Siewerdsen JH, Wong JW, Martinez AA. Flat-panel cone-beam computed tomography for image-guided radiation therapy. Int J Radiat Oncol Biol Phys. 2002;53:1337–49.
3. Gurney-Champion OJ, Mahmood F, van Schie M, Julian R, George B, Philippens MEP, van der Heide UA, Thorwarth D, Redalen KR. Quantitative imaging for radiotherapy purposes. Radiother Oncol. 2020;146:66–75.
4. Gunnlaugsson A, Persson E, Gustafsson C, Kjellén E, Ambolt P, Engelholm S, Nilsson P, Olsson LE. Definition of the prostate in CT and MRI: A multi-observer study. Phys Imaging Radiat Oncol. 2019;43:57–66.

5. Rasch C, Barillot I, Remeijer P, Touw A, Van Herk M, Lebesque JV. A general methodology for three-dimensional analysis of variation in target volume delineation. Int J Radiat Oncol Biol Phys. 1999;26:931–40.
6. Rasch CRN, Steenbakkers RJHM, Fitton I, Duppen JC, Nowak PJCM, Pameijer FA, Eisbruch A, Kaanders JHAM, Paulsen F, van Herk M. Decreased 3D observer variation with matched CT-MRI, for target delineation in nasopharynx cancer. Radiat Oncol. 2010;5:93–9.
7. Ruiz B, Feng Y. Phys Clinical and radiobiological evaluation of a method for planning target volume generation dependent on organ-at-risk exclusions in magnetic resonance imaging-based prostate radiotherapy. Imaging Radiat Oncol. 2018;8:51–6.
8. Groenendaal G, Borren A, Moman MR, Monninkhof E, Van Diest PJ, Philippens MEP, Van Vulpen M, Van Der Heide UA. Target definition in radiotherapy of prostate cancer using magnetic resonance imaging only workflow. Int J Radiat Oncol Biol Phys. 2012;9:89–91.
9. Groenendaal G, Moman MR, Korporaal JG, van Diest PJ, van Vulpen M, Philippens MEP, van der Heide UA. Validation of functional imaging with pathology for tumor delineation in the prostate. Radiother Oncol. 2010;94:145–50.
10. Fallone BG. Semin Radiat. Oncol. 2014; The rotating biplanar linac-magnetic resonance imaging system; 24:200–2.
11. Keall PJ, Barton M, Crozier S. The Australian magnetic resonance imaging-linac program. Semin Radiat Oncol. 2014;24:203–6.
12. Mutic S, Dempsey JF. The viewray system: magnetic resonance-guided and controlled radiotherapy. Semin Radiat Oncol. 2014;24:196–9.
13. Henke LE, Kashani R, Yang D, Zhao T, Green OL, Wooten H, Li H, Hu Y, Rodriguez VL, Olsen LA, Robinson CG, Parikh PJ, Michalski JM, Mutic S, Olsen JR. Online adaptive MR guided stereotactic body radiation therapy for the treatment of oligometastatic disease of the abdomen and central thorax: characterization of potential advantages. Int. J. Radiat. Oncol. 2015;93:S20–1.
14. Mutic S, Low D, Chmielewski T, Fought G, Gerganov G, Hernandez M, Kawrakow I, Kishawi E, Kuduvalli G, Sharma A, Shvartsman S, Tabachnik J, Kashani R, Green OL, Dempsey JF. The design and implementation of a novel compact linear accelerator–based magnetic resonance imaging–guided radiation therapy (MR-IGRT) system. Int. J. Radiat. Oncol. 2016;96:E641.
15. Lagendijk JJ, Raaymakers BW, van Der Heide UA, Topolnjak R, Dehnad H, Hofman P, Nederveen AJ, Schulz IM, Welleweerd J, Bakker CJ. MRI guided radiotherapy: MRI as position verification system for IMRT. Radiother Oncol. 2002;64:S75–6.
16. Lagendijk JJW, Raaymakers BW, van Vulpen M. The magnetic resonance imaging-linac system. Semin Radiat Oncol. 2014;24:207–9.
17. Raaymakers BW, Lagendijk JJW, Overweg J, Kok JGM, Raaijmakers AJE, Kerkhof EM, Van Der Put RW, Meijsing I, Crijns SPM, Benedosso F, Van Vulpen M, De Graaff CHW, Allen J, Brown KJ. Integrating a 1.5 T MRI scanner with a 6 MV accelerator: Proof of concept. Phys Med Biol. 2009;24–9.
18. Raaymakers BW, Jürgenliemk-Schulz IM, Bol GH, Glitzner M, Kotte ANTJ, Van Asselen B, De Boer JCJ, Bluemink JJ, Hackett SL, Moerland MA, Woodings SJ, Wolthaus JWH, Van Zijp HM, Philippens MEP, Tijssen R, Kok JGM, De Groot-Van Breugel EN, Kiekebosch I, Meijers LTC, Nomden CN, Sikkes GG, Doornaert PAH, Eppinga WSC, Kasperts N, Kerkmeijer LGW, Tersteeg JHA, Brown KJ, Pais B, Woodhead P, Lagendijk JJW. First patients treated with a 1.5 T MRI-Linac: Clinical proof of concept of a high-precision, high-field MRI guided radiotherapy treatment. Phys Med Biol. 2017;62:194–7.
19. Keyvanloo A, Burke B, Warkentin B, Tadic T, Rathee S, Kirkby C, Santos DM, Fallone BG. Skin dose in longitudinal and transverse linac-MRIs using monte carlo and realistic 3D MRI field models. Med Phys. 2012;39:6509–21.
20. Oborn BM, Metcalfe PE, Butson MJ, Rosenfeld AB, Keall PJ. Electron contamination modeling and skin dose in 6 MV longitudinal field MRIgRT: impact of the MRI and MRI fringe field. Med Phys. 2012;39:874–90.
21. Hackett SL, Van Asselen B, Wolthaus JWH, Bluemink JJ, Ishakoglu K, Kok J, Lagendijk JJW, Raaymakers BW. Spiraling contaminant electrons increase doses to surfaces outside the photon beam of an MRI-linac with a perpendicular magnetic field. Phys Med Biol. 2018;63:166–71.

22. Malkov VN, Hackett SL, van Asselen B, Raaymakers BW, Wolthaus JWH. Monte Carlo simulations of out-of-field skin dose due to spiralling contaminant electrons in a perpendicular magnetic field. Med Phys. 2019a;46:223–6.
23. Oborn BM, Metcalfe PE, Butson MJ, Rosenfeld AB. High resolution entry and exit Monte Carlo dose calculations from a linear accelerator 6 MV beam under the influence of transverse magnetic fields. Med Phys. 2009;36:3549–59.
24. Raaijmakers AJE, Raaymakers BW, Lagendijk JJW. Magnetic-field-induced dose effects in MR-guided radiotherapy systems: dependence on the magnetic field strength. Phys Med Biol. 2008;53:909–23.
25. Ahmad SB, Sarfehnia A, Paudel MR, Kim A, Hissoiny S, Sahgal A, Keller A and Keller B. Evaluation of a commercial MRI linac based monte carlo dose calculation algorithm with GEANT. Med Phys. 2016;43:894–907.
26. Raaijmakers AJE, Raaymakers BW, Van Der Meer S, Lagendijk JJW. Integrating a MRI scanner with a 6 MV radiotherapy accelerator: Impact of the surface orientation on the entrance and exit dose due to the transverse magnetic field. Phys Med Biol. 2007;52:929–39.
27. Malkov VN, Hackett SL, Wolthaus JWH, Raaymakers BW, Van Asselen B. Monte Carlo simulations of out-of-field surface doses due to the electron streaming effect in orthogonal magnetic fields. Phys Med Biol. 2019b;64:101–6.
28. Raaymakers BW, Raaijmakers AJE, Kotte ANTJ, Jette D, Lagendijk JJW. Integrating a MRI scanner with a 6 MV radiotherapy accelerator: dose deposition in a transverse magnetic field. Phys Med Biol. 2004;49:4109–18.
29. Woodings SJ, Bluemink JJ, De Vries JHW, Niatsetski Y, Van Veelen B, Schillings J, Kok JGM, Wolthaus JWH, Hackett SL, Van Asselen B, Van Zijp HM, Pencea S, Roberts DA, Lagendijk JJW, Raaymakers BW. Beam characterisation of the 1.5 T MRI-linac. Phys Med Biol. 2018;63:118–24.
30. Van Asselen B, Woodings SJ, Hackett SL, Van Soest TL, Kok JGM, Raaymakers BW, Wolthaus JWH. A formalism for reference dosimetry in photon beams in the presence of a magnetic field. Phys Med Biol. 2018;63:188–94.
31. O'Brien DJ, Roberts DA, Ibbott GS, Sawakuchi GO. Reference dosimetry in magnetic fields: formalism and ionization chamber correction factors. Med Phys. 2016;43:4915–27.
32. Agnew J, O'Grady F, Young R, Duane S, Budgell GJ. Quantification of static magnetic field effects on radiotherapy ionization chambers. Phys Med Biol. 2017;62:1731–43.
33. Hackett SL, Van Asselen B, Wolthaus JWH, Kok JGM, Woodings SJ, Lagendijk JJW, Raaymakers BW. Consequences of air around an ionization chamber: are existing solid phantoms suitable for reference dosimetry on an MR-linac? Med Phys. 2016;43:82–95.
34. Van Esch A, Clermont C, Devillers M, Iori M, Huyskens DP. On-line quality assurance of rotational radiotherapy treatment delivery by means of a 2D ion chamber array and the Octavius phantom. Med Phys. 2007;34:10–18.
35. Houweling AC, De Vries JHW, Wolthaus J, Woodings S, Kok JGM, Van Asselen B, Smit K, Bel A, Lagendijk JJW, Raaymakers BW. Performance of a cylindrical diode array for use in a 1.5 T MR-linac. Phys Med Biol. 2016;61:N80.
36. Smit K, Kok JGM, Lagendijk JJW, Raaymakers BW. Performance of a multi-axis ionization chamber array in a 1.5 T magnetic field. Phys Med Biol. 2014a;59:1845–50.
37. Smit K, Sjöholm J, Kok JGM, Lagendijk JJW, Raaymakers BW. Towards reference dosimetry for the MR-linac: magnetic field correction of the ionization chamber reading. Phys Med Biol. 2014b;58:5945–57.
38. De Vries JHW, Seravalli E, Houweling AC, Woodings SJ, Van Rooij R, Wolthaus JWH, Lagendijk JJW, Raaymakers BW. Characterization of a prototype MR-compatible delta4 QA system in a 1.5 tesla MR-linac. Phys Med Biol. 2018;63:118–25.
39. Meijsing I, Raaymakers BW, Raaijmakers AJE, Kok JGM, Hogeweg L, Liu B, Lagendijk JJW. Dosimetry for the MRI accelerator: The impact of a magnetic field on the response of a farmer NE2571 ionization chamber. Phys Med Biol. 2009;54:2993–3002.
40. Smit K, Van Asselen B, Kok JGM, Aalbers AHL, Lagendijk JJW, Raaymakers BW. Towards reference dosimetry for the MR-linac: magnetic field correction of the ionization chamber reading. Phys Med Biol. 2013;58:5945–57.

41. O'Brien DJ, Dolan J, Pencea S, Schupp N, Sawakuchi GO. Relative dosimetry with an MR-linac: Response of ion chambers, diamond, and diode detectors for off-axis, depth dose, and output factor measurements: response. Med Phys. 2018;45:884–97.
42. Lehmann J, Beveridge T, Oliver C, Bailey TE, Lye JE, Livingstone J, Stevenson AW, Butler DJ. Impact of magnetic fields on dose measurement with small ion chambers illustrated in high-resolution response maps. Med Phys. 2019;46:3298–305.
43. Malkov VN, Rogers DWO. Sensitive volume effects on Monte Carlo calculated ion chamber response in magnetic fields. Med Phys. 2017;44:4854–8.
44. O'Brien DJ, Schupp N, Pencea S, Dolan J, Sawakuchi GO. Dosimetry in the presence of strong magnetic fields. J Phys Conf Ser. 2017;847:012055.
45. Perik TJ, Kaas JJ, Greilich S, Wolthaus JWH, Wittkamper FW. The characterization of a large multi-axis ionization chamber array in a 1.5 T MRI linac. Phys Med Biol. 2018;62:225007.
46. De Prez L, Woodings S, De Pooter J, Van Asselen B, Wolthaus J, Jansen B, Raaymakers B. Direct measurement of ion chamber correction factors, k Q and k B, in a 7 MV MRI-linac. Phys Med Biol. 2019b;64:223–32.
47. De Prez L, De Pooter J, Jansen B, Woodings S, Wolthaus J, Van Asselen B, Van Soest T, Kok J, Raaymakers B. Commissioning of a water calorimeter as a primary standard for absorbed dose to water in magnetic fields. Phys Med Biol. 2019a;64:102–18.
48. Billas I, Bouchard H, Gouldstone C, Duane S. The effect of magnetic field strength on the response of Gafchromic EBT-3 film. Radiother Oncol. 2018;64:212–20.
49. Malkov VN, Rogers DWO. Monte Carlo study of ionization chamber magnetic field correction factors as a function of angle and beam quality. Med Phys. 2018;45:908–25.
50. Reynolds M, Fallone BG, Rathee S. Technical Note: Ion chamber angular dependence in a magnetic field. Med Phys. 2013;44:4322–8.
51. Spindeldreier CK, Schrenk O, Bakenecker A, Kawrakow I, Burigo L, Karger CP, Greilich S, Pfaffenberger A. Radiation dosimetry in magnetic fields with Farmer-type ionization chambers: determination of magnetic field correction factors for different magnetic field strengths and field orientations. Phys Med Biol. 2017;62:6708–28.
52. Woodings SJ, van Asselen B, van Soest TL, de Prez LA, Lagendijk JJW, Raaymakers BW, Wolthaus JWH. Technical note: consistency of PTW30013 and FC65-G ion chamber magnetic field correction factors. Med Phys. 2019;46:3739–45.
53. Reynolds M, Rathee S, Fallone BG. Technical Note: Ion chamber angular dependence in a magnetic field. Med Phys. 2017;44:4322–8.
54. Billas I, Bouchard H, Oelfke U, Duane S. The effect of magnetic field strength on the response of Gafchromic EBT-3 film. Phys Med Biol. 2019;64:06NT03.
55. Van Zijp HM, Van Asselen B, Wolthaus JWH, Kok JMG, De Vries JHW, Ishakoglu K, Beld E, Lagendijk JJW, Raaymakers BW. Minimizing the magnetic field effect in MR-linac specific QA-tests: the use of electron dense materials. Phys Med Biol. 2016;61:N50–9.
56. Raaymakers BW, De Boer JCJ, Knox C, Crijns SPM, Smit K, Stam MK, Den Bosch MRV, Kok JGM, Lagendijk JJW. Integrated megavoltage portal imaging with a 1.5 T MRI linac. Phys Med Biol. 2011;56:331–40.
57. Torres-Xirau I, Olaciregui-Ruiz I, Baldvinsson G, Mijnheer BJ, Van Der Heide UA, Mans A. Characterization of the a-Si EPID in the unity MR-linac for dosimetric applications. Phys Med Biol. 2018;63:81–90.
58. Park JM, Shin KH, Kim J, Park S-Y, Jeon SH, Choi N, Kim JH, Wu H-G. Air–electron stream interactions during magnetic resonance IGRT: skin irradiation outside the treatment field during accelerated partial breast irradiation. Strahlenther Onkol. 2017;194:50–9.
59. Dawson LA, Ménard C. Imaging in radiation oncology: a perspective. Oncologist. 2010;15:338–49.
60. Calamante F, Ittermann B, Kanal E, Norris D. Recommended responsibilities for management of MR safety. J Magn Reson Imaging. 2016;44:1067–9.
61. Shellock FG, Crues JV. MRI bioeffects, safety and patient management. Los Angeles, CA: Biomedical Research Publishing Group; 2014.
62. Panych LP, Madore B. The physics of MRI safety. J Magn Reson Imaging. 2018;47:28–43.

63. Collins CM, Smith MB. Signal-to-noise ratio and absorbed power as functions of main magnetic field strength, and definition of "90°" RF pulse for the head in the birdcage coil. Magn Reson Med. 2001;45:684–91.
64. Doran SJ, Charles-Edwards L, Reinsberg SA, Leach MO. A complete distortion correction for MR images: I. Gradient warp correction. Phys Med Biol. 2005;50:1343–61.
65. Moerland MA, Beersma R, Bhagwandien R, Wijrdeman HK, Bakker CJG. Analysis and correction of geometric distortions in 1.5 T magnetic resonance images for use in radiotherapy treatment planning. Phys Med Biol. 1995;40:1651–64.
66. Walker A, Liney G, Metcalfe P, Holloway L. MRI distortion: Considerations for MRI based radiotherapy treatment planning. Australas. Phys Eng Sci Med. 2014;37:103–13.
67. Schakel T, Hoogduin JM, Terhaard CHJ, Philippens MEP. Technical Note: Diffusion-weighted MRI with minimal distortion in head-and-neck radiotherapy using a turbo spin echo acquisition method. Med Phys. 2017;44:4188–93.
68. Wu W, Miller KL. Image formation in diffusion MRI: a review of recent technical developments. J Magn Reson Imaging. 2017;46:646–62.
69. Adjeiwaah M, Bylund M, Lundman JA, Karlsson CT, Jonsson JH, Nyholm T. Quantifying the effect of 3t magnetic resonance imaging residual system distortions and patient-induced susceptibility distortions on radiation therapy treatment planning for prostate cancer. Int J Radiat Oncol Biol Phys. 2018;100:317–24.
70. Bieri O, Scheffler K. Fundamentals of balanced steady state free precession MRI. J Magn Reson Imaging. 2013;38:2–11.
71. Green OL, Rankine LJ, Cai B, Curcuru A, Kashani R, Rodriguez V, Li HH, Parikh PJ, Robinson CG, Olsen JR, Mutic S, Goddu SM, Santanam L. First clinical implementation of real-time, real anatomy tracking and radiation beam control. Med Phys. 2018;45:3728–40.
72. Tijssen RHN, Philippens MEP, Paulson ES, Glitzner M, Chugh B, Wetscherek A, Dubec M, Wang J, van der Heide UA. MRI commissioning of 1.5T MR-linac systems – a multi-institutional study. Radiother Oncol. 2019;132:114–20.
73. Borman PTS, Tijssen RHN, Bos C, Moonen CTW, Raaymakers BW, Glitzner M. Characterization of imaging latency for real-time MRI-guided radiotherapy. Phys Med Biol. 2018;63:155023.
74. Kawrakow I, Rogers DWO. The EGSnrc code system: monte carlo simulation of electron and photon transport. System. 2003;2001–3.
75. Salvat F, Fernández-Vera J, Sempau J. PENELOPE-2008: a code system for monte carlo simulation of electron and photon transport. Work Proc. 2009;324.
76. Agostinelli S, Allison J, Amako K, Apostolakis J, Araujo H, Arce P, Asai M, Axen D, Banerjee S, Barrand G, Behner F, Bellagamba L, Boudreau J, Broglia L, Brunengo A, Burkhardt H, Chauvie S, Chuma J, Chytracek R, Cooperman G, Cosmo G, Degtyarenko P, Dell'Acqua A, Depaola G, Dietrich D, Enami R, Feliciello A, Ferguson C, Fesefeldt H, Folger G, Foppiano F, Forti A, Garelli S, Giani S, Giannitrapani R, Gibin D, Gomez Cadenas JJ, Gonzalez I, Gracia Abril G, Greeniaus G, Greiner W, Grichine V, Grossheim A, Guatelli S, Gumplinger P, Hamatsu R, Hashimoto K, Hasui H, Heikkinen A, Howard A, Ivanchenko V, Johnson A, Jones FW, Kallenbach J, Kanaya N, Kawabata M, Kawabata Y, Kawaguti M, Kelner S, Kent P, Kimura A, Kodama T, Kokoulin R, Kossov M, Kurashige H, Lamanna E, Lampen T, Lara V, Lefebure V, Lei F, Liendl M, Lockman W, Longo F, Magni S, Maire M, Medernach E, Minamimoto K, Mora de Freitas P, Morita Y, Murakami K, Nagamatu M, Nartallo R, Nieminen P, Nishimura T, Ohtsubo K, Okamura M, O'Neale S, Oohata Y, Paech K, Perl J, Pfeiffer A, Pia MG, Ranjard F, Rybin A, Sadilov S, di Salvo E, Santin G, Sasaki T, Savvas N, Sawada Y, Scherer S, Sei S, Sirotenko V, Smith D, Starkov N, Stoecker H, Sulkimo J, Takahata M, Tanaka S, Tcherniaev E, Safai Tehrani E, Tropeano M, Truscott P, Uno H, Urban L, Urban P, Verderi M, Walkden A, Wander W, Weber H, Wellisch JP, Wenaus T, Williams DC, Wright D, Yamada T, Yoshida H, Zschiesche D. GEANT4 - A simulation toolkit, nucl instruments methods phys res sect a accel spectrometers. Detect Assoc Equip. 2003;506:250–303.
77. Hissoiny S, Ozell B, Bouchard H, Despfs P. GPUMCD: a new GPU-oriented monte carlo dose calculation platform. Med Phys. 2011a;38:754–64.

78. Sempau J, Wilderman SJ, Bielajew AF. DPM, a fast, accurate monte carlo code optimized for photon and electron radiotherapy treatment planning dose calculations. Phys Med Biol. 2000;45:2263–91.
79. Hissoiny S, Raaijmakers AJE, Ozell B, Després P, Raaymakers BW. Fast dose calculation in magnetic fields with GPUMCD. Phys Med Biol. 2011b;56:5119–29.
80. Kawrakow I, Fippel M. Investigation of variance reduction techniques for Monte Carlo photon dose calculation using XVMC. Phys Med Biol. 2000;45:2163–83.
81. Tetar SU, Bruynzeel AME, Lagerwaard FJ, Slotman BJ, Bohoudi O, Palacios MA. Clinical implementation of magnetic resonance imaging guided adaptive radiotherapy for localized prostate cancer. Phys Imaging Radiat Oncol. 2019;9:69–76.
82. Werensteijn-Honingh AM, Kroon PS, Winkel D, Aalbers EM, van Asselen B, Bol GH, Brown KJ, Eppinga WSC, van Es CA, Glitzner M, de Groot-van Breugel EN, Hackett SL, Intven M, Kok JGM, Kontaxis C, Kotte AN, Lagendijk JJW, Philippens MEP, Tijssen RHN, Wolthaus JWH, Woodings SJ, Raaymakers BW, Jürgenliemk-Schulz IM. Feasibility of stereotactic radiotherapy using a 1.5 T MR-linac: multi-fraction treatment of pelvic lymph node oligometastases. Radiother Oncol. 2019;34:50–54.
83. Winkel D, Bol GH, Werensteijn-Honingh AM, Kiekebosch IH, van Asselen B, Intven MPW, Eppinga WSC, Raaymakers BW, Jürgenliemk-Schulz IM, Kroon PS. Evaluation of plan adaptation strategies for stereotactic radiotherapy of lymph node oligometastases using online magnetic resonance image guidance. Phys Imaging Radiat Oncol. 2019;9:58–64.
84. Wang Y, Mazur TR, Park JC, Yang D, Mutic S, Harold Li H. Development of a fast Monte Carlo dose calculation system for online adaptive radiation therapy quality assurance. Phys Med Biol. 2017;62:4970–90.
85. Chen X, Ahunbay E, Paulson ES, Chen G, Li XA. A daily end-to-end quality assurance workflow for MR-guided online adaptive radiation therapy on MR-Linac. J Appl Clin Med Phys. 2020;21:205–12.
86. Agnew A, Agnew CE, Grattan MWD, Hounsell AR, McGarry CK. Monitoring daily MLC positional errors using trajectory log files and EPID measurements for IMRT and VMAT deliveries. Phys Med Biol. 2014;59.
87. Dinesh Kumar M, Thirumavalavan N, Venugopal Krishna D, Babaiah M. QA of intensity-modulated beams using dynamic MLC log files. J Med Phys. 2006;31:36–41.
88. Teke T, Bergman AM, Kwa W, Gill B, Duzenli C, Popescu IA. Monte carlo based, patient-specific rapidarc qa using linac log files. Med Phys. 2010;37:116–23.
89. Li HH, Rodriguez VL, Green OL, Hu Y, Kashani R, Wooten HO, Yang D, Mutic S. Patient-specific quality assurance for the delivery of60Co intensity modulated radiation therapy subject to a 0.35-T lateral magnetic field. Int J Radiat Oncol Biol Phys. 2015;91:65–72.
90. Denis De Senneville B, Zachiu C, Ries M, Moonen C. EVolution: An edge-based variational method for non-rigid multi-modal image registration. Phys Med Biol. 2016;61:7377.
91. Heinrich MP, Jenkinson M, Bhushan M, Matin T, Gleeson FV, Brady SM, Schnabel JA. MIND: Modality independent neighbourhood descriptor for multi-modal deformable registration. Med Image Anal. 2012;16:1423–35.
92. Lamb J, Cao M, Kishan A, Agazaryan N, Thomas DH, Shaverdian N, Yang Y, Ray S, Low DA, Raldow A, Steinberg ML, Lee P. Online adaptive radiation therapy: implementation of a new process of care. Cureus. 2017;9:e1618.
93. Beasley WJ, McWilliam A, Slevin NJ, Mackay RI, Van Herk M. An automated workflow for patient-specific quality control of contour propagation. Phys Med Biol. 2016;61:8577–86.
94. Liang F, Qian P, Su KH, Baydoun A, Leisser A, Van Hedent S, Kuo JW, Zhao K, Parikh P, Lu Y, Traughber BJ, Muzic RF. Abdominal, multi-organ, auto-contouring method for online adaptive magnetic resonance guided radiotherapy: an intelligent, multi-level fusion approach. Artif Intell Med. 2018;90:34–41.
95. Lustberg T, van Soest J, Gooding M, Peressutti D, Aljabar P, van der Stoep J, van Elmpt W, Dekker A. Clinical evaluation of atlas and deep learning based automatic contouring for lung cancer. Radiother Oncol. 2018;126:312–7.

96. Vaassen F, Hazelaar C, Vaniqui A, Gooding M, van der Heyden B, Canters R, van Elmpt W. Evaluation of measures for assessing time-saving of automatic organ-at-risk segmentation in radiotherapy. Phys Imaging Radiat Oncol. 2020;13:1–6.
97. Ahunbay EE, Peng C, Chen GP, Narayanan S, Yu C, Lawton C, Li XA. An on-line replanning scheme for interfractional variations. Med Phys. 2008;35:3607–15.
98. Ahunbay EE, Peng C, Holmes S, Godley A, Lawton C, Li XA. Online adaptive replanning method for prostate radiotherapy. Int J Radiat Oncol Biol Phys. 2010;77:1561–72.
99. Li T, Wu Q, Zhang Y, Vergalasova I, Lee WR, Yin FF, Wu QJ. Strategies for automatic online treatment plan reoptimization using clinical treatment planning system: a planning parameters study. Med Phys. 2013;40:11.
100. van Herk M, McWilliam A, Dubec M, Faivre-Finn C, Choudhury A. Magnetic resonance imaging–guided radiation therapy: a short strengths, weaknesses, opportunities, and threats analysis. Int J Radiat Oncol Biol Phys. 2018;101:1057–60.
101. Coolens C, White MJ, Crum WR, Charles-Edwards L, O'Neill B, Tait D, Hawkins M. Feasibility of free-breathing respiratory gated liver radiotherapy with mri-derived models. Clin Oncol. 2007;19:S13.
102. Kirilova A, Lockwood G, Choi P, Bana N, Haider MA, Brock KK, Eccles C, Dawson LA. Three-dimensional motion of liver tumors using cine-magnetic resonance imaging. Int J Radiat Oncol Biol Phys. 2008;71:1189–95.
103. van Sörnsen de Koste JR, Palacios MA, Bruynzeel AME, Slotman BJ, Senan S, Lagerwaard FJ. Gated stereotactic radiation therapy delivery for lung, adrenal, and pancreatic tumors: a geometric analysis. Int J Radiat Oncol Biol Phys. 2018;02:858–66.
104. Crijns SPM, Kok JGM, Lagendijk JJW, Raaymakers BW. Towards mri-guided linear accelerator control: gating on an MRI accelerator. Phys Med Biol. 2011;56:4815–25.
105. Crijns SPM, Raaymakers BW, Lagendijk JJW. Proof of concept of MRI-guided tracked radiation delivery: tracking one-dimensional motion. Phys Med Biol. 2012;57:7863–72.
106. Yun J, Wachowicz K, Mackenzie M, Rathee S, Robinson D, Fallone BG. First demonstration of intrafractional tumor-tracked irradiation using 2D phantom MR images on a prototype linac-MR. Med Phys. 2013;40.
107. Fast MF, Nill S, Bedford JL, Oelfke U. Dynamic tumor tracking using the elekta agility MLC. Med Phys. 2014;40.
108. Menten MJ, Fast MF, Nill S, Kamerling CP, McDonald F, Oelfke U. Lung stereotactic body radiotherapy with an MR-linac – quantifying the impact of the magnetic field and real-time tumor tracking the impact of a magnetic field and real-time MLC tumor tracking on lung SBRT. Radiother Oncol. 2016;119:461–6.
109. Al-Ward S, Wronski M, Ahmad SB, Myrehaug S, Chu W, Sahgal A, Keller BM. The radiobiological impact of motion tracking of liver, pancreas and kidney SBRT tumors in a MR-linac. Phys Med Biol. 2018;63.
110. Lagerwaard F, Bohoudi O, Tetar S, Admiraal MA, Rosario TS, Bruynzeel A. Combined inter- and intrafractional plan adaptation using fraction partitioning in magnetic resonance-guided radiotherapy delivery. Cureus. 2018;10:e2434.
111. Zou W, Dong L, Kevin Teo BK. Current state of image guidance in radiation oncology: implications for PTV margin expansion and adaptive therapy. Semin Radiat Oncol. 2018;28:238–47.
112. Bainbridge HE, Menten MJ, Fast MF, Nill S, Oelfke U, McDonald F. Treating locally advanced lung cancer with a 1.5 T MR-linac – effects of the magnetic field and irradiation geometry on conventionally fractionated and isotoxic dose-escalated radiotherapy. Radiother Oncol. 2017;25:280–5.
113. Henke LE, Kashani R, Hilliard J, DeWees TA, Curcuru A, Przybysz D, Green O, Robinson CG, Bradley JD. In silico trial of mr-guided midtreatment adaptive planning for hypofractionated stereotactic radiation therapy in centrally located thoracic tumors. Int J Radiat Oncol Biol Phys. 2018;102:987–95.
114. Padgett KR, Simpson GN, Llorente R, Samuels MA, Dogan N. Feasibility of adaptive mr-guided stereotactic body radiotherapy (SBRT) of lung tumors. Cureus. 2018;10:e2423.

MR-Integrated Linear Accelerators: First Clinical Results

7

Olga Pen, Borna Maraghechi, Lauren Henke,
and Olga Green

7.1 Introduction

Harold Johns from Ontario Cancer Institute once said, "If you can't see it, you can't hit it, and if you can't hit it, you can't cure it". No truer words have been spoken in the world of radiation therapy when it comes to cancer, and the paradigm of improving the imaging techniques as the means of narrowing down the target that needs to be irradiated in order to reliably cure cancer has been the moving force behind the invention of the adaptive treatment workflow. After all, by accounting for the changes in the patient's anatomy on the day-to-day basis, both the precise delivery of the maximum dose to the target with the simultaneous significant reduction of the dose to the surrounding tissue can be achieved, providing for both the reduced toxicity and a possibility of the dose escalation and shorter treatment times. The majority of the radiation treatment system employs computed tomography (CT)-based imaging in order to delineate the target and calculate the necessary radiation dose; however, it comes with certain limitations. Photon scattering has been long plaguing the quality of the CT images, providing for the poor contrast between the different soft tissues and necessitating the reliance on the implanted fiducial markers when considering the target for adaptive treatment prospects. Utilizing other imaging modalities might prove to the key to solving that particular problem, with magnetic resonance imaging (MRI) in particular coming to mind as a versatile tool in providing us with deeper information about the soft tissue contrast. Currently, there are several commercially available linear accelerator (LINAC) systems incorporating

O. Pen (✉)
Atrium Health, Huntersville, NC, USA

Washington University in St Louis, St Louis, MO, USA

B. Maraghechi · L. Henke · O. Green
Washington University in St Louis, St Louis, MO, USA
e-mail: borna.maraghechi@wustl.edu; henke.lauren@wustl.edu; ogreen@wustl.edu

E. G. C. Troost (ed.), *Image-Guided High-Precision Radiotherapy*,
https://doi.org/10.1007/978-3-031-08601-4_7

an MRI scanner (MR-LINAC), with the magnetic field strength ranging from 0.35 Tesla (T) to 1.5 T (see Chap. 6). Lower magnetic strength allows for the normal operation of linear accelerator, preventing the electron path distortion and allowing for a precise calculation of the radiation dose; however, it inevitably affects the image quality. A compromise must be reached so that the image quality is still sufficient for the purpose of target and organs-at-risk (OAR) delineation in real time, allowing for fraction-to-fraction adaptation with patient never leaving the treatment table while the new plan based on the day-to-day anatomical variation is devised. Several problems need to be solved in order to make it a possibility, with key elements of the adaptive treatment being subdivided into imaging, assessment, replanning, and quality assurance. Overall the workflow of the adaptive radiation treatment can be summarized by the following diagram [1] (Fig. 7.1).

When it comes to imaging, the problem can be further subdivided into the image quality assurance in general and ensuring the imaging suitability for the purposes of the adaptive treatment in particular. For instance, gating is a powerful tool that allows to incorporate the natural breathing pattern and associated anatomical variations and target movement. Incorporating the gating capabilities in the operation of MR-LINAC is an important step of making the adaptive treatment a reality. Significant effort is devoted to develop real-time three-dimensional MRI techniques that minimize the imaging latency and allow decreasing the computational time required to adapt the treatment pattern to the current anatomy. One of the unique challenges of the adaptive radiation treatment is the need to immobilize patient for the duration of the full workflow, which can be further exacerbated by the claustrophobia and discomfort associated with the extremely limited space inside the MR-LINAC bore. Thus, the imaging strategy has to be robust in order to account for patient's involuntary movement [2].

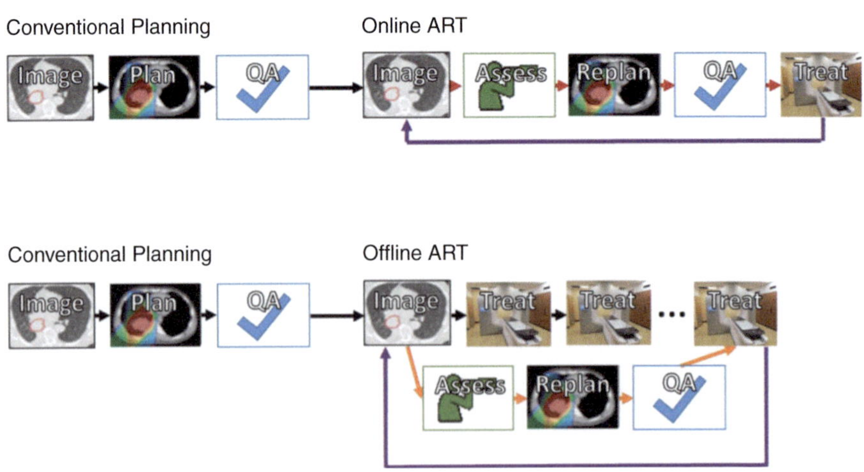

Fig. 7.1 Adaptive workflow—online and offline [1]. Image used with permission

The next question to be considered when devising the strategy for online adaptive treatment with the use on MR-LINAC is the exact imaging technique to use for the target and OAR assessment to determine if radiation treatment adaptation is even required. A wide variety of different sequences exist in the world of diagnostic MRI; however, due to the time constraints, not all of them are well adapted for the time-constrained environment of the online adaptive radiation therapy. The common techniques used these days include T1- and T2-weighted images, dynamic contrast-enhanced MRI for vasculature visualization, chemical effect saturation transfer (CEST) MRI for mobile protein and peptide content, as well as tumor hypoxia tracing, diffusion-weighted imaging, as well as many other less common modalities [3]. As of this moment, however, T1- and T2-weighted images remain to be most commonly used for the purposes of radiation treatment adaptation, though that might change as the technology of image acquisition and reconstruction continues to improve. The emergence of radiogenomics and imaging genomics is also a developing field that might be particularly helpful in the future with devising the adaptive radiation treatment for patients with glioblastoma, as well as other sites, as the field continues to develop. MRI fingerprinting for the multiple biomarker mapping might become a reality in the nearest future.

When it comes to replanning, several unique challenges arise. One such concern specific to radiation treatment in MR-LINACs in particular is the electron return effect that adds to the computational burden when assessing the dose at the interface of the tissues with highly varying electron densities. Monte Carlo simulation solution seems to be the most accurate from the calculation algorithms currently present on the market; however, the time constraints are imminent when considering the MR-LINAC application for the online adaptive radiation treatment, and not as much time can be devoted to recalculating the dose and optimizing the multileaf collimator (MLC) leaf pattern as would be common for the offline radiation treatment planning.

The real-time quality assurance has to rely on the extensive use of the Monte Carlo simulation as well as the customary dose measurement common to the intensity-modulated radiation therapy (IMRT)-based treatment is unavailable with the adaptive treatment workflow. Portal dosimetry and exit dose analysis, as well as extensive machine logs, become an absolute necessity.

7.2 Clinical Sites

All of these challenges contribute to the necessity to improve and develop better adaptive treatment protocols and strategies. Nevertheless, the movement to use MR-LINACs for adaptive treatment is gaining momentum in the field of radiation oncology, with new reports of a successful implementation appearing in the literature. Numerous clinical trials are being conducted on various anatomical sites to assess the suitability of using the MRI-guided adaptive radiation treatment at this moment, and summary of some of these trials and clinical cases is presented in this chapter in the form of review on site-by-site basis [1, 4].

7.2.1 Brain and Spine

Radiation treatment is a common strategy for dealing with the tumors of the central nervous system in general and brain tumors in particular. Both primary and metastatic tumors of the brain have long been benefiting from MRI imaging for target delineation and OAR sparing. MRI scan obtained via a diagnostic scanner is typically registered to the CT scan via bony anatomy with high degree of confidence and can then be used for contouring. As the target is unlikely to move within the rigid structure of the brain, the most common consideration for the need for the adaptive treatment comes from the target size change postresection, if a significant time has passed between the diagnostic scan and the day of treatment, or the target size assessment of the fraction to fraction basis in case of multifraction stereotactic body radiotherapy (SBRT; typically 3–5 fractions; fx). Mehta et al. [5] present a study on several cases of grade 4 glioblastoma patients postresection, with the changes of the resection cavity size, tumor volume and cerebral edema being tracked via MR-LINAC imaging capabilities. The daily decrease in the cavity measurement was observed in all patients and was significant enough to justify the additional costs of the adaptive treatment for the improved tumor control and toxicity decrease. These results are consistent with results previously obtained with the help of diagnostic MRI scans mid-treatment by Tsien et al. [6], Shukla et al. [7], and Yang et al. [8]. Another study was performed by Maziero et al. [9] on conventionally fractionated RT conducted on MR-LINAC with the MRgRT (MR-guided radiotherapy) scans obtained to identify serious pathologies and edema changes during the course of treatment, highlighting the evolution in the tumor volume following the course of radiation treatment and providing recommendations for gross tumor volume (GTV) adaptation. The authors discuss the possibility of physiologic adaptive radiotherapy as the future venue for the treatment of brain tumors. In addition, a presentation of the cases of the spine adaptive treatment, with a focus on bowel OAR migration, has been presented. Another study by Spieler et al. [10] also presents the cases of the SBRT treatment of the spinal metastases conducted on 0.35 T MRI-RT Co-60 system. In addition to the advantages of more precise target delineation and OAR sparing, authors noted that MR-LINAC-generated images had the additional advantages of using the low-field MRI to mitigate the magnetic susceptibility artifacts caused by the spinal hardware.

7.2.2 Head and Neck

The first studies related to the use of MR-LINAC on head and neck patients date back to 2016, when six patients were observed during the course of IMRT treatment by Raghavan et al. [11]. At that time, the pretreatment MRIs on selected fractions were performed and the changes in the GTV and parotid glands were delineated. A significant shrinkage of GTV and parotid gland volume was observed, establishing the need for the treatment planning adaptation in the future. In 2017, a more thorough clinical trial involving the use of the Co-60 Viewray MR-LINAC on head and neck patients was performed by Chen et al. [12]. At that time, 18 patients received the standard IMRT radiation courses with the target and OAR delineation being manually adjusted by the attending physician on the day-to-day basis. Two of the patients also had functional MRI data obtained via diffusion-weighted sequences on a weekly basis. All of the patients were followed up for 18-month postcompletion, with positron emission tomography (PET) scans obtained approximately 3-months postcompletion, and quality of life assessments performed periodically. All of the patients demonstrated the treatment results comparable to one with the conventional IMRT treatment, with quality of life being rated either very good or outstanding for 70% of the patients, thus validating the feasibility of the MR-guided radiation therapy [12]. This study was followed by several other studies exploring different aspects of the adaptive treatment planning and delivery process when performed on the head and neck cases. A study performed by Chamberlain et al. [13] established that increasing the number of segments and beams increased the dose conformality without prolonging the overall treatment time. A study by Gurney-Champion et al. [14] helped to determine the extent of the 3D intrafractional motion of the head and neck patients to determine the effect of the increased treatment time for the adaptive treatment on the patient's ability to retain the position for the minimal movement of the tumor. The results of the assessment showed that both the systematic and random motions were well within the clinical safety margins. Another study to determine the radiation treatment margins for head and neck tumors was performed by Bruijen et al. [15]. A first adaptive radiation treatment study using 1.5 T Elekta Unity MR-LINAC was performed by McDonald et al. [16] and confirmed the feasibility of the previously established margins. At that time, 10 patients received treatment. Seven patients received at least one treatment with the backup plan on a conventional LINAC owing to the machine downtime or admittance to inpatient facilities. All patients were treated with online adaptive treatment workflow. Doses to all OARs were consistent between the reference plan and summation plan. Significant tumor shrinkage, weight loss, and anatomical deformations were observed but were able to be accounted for with the use of adaptive treatment workflow. Parotid glands and spinal cord were specifically benefited from the treatment adaptation. Treatment times were less than an hour in 91% of the cases. These results were consisted with the similar online adaptation workflow results performed on the ViewRay 0.35 T MR-LINAC. Several other studies are currently being performed in order to establish the protocols for safe dose reduction without the sacrifice in tumor control.

7.2.3 Thoracic Tumors

The thoracic region presents unique challenges when it comes to MRI. The respiratory motion introduces an uncertainty that often requires increased planning target volume (PTV) margins, and the variability of the anatomy in the region on the day-to-day basis introduces the possibility of the high degree of toxicity. Technical challenges and solutions associated with MR-guided radiation treatment in the thorax include, e.g., low proton density in the lungs producing low MR signal, respiratory and cardiac motion during image acquisition, lack of intrinsic electron density information requiring bulk overrides for the synthetic CT generation, electron return effect being especially pronounced at air-tissue interfaces, and physiological motion during patient setup and treatment. Breath hold imaging, 4D-MRI, gating, and tracking become paramount in order to ensure the tight margins of the PTV and OAR sparing, especially in the cases of the tumors located in the central portion of the thoracic cavity.

Lung tumors have long been a target of SBRT-type treatment that requires increasingly precise delineation of the target and OARs. For instance, the suitability of using the stereotactic magnetic-resonance-guided radiation therapy (SMART) has been investigated by Finazzi et al. [17] on 25 patients with centrally located lung tumors where soft tissue delineation is especially important due to proximity of the heart, esophagus, bronchial tree, and major vessels. MRIdian ViewRay 0.35 T LINAC has been used in these studies. Before each fraction, a breath-hold 3D MR scan was acquired to define the anatomy of the day. The registration would be performed and the physician could then adjust the GTV and the OAR contours as needed. Online plans were reoptimized with the MRIdian planning software using the same beam parameters and optimization objectives. In 92% of cases, the physician chose to proceed with the adapted plans. Treatment delivery occurred during the breath-holds. The optimized plans provided clinically meaningful improvement in the PTV coverage and were able to avoid high doses in the stomach, vertebral bodies, and brachial plexus. PTV dose escalation with the simultaneous OAR sparing was feasible with the provided SMART workflow. A longer study performed by the same group on 54 patients was followed up by 2-year observation period [18]. The use of the SMART workflow did not compromise the tumor control while significantly reducing the toxicity of the treatment, including for patients with previous radiation treatment or resection. No high-grade bronchial toxicity common for the patients with central lung tumor was observed. Much smaller tumor volumes could be used. The results were used to devise a single fraction stereotactic ablative body radiotherapy (SABR) approach for early stage cancer [19]. Ten patients were selected for the study. On the day of treatment, the GTV contours were adjusted by the physicians. On mid-treatment 3D-MR scans, the plans were reoptimized in order to better control dose to the OARs and decrease the hotspot. The patients were observed for 1-year post-SABR, with one patient developing a myocardial infraction. For the remaining nine patients, no grade 3–5 toxicities (according to Common Terminology Criteria for Adverse Effects; CTCAE) and no local recurrences have been observed. Similar results were observed for a single fraction 34 Gy SBRT treatment performed by Chuong et al. [20]. When it comes to Elekta Unity MR-Linac system, Winkel et al. [21] performed a study on 10 patients with ultracentral tumors treated with a hypofractionated schema of 60 Gy in 8–12 fx. All treatments have been well tolerated by patients. A summary of the clinical experience to date has been presented by Crockett et al. [22] (Table 7.1):

The heart provides an even harder target to irradiate as the rapid nature of the human heartbeat makes gating difficult. Nevertheless, several groups have made the attempts to utilize MRI-guided radiation therapy for the treatment of various conditions of the heart. For instance, Pomp et al. [28] report the treatment of the sarcoma

Table 7.1 MRgRT of primary lung tumors and pulmonary metastases, clinical experience to date

Team	Machine	No. of patients	Tumor location	Fractionation schedule	Adaptation	Gating/tracking	Couch time (min)
Thomas et al. [23]	MRIdian Cobalt-60	5	Peripheral and central	50–54 Gy/3–4 fx	NR	Tracking	>20
Padgett et al. [24]	MRIdian Cobalt-60	3 (one primary lung)	Peripheral	50 Gy/5 fx	To anatomy	NR	NR
De Costa et al. [25]	MRIdian Cobalt-60	14 (11 primary lung)	NR	40–50 Gy/5 fx	NR	Both	NR
Henke et al. [26]	MRIdian Cobalt-60	5 (one primary lung)	Ultra-central	50 Gy/5 fx	To anatomy	Gating	Median = 69
Finazzi et al. [27]	MRIdian Cobalt-60 or MR-Linac	23 (25 tumors, 14 primary lung)	Peripheral	54–60 Gy/3–8 fx	To anatomy	Gating	Median Cobalt-60 = 62; MR-Linac = 48
Finazzi et al. [19]	MRIdian MR-Linac	10 (eight primary lung)	Peripheral	34 Gy/1 fx	To anatomy	Both	Median = 120 min
Finazzi et al. [18]	MRIdian Cobalt-60 or MRI Linac	50 (29 primary lung)	Peripheral and central	54–60 Gy/3–12 fx	To anatomy	Both	Median Cobalt-60 = 60; MR-Linac = 49
Lung metastases							
Henke et al. [26]	MRIdian Cobalt-60	5 (four oligometastases)	Ultra-central	50 Gy/5 fx	To anatomy	Gating	Median = 69
Finazzi et al. [27]	MRIdian Cobalt-60 or MR- Linac	23 (25 tumors, 11 oligometastases)	Peripheral	54–60 Gy/3–8 fx	To anatomy	Gating	Median Cobalt-60 = 62, MR-Linac = 48
Finazzi et al. [19]	MRIdian MR-Linac	10 (two oligometastases)	Peripheral	34 Gy/1 fx	To anatomy	Both	Median = 120
Finazzi et al. [18]	MRIdian Cobalt-60 or MRI Linac	50 (21 oligometastases)	Peripheral and central	54–60 Gy/3–12 fx	To anatomy	Both	Median Cobalt-60 = 60; MR-Linac = 49

Adapted from: Crockett, C. B., Samson, P., Chuter, R., Dubec, M., Faivre-Finn, C., Green, O. L., & Cobben, D. (2021). Initial clinical experience of MR-guided radiotherapy (MRgRT) for nonsmall cell lung cancer (NSCLC). Frontiers in Oncology, 11, 157 of the heart. The patient had already experienced recurrent strokes and a cardiac surgery before the radiation treatment took place to control a recurrent nonresectable tumor. As only the portion of the heart containing tumor was irradiated, the remaining healthy heart, along with lungs, esophagus, and bronchi were treated as OARs. SBRT-type treatment with 60 Gy delivered in 12 fx with online adaptation was performed and well tolerated. Another case study was described by Gach et al. [29]. The patient in question had cardiac fibroma, as well as an implantable cardioverter defibrillator, making treatment planning and delivery an additional challenge. The patient had an MR-compatible Medtronic Evera Surescan ICD, and, according to the cardiologist assessment, was not device-dependent, presenting standard medium-risk. All the MRI conditions were confirmed with a vendor, with all of them being met with the exception of the use of the device in the presence of the 0.35-T magnetic field, as the device was tested in 1.5-T field conditions. The off-label use of the device was assessed by the medical physicist and discussed with the patient, and several adjustments to the device operation mode were made based on vendor's recommendations. The presence of the ICD on the MR images caused null band artifacts that ran through the heart. Nevertheless, the attending physician was able to successfully identify the target and make the GTV adjustments as needed for the gating purposes. The patient reported no pain during the treatment and was not in cardiac distress. The device appeared to be undamaged by the MRI scans or the radiation.

A separate study was presented by Sim et al. [30] where the MR-guided radiation therapy was considered for the treatment of intracardiac and pericardial metastases. Five patients were selected for the study, including two with pre-existent cardiac disease. SBRT-type treatment with 40–50 Gy delivered over the course of 5 fx was prescribed. In this scenario, the representative slice of the lesion was contoured on each day and used for the gating purposes. No plan adaptation was used for the patients. All symptomatic patients experienced some relief postirradiation, and there were no acute adverse effects; however, one of the patients without prior cardiac disease ended up developing atrial defibrillation 6 months after treatment. An adaptation of the treatment plan was considered to be a viable plan as a result of the study based on the observed workflow.

Esophageal tumors in the thoracic cavity also present a unique challenge. Boekhoff et al. [31] discuss the reduction of the dose to the heart, large vessels, trachea, bronchial tree, and lungs with the help of the adaptive MR-guided radiation therapy on a study consisting of 32 patients with the esophageal cancers. This study did not contain any cases of the prior irradiation and surgery. Daily GTV changes were evaluated based on the acquired on-board MR imaging. Considerable day-to-day shape changes of the clinical target volume (CTV) were observed. The target coverage was most often compromised on the distal part of the CTV, near the gastroesophageal junction and into the cardia. The changes could not be accounted for by translation and rotation only, and required on-table adaptive workflow with daily regeneration of the new plans. Winkel et al. [21] and Lee at al [32]. reach similar conclusion. In addition to the day-to-day positional variation of the location of the GTV and CTV, the esophageal cancer GTV tends to shrink significantly as the treatment progresses, with the tumors decreasing up to 28% by the fifth week, thus also necessitating the radiation treatment plan adjustment [33]. When it comes to respiratory gating management, lower esophageal tumors experience the largest range of motion associated with breathing pattern due to the proximity of the diaphragm.

7.2.4 Abdominal Tumors

Abdominal structures have long been a challenge to a traditional CT-based approach due to the low soft tissue contrast. MR-guided radiation treatment provides a unique opportunity to differentiate between the abdominal structures, allowing for the better OAR sparing and potential dose escalation to the mobile tumors in abdomen. Various treatment sites in the abdominal cavity have been considered for MR-guided radiation therapy, with liver and pancreas being the most attractive targets. Bohoudi et al. [34] suggested the adaptive workflow and evaluated the margins within which the recountouring was required in order to ensure the same or better OAR sparing and target control as with the full contouring, determining that a 3-cm ring around the PTV was sufficient for the clinical purposes for the abdominal targets. In their later publication, Bohoudi et al. [35] also presented the analysis of the criteria of patient selection for the adaptive radiation therapy. Plan adaptation appeared to be relevant mainly in cases where the GTV to adjacent OAR distance was <3 mm. These criteria were evaluated on the example of pancreatic cancer but were later adopted as a strategy for all abdominal cancers. One of the earliest studies has been conducted by Henke et al. [36] in 2017 on the MRIdian ViewRay Linac system. Twenty patients with oligometastatic or unresectable primary abdominal malignancies, including 10 patients with liver tumors, and 10 patients with nonliver tumors, received 50 Gy in 5 fx, with each fraction following the adapt-to-shape workflow that allowed for the complete plan adaptation based on the daily anatomy variation. The patients were observed for 6 months, with zero grade 3 (acc. To CTCAE) acute treatment-related toxicities observed. Several years later, a similar study was repeated for the Elekta Unity MR-LINAC machine, this time with free-breathing abdominal SBRT [37]. Both adapt-to-shape and adapt-to-position workflows were considered. Due to software limitation, an offline Monaco system was used for adaptive plan generation in Adapt-To-Shape (ATS) workflow. Likewise, the study confirmed the feasibility of the MR-guided radiation therapy adaptive workflow for the abdominal cases. Palliative abdominal cases have also been at attractive target for the adaptive radiation therapy. Green et al. [38] presented a case of a nonsmall metastatic lung cancer patient who has experienced a gastrointestinal hemorrhage requiring transfusion. Patient was ineligible for surgery, and an urgent course of radiation treatment of 25 Gy in 5 fx was prescribed. Due to urgency, simulation and the first fraction of treatment occurred on the same day, with 30-min, free breathing, volumetric MRI being acquired and used as the primary planning image. Daily image acquisition and plan adaption based on the anatomy variation were conducted. After completion of the treatment, the patient reported resolution of melena, his hemoglobin improved without subsequent transfusion required, and no toxicity following 3 month was reported. Another case presented in the same report concerns an omental metastatic lesion with high degree of movement in extremely short periods of time. The CT scans taken in the morning and in the afternoon showed a different location of the lesion, and a decision has been made to perform an MRI simulation with a moving field of view from upper mid-abdomen to pelvis, and to adapt plan “on the fly”. The location of the nodule was finally identified, allowing to proceed with treatment. The lesion exhibited a significant change in the position throughout all five fractions, moving at least 2 cm a day (3 cm average) and had a maximum lateral movement of 5 cm. Thus, it would be nearly impossible to treat the patient without daily adaptation. One year after treatment completion, patient exhibited no further growth of the omental lesion and no acute or late abdominopelvic toxicities. Both of these cases presented the motion of the tumors far beyond the boundary of the commonly used PTVs, especially for SBRT-type treatment. Similar case was reported for a stomach cancer by Chun et al. [39]. Stomach is one of the most deforming organs due to respiratory motion and differences in food intake on day-to-day basis. A patient with multiple comorbidities, including end-stage renal disease and liver cirrhosis, and a history of prior distal gastrectomy thus presented a challenging case. Due to the high anatomical variability, daily adjustments of the target volume and OARs were required. The adaptive treatment process took less than 30 min overall. Patient only experienced CTCAE grade 1 nausea throughout the treatment sessions, and the tumor was nearly resolved on post real-time endoscopic evaluation.

An example of the typical isodose coverage for the abdominal tumor treatment is presented on the following figure (Fig. 7.2).

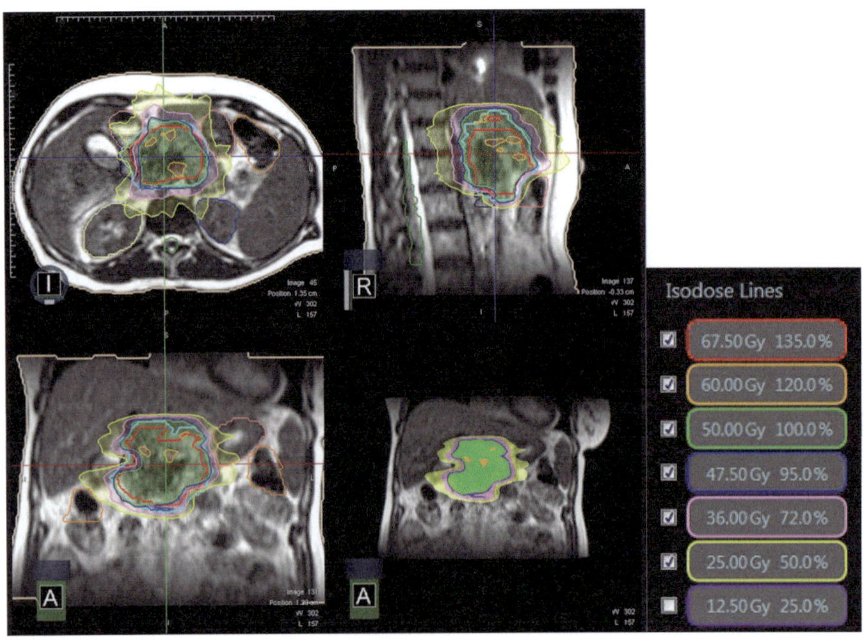

Fig. 7.2 Isodose lines of a radiation treatment plan for a pancreatic adenocarcinoma patient delivered on an MR-LINAC. The plan is depicted in transverse, sagittal, and frontal view, and isodose lines presented in various colors

As can be seen on Fig. 7.2, typical OARs of particular concern usually include duodenum, bowel, stomach, and kidneys. Spinal cord is usually less affected, but nevertheless care should be taken not to let the static beams go directly through the cord during the planning process.

When it comes to the particular organs, liver perhaps takes the lead of being the most common target for the adaptive treatment. For patient with compromised liver function, few local treatment options are available, with chemoembolization and radioembolization being highly dependent on the liver function and lung shunting percentage, with external radiation treatment being left as an only option. Numerous studies confirm the feasibility of using MR-guided radiation treatment for liver lesions, including hepatocellular carcinoma, cholangiosarcomas, metastasis of the neuroendocrine tumors, colorectal carcinomas, and gastrointestinal stroma tumors [40–44]. Boldrini et al. [45] provide a summary of the recent clinical studies on the role of MR-guided radiation therapy in various institutions (Table 7.2).

For the illustrative purposes, an example of the treatment plan for the tumor located in the liver is provided in Fig. 7.3.

Table 7.2 Recent clinical studies on the role of MRgRT in hepatic malignancies

Reference	Year	Dose	No. of patients	Response
Henke et al. [36]	2018	50 Gy/5 fx	Ten nonliver abdomen lesions, six MLL, four HCC	3 months LPFS 95%, 6 months LPFS 89.1%, 1 year OS 75%
Feldman et al. [42]	2019	45–50 Gy/5 fx	26 HCC, two cholangiocarcinoma	1 year LC 96.5%, 1 year OS 92.8%
Rosenberg et al. [43]	2019	Median dose 50 (30–60) Gy/3–5 fx	Six MLL, six HCC, 20 MLL	1 year OS 69%, 2 year OS 60%
Hal et al. [44]	2020	Median dose 45 (25–60 Gy)/3–5 fx	Three pancreatic cancer, two HCC, one pancreatic metastasis, four MLL	7.2 months LC 100%
Luterstein et al. [46]	2020	40 Gy/5 fx	17 cholangiocarcinoma	1 year OS 76%, 2 year OS 46.1%, 1 year LC 85.6%, 2 year LC 73.3%
Boldrini et al. [40]	2021	50–55 Gy/5 fx	Ten HCC	6.5 months LC 90%
ClinicalTrials.gov. NCT0424342 [47]	2019-recruiting	50–60 Gy/5–6 fx	46 primary or secondary liver tumors	2 year LC lack of progression according to RECIST criteria

Adapted from: Boldrini, L., Corradini, S., Gani, C., Henke, L., Hosni, A., Romano, A., & Dawson, L. (2021). MR-guided radiotherapy for liver malignancies. Frontiers in Oncology, 11, 1053

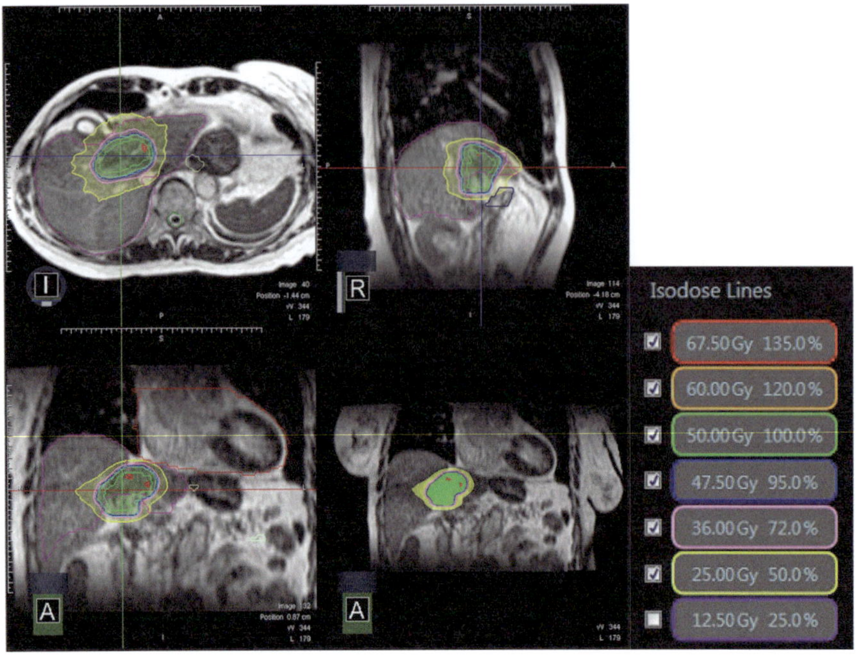

Fig. 7.3 Isodose lines of a radiation treatment plan for a liver tumor patient delivered on an MR-LINAC. The plan is depicted in transverse, sagittal, and frontal view, and isodose lines presented in various colors

An atlas of OAR contouring in the upper abdomen has been published by Lukovic et al. [48] to provide the reference for adaptive radiation therapy for liver malignancies. The use of contrast agents, especially gadoxetic acid, is especially advantageous as it highlights the liver, improving the contrast between healthy and tumorous tissue [49]. Superparamagnetic iron oxide (SPIO) also provides superior liver tumor contrast, particularly in 0.35 T field, as described by Hama et al. [50]. MR compatible fiducial markers, particularly platinum-based, might also be advantageous. In addition, various sequences can be used depending on the type of malignancy, as noted by Namasivayam et al. [51]. Will et al. [52] provide a thorough review of the current state of various approaches to the treatment of liver malignancies, highlighting the importance of the MRI-guided workflow with online adaptation in dose escalation and OAR sparing when facing large anatomical changes on the day-to-day basis. The reduction in toxicity due to online adaptation has been remarkable. In addition, authors suggest that the future venues of research might enable the use of learning neural networks to predict the probability of toxicity, extract the radiomic features, and thus reduce the need for biopsies, and, when combined with genetic factors and tumor microenvironment information, allow to customize radiation dose to different portions of the tumor and allow for prescription variation on the day-to-day basis.

Pancreas is another target of the adaptive radiation treatment that has been attracting a lot of attention in the recent years. Notoriously difficult to detect and often unresectable, it has long been characterized by high lethality and difficulties in finding a treatment approach. Decreased toxicity and improved accuracy offered by the adaptive MR-guided workflow provide a treatment solution to previously untreatable cases. Hassandazeh et al. [53] presented a study on 44 patients with inoperable pancreatic cancer treated over the course of five years (2014–2019) with 50 Gy in 5 fx. Majority of the patients had the tumor either abutting or invading the OARs. Late toxicity was limited to two grade 3 and three grade 2 (acc. to CTCAE) toxicities. Median overall survival was 15.7 months, with one-year local control reaching 84.3%. The minimization of toxicity allowed for significant dose escalation and improved tumor control. Similar results were reported by Rudra et al. [54], with higher overall survival being reported for patients with escalated dose regimen.

Adrenal and renal metastases are also a frequent target of MR-guided adaptive radiotherapy. In a study by Palacios et al. [55], 17 patients who were deemed poor candidates for a traditional surgical approach were evaluated, with plan adaptation required due to significant OAR displacement. Primary renal cell cancer treatment with the use of MR-guided adaptive radiation therapy has been reported by Rudra et al. [56], Tetar et al. [57], Kutuk et al. [58], with varying doses, all demonstrating good tumor control in addition to decreased toxicity to the OARs. This is consistent with the treatment results observed for other abdominal sites.

7.2.5 Pelvic Tumors

The anatomy of the pelvis, while undergoing less changes on the day-to-day basis than the abdominal cavity, and not susceptible to the breathing-induced movement, can nevertheless present a challenge for the daily positioning. Soft tissue contrast provided by the MR-based imaging allows for better target localization. Several sites have been considered for the feasibility of using MR-guided radiation therapy with adapted workflow, with prostate being the most promising candidate. Improved local control and decreased toxicity allow for hypofractionated treatment with a significant dose escalation. Bruynzeel et al. [59] presented one of the first comprehensive studies conducted on 101 patients with T1-3bN0M0 prostate cancer, with no fiducial markers implanted, requiring daily adaptation of the OARs and the PTV localization. Clinically comparable local control and significantly reduced GI toxicity were observed. Urethral sparing was particularly noticeable compared to the normal workflow. A later study on the same patient study was performed to investigate the possible late-term toxicity [60]. All of the urinary and bowel syndromes resolved within 12 months. The same group later investigated the drift of the extent of the intrafractional prostate drift, which was exhibited in 20% of the cases [61]. Similar results were reported by Mazolla et al. [62] for oligometastatic cancer. Several groups have attempted to implement MR-guided SBRT regimen, with the results summarized in the following table [63] (Table 7.3).

Table 7.3 Literature experience of MRgRT for prostate cancer

Author	No. of patients	MR-Linac device	Fractionation schedule	Endpoint of the study	Results
Alongi et al. [64]	20	Elekta Unity	35 Gy/5 fx	Dosimetric analysis and preliminary PROMs report	Hydrogel improves rectal sparing with minimal impact on QoL
Bruynzeel et al. [59]	101	ViewRay MRIdian	36.25 Gy/5 fx	Early toxicity analysis	G > 2 GU = 23.8%, ≥2 GI = 5%
Cuccia et al. [65]	20	Elekta Unity	35 Gy/5 fx	Assessment of the impact of rectal spacer on prostate motion	Significant impact on rotational antero-posterior shifts with consequently reduced prostate motion
Tetar et al. [60]	101	ViewRay MRIdian	36.25 Gy/5 fx	PROMs analysis	After one year, only 2.25 of cases reported relevant impact to daily activities due to GU toxicity
Nicosia et al. [66]	10	Elekta Unity	35 Gy/5 fx	Dosimetric comparison between MR-guided SBRT and conventional LINAC SBRT	MR-guided SBRT resulted in lower constraint violation rates
Sahin et al. [67]	24	ViewRay MRIdian	36.25 Gy/5 fx	Preliminary report of feasibility	Substantial feasibility of MR-adaptive SBRT with acceptable time schedules
Ugurluer at al [68]	50	ViewRay MRIdian	36.25 Gy/5 fx	Early toxicity analysis	Acute G2 GU = 28%, late G2 GU = 6%, late GI GU = 2%

Adapted from: Cuccia, F., Corradini, S., Mazzola, R., Spiazzi, L., Rigo, M., Bonù, M. L., ... & Alongi, F. (2021). MR-guided hypofractionated radiotherapy: current emerging data and promising perspectives for localized prostate cancer. Cancers, 13(8), 1791

The possibility of further margin reduction and single-shot treatment is currently being considered in prostate cancer. Possibility of the sexual function preservation might also become possible as the MR-guided radiation therapy provides a better sparing of the healthy tissue. This can also be an exciting prospect for the re-irradiation cases.

Cervical cancer can also benefit from MR-guided radiation therapy. Boldrini et al. [69] presented the first study conducted on eight patients that was compared to the results of the treatment on a conventional linear accelerator. A significant reduction in both gastrointestinal and genitourinary toxicities was observed for the patients undergoing MR-guided radiation treatment, with no difference in pathological response observed between the two groups. This is consistent with the results observed for prostate cancer treatment.

Ovarian cancer can also benefit from MR-guided radiation therapy. A study presented by Henke et al. [70] covers ten patients, initially prescribed 35 Gy in 5 fx, with dose escalation permitted subject to strict OAR dose constraints. Only a single grade 3 toxicity was observed. Local control at 3 months reached 94%.

Rectum is an organ that experiences significant day-to-day deformation, and rectal wall can also be difficult to trace exactly on the cone-beam computed tomography (CBCT). MRI provides better soft tissue contrast and enables exact GTV localization. While the speculation of the use of MR-guided workflow has been present in the literature, as of this moment, only one study has been presented. Chiloiro et al. [71] conducted a study on 22 patients with colorectal cancer, with 86% exhibiting nodal involvement. As a result of the therapy, five patients reached grade 3 gastrointestinal toxicity. No grade 3 hematologic or genitourinary toxicity was observed. Improved local tumor control was observed.

Bladder is another target that is susceptible to significant anatomical changes. In addition, MR imaging allows the visualization of the bladder muscle layer otherwise invisible on the CT. Hijab et al. [72] discuss the potential MR-guided adaptive workflow for bladder cancers, though as of this moment, no thorough study has been conducted on a patient set.

Overall, the MR-guided radiation therapy presents a promising venue for the exploration of new treatment regimens. Additional studies with a larger number of patients are being conducted on various sites across the world, and with MR-equipped linear accelerators becoming more and more widely spread, it can soon become a standard of care. New developments are highly anticipated in the upcoming years.

References

1. Green OL, Henke LE, Hugo GD. Practical clinical workflows for online and offline adaptive radiation therapy. Semin Radiat Oncol. 2019;29(3). WB Saunders
2. Hall WA, Paulson ES, van der Heide UA, Fuller CD, Raaymakers BW, Lagendijk JJ, et al. The transformation of radiation oncology using real-time magnetic resonance guidance: a review. Eur J Cancer. 2019;122:42–52.
3. Otazo R, Lambin P, Pignol JP, Ladd ME, Schlemmer HP, Baumann M, Hricak H. MRI-guided radiation therapy: an emerging paradigm in adaptive radiation oncology. Radiology. 2021;298(2):248–60.
4. Glide-Hurst CK, Lee P, Yock AD, Olsen JR, Cao M, Siddiqui F, et al. Adaptive radiation therapy (art) strategies and technical considerations: a state of the art review from nrg oncology. Int J Radiat Oncol Biol Phys. 2021;109(4):1054–75.
5. Mehta S, Gajjar SR, Padgett KR, Asher D, Stoyanova R, Ford JC, Mellon EA. Daily tracking of glioblastoma resection cavity, cerebral edema, and tumor volume with MRI-guided radiation therapy. Cureus. 2018;10(3):e2346.
6. Tsien C, Gomez-Hassan D, Ten Haken RK, Tatro D, Junck L, Chenevert TL, Lawrence T. Evaluating changes in tumor volume using magnetic resonance imaging during the course

of radiotherapy treatment of high-grade gliomas: implications for conformal dose-escalation studies. Int J Radiat Oncol Biol Phys. 2005;62(2):328–32.
7. Shukla D, Huilgol NG, Trivedi N, Mekala C. T2-weighted MRI in assessment of volume changes during radiotherapy of high-grade gliomas. J Cancer Res Ther. 2005;1(4):235.
8. Yang Z, Zhang Z, Wang X, Hu Y, Lyu Z, Huo L, et al. Intensity-modulated radiotherapy for gliomas: dosimetric effects of changes in gross tumor volume on organs at risk and healthy brain tissue. Onco Targets Ther. 2016;9:3545.
9. Maziero D, Straza MW, Ford JC, Bovi JA, Diwanji T, Stoyanova R, et al. MR-guided radiotherapy for brain and spine tumors. Front Oncol. 2021;11:600.
10. Spieler B, Samuels SE, Llorente R, Yechieli R, Ford JC, Mellon EA. Advantages of radiation therapy simulation with 0.35 tesla magnetic resonance imaging for stereotactic ablation of spinal metastases. Pract Radiat Oncol. 2020;10(5):339–44.
11. Boeke S, Mönnich D, Van Timmeren JE, Balermpas P. MR-guided radiotherapy for head and neck cancer: current developments, perspectives, and challenges. Front Oncol. 2021;11:429.
12. Chen AM, Hsu S, Lamb J, Yang Y, Agazaryan N, Steinberg ML, et al. MRI-guided radiotherapy for head and neck cancer: initial clinical experience. Clin Transl Oncol. 2018;20(2):160–8.
13. Chamberlain M, Krayenbuehl J, van Timmeren JE, Wilke L, Andratschke N, Schüler HG, et al. Head and neck radiotherapy on the MR linac: a multicenter planning challenge amongst MRIdian platform users. Strahlenther Onkol. 2021:1–11.
14. Gurney-Champion OJ, McQuaid D, Dunlop A, Wong KH, Welsh LC, Riddell AM, et al. MRI-based assessment of 3D Intrafractional motion of head and neck cancer for radiation therapy. Int J Radiat Oncol Biol Phys. 2018;100(2):306–16.
15. Bruijnen T, Stemkens B, Terhaard CH, Lagendijk JJ, Raaijmakers CP, Tijssen RH. Intrafraction motion quantification and planning target volume margin determination of head-and-neck tumors using cine magnetic resonance imaging. Radiother Oncol. 2019;130:82–8.
16. McDonald BA, Vedam S, Yang J, Wang J, Castillo P, Lee B, et al. Initial feasibility and clinical implementation of daily MR-guided adaptive head and neck cancer radiation therapy on a 1.5 T MR-Linac system: prospective R-IDEAL 2a/2b systematic clinical evaluation of technical innovation. Int J Radiat Oncol Biol Phys. 2021;109(5):1606–18.
17. Finazzi T, Palacios MA, Spoelstra FO, Haasbeek CJ, Bruynzeel AM, Slotman BJ, et al. Role of on-table plan adaptation in MR-guided ablative radiation therapy for central lung tumors. Int J Radiat Oncol Biol Phys. 2019;104(4):933–41.
18. Finazzi T, Haasbeek CJ, Spoelstra FO, Palacios MA, Admiraal MA, Bruynzeel AM, et al. Clinical outcomes of stereotactic MR-guided adaptive radiation therapy for high-risk lung tumors. Int J Radiat Oncol Biol Phys. 2020;107(2):270–8.
19. Finazzi T, de Koste JRVS, Palacios MA, Spoelstra FO, Slotman BJ, Haasbeek CJ, Senan S. Delivery of magnetic resonance-guided single-fraction stereotactic lung radiotherapy. Phys Imaging Radiat Oncol. 2020;14:17–23.
20. Chuong MD, Kotecha R, Mehta MP, Adamson S, Romaguera T, Hall MD, et al. Case report of visual biofeedback-driven, magnetic resonance-guided single-fraction SABR in breath hold for early stage non–small-cell lung cancer. Med Dosim. 2021;46(3):247–52.
21. Winkel D, Bol GH, Kroon PS, van Asselen B, Hackett SS, Werensteijn-Honingh AM, et al. Adaptive radiotherapy: the Elekta Unity MR-linac concept. Clin Translat Radiat Oncol. 2019;18:54–9.
22. Crockett CB, Samson P, Chuter R, Dubec M, Faivre-Finn C, Green OL, et al. Initial clinical experience of MR-guided radiotherapy (MRgRT) for non-small cell lung cancer (NSCLC). Front Oncol. 2021;11:157.
23. Thomas DH, Santhanam A, Kishan AU, Cao M, Lamb J, Min Y, et al. Initial clinical observations of intra-and interfractional motion variation in MR-guided lung SBRT. Br J Radiol. 2018;91(xxxx):20170522.
24. Padgett KR, Simpson GN, Llorente R, Samuels MA, Dogan N. Feasibility of adaptive MR-guided stereotactic body radiotherapy (SBRT) of lung tumors. Cureus. 2018;10(4):e2423.

25. De Costa AMA, Mittauer KE, Hill PM, Bassetti MF, Bayouth J, Baschnagel AM. Outcomes of real-time MRI-guided lung stereotactic body radiation therapy. Int J Radiat Oncol Biol Phys. 2018;102(3):e679–80.
26. Henke LE, Olsen JR, Contreras JA, Curcuru A, DeWees TA, Green OL, et al. Stereotactic MR-guided online adaptive radiation therapy (SMART) for ultracentral thorax malignancies: results of a phase 1 trial. Adv Radiat Oncol. 2019;4(1):201–9.
27. Finazzi T, Palacios MA, Haasbeek CJ, Admiraal MA, Spoelstra FO, Bruynzeel AM, et al. Stereotactic MR-guided adaptive radiation therapy for peripheral lung tumors. Radiother Oncol. 2020;144:46–52.
28. Pomp J, van Asselen B, Tersteeg RH, Vink A, Hassink RJ, van der Kaaij NP, et al. Sarcoma of the heart treated with stereotactic MR-guided online adaptive radiation therapy. Case Rep Oncol. 2021;14(1):453–8.
29. Michael Gach H, Curcuru AN, Wittland EJ, Maraghechi B, Cai B, Mutic S, Green OL. MRI quality control for low-field MR-IGRT systems: lessons learned. J Appl Clin Med Phys. 2019;20(10):53–66.
30. Sim AJ, Palm RF, DeLozier KB, Feygelman V, Latifi K, Redler G, et al. MR-guided stereotactic body radiation therapy for intracardiac and pericardial metastases. Clin Translat Radiat Oncol. 2020;25:102–6.
31. Boekhoff MR, Defize IL, Borggreve AS, Takahashi N, van Lier ALHMW, Ruurda JP, et al. 3-Dimensional target coverage assessment for MRI-guided esophageal cancer radiotherapy. Radiother Oncol. 2020;147:1–7.
32. Lee SL, Bassetti M, Meijer GJ, Mook S. Review of MR-guided radiotherapy for esophageal cancer. Front Oncol. 2021;11:468.
33. Defize IL, Boekhoff MR, Borggreve AS, van Lier AL, Takahashi N, Haj Mohammad N, et al. Tumor volume regression during neoadjuvant chemoradiotherapy for esophageal cancer: a prospective study with weekly MRI. Acta Oncol. 2020;59(7):753–9.
34. Bohoudi O, Bruynzeel AME, Senan S, Cuijpers JP, Slotman BJ, Lagerwaard FJ, Palacios MA. Fast and robust online adaptive planning in stereotactic MR-guided adaptive radiation therapy (SMART) for pancreatic cancer. Radiother Oncol. 2017;125(3):439–44.
35. Bohoudi O, Bruynzeel AM, Meijerink MR, Senan S, Slotman BJ, Palacios MA, Lagerwaard FJ. Identification of patients with locally advanced pancreatic cancer benefitting from plan adaptation in MR-guided radiation therapy. Radiother Oncol. 2019;132:16–22.
36. Henke L, Kashani R, Robinson C, Curcuru A, DeWees T, Bradley J, et al. Phase I trial of stereotactic MR-guided online adaptive radiation therapy (SMART) for the treatment of oligometastatic or unresectable primary malignancies of the abdomen. Radiother Oncol. 2018;126(3):519–26.
37. Paulson ES, Ahunbay E, Chen X, Mickevicius NJ, Chen GP, Schultz C, et al. 4D-MRI driven MR-guided online adaptive radiotherapy for abdominal stereotactic body radiation therapy on a high field MR-Linac: implementation and initial clinical experience. Clin Translat Radiat Oncol. 2020;23:72–9.
38. Green OL, Henke LE, Price A, Marko A, Wittland EJ, Rudra S, et al. The role of MRI-guided radiation therapy for palliation of Mobile abdominal cancers: a report of two cases. Adv Radiat Oncol. 2021;6(4):100662.
39. Chun SJ, Jeon SH, Chie EK. A case report of salvage radiotherapy for a patient with recurrent gastric cancer and multiple comorbidities using real-time MRI-guided adaptive treatment system. Cureus. 2018;10(4):e2471.
40. Boldrini L, Romano A, Mariani S, Cusumano D, Catucci F, Placidi L, et al. MRI-guided stereotactic radiation therapy for hepatocellular carcinoma: a feasible and safe innovative treatment approach. J Cancer Res Clin Oncol. 2021;147(7):2057–68.
41. Rogowski P, von Bestenbostel R, Walter F, Straub K, Nierer L, Kurz C, et al. Feasibility and early clinical experience of online adaptive MR-guided radiotherapy of liver tumors. Cancers. 2021;13(7):1523.

42. Feldman AM, Modh A, Glide-Hurst C, Chetty IJ, Movsas B. Real-time magnetic resonance-guided liver stereotactic body radiation therapy: an institutional report using a magnetic resonance-linac system. Cureus. 2019;11(9):e5774.
43. Rosenberg SA, Henke LE, Shaverdian N, Mittauer K, Wojcieszynski AP, Hullett CR, et al. A multi-institutional experience of MR-guided liver stereotactic body radiation therapy. Adv Radiat Oncol. 2019;4(1):142–9.
44. Hal WA, Straza MW, Chen X, Mickevicius N, Erickson B, Schultz C, et al. Initial clinical experience of Stereotactic Body Radiation Therapy (SBRT) for liver metastases, primary liver malignancy, and pancreatic cancer with 4D-MRI-based online adaptation and real-time MRI monitoring using a 1.5 Tesla MR-Linac. PLoS One. 2020;15(8):e0236570.
45. Boldrini L, Corradini S, Gani C, Henke L, Hosni A, Romano A, Dawson L. MR-guided radiotherapy for liver malignancies. Front Oncol. 2021;11:1053.
46. Luterstein E, Cao M, Lamb JM, Raldow A, Low D, Steinberg ML, Lee P. Clinical outcomes using magnetic resonance–guided stereotactic body radiation therapy in patients with locally advanced cholangiocarcinoma. Adv Radiat Oncol. 2020;5(2):189–95.
47. Centre Georges Francois Leclerc. Phase II of Adaptative Magnetic Resonance-Guided Stereotactic Body Radiotherapy (SBRT) for Treatment of Primary or Secondary Progressive Liver Tumors. clinicaltrials.gov (2020). https://clinicaltrials.gov/ct2/show/NCT04242342. Accessed 20 Dec 2021.
48. Lukovic J, Henke L, Gani C, Kim TK, Stanescu T, Hosni A, et al. MRI-based upper abdominal organs-at-risk atlas for radiation oncology. Int J Radiat Oncol Biol Phys. 2020;106(4):743–53.
49. Goodwin MD, Dobson JE, Sirlin CB, Lim BG, Stella DL. Diagnostic challenges and pitfalls in MR imaging with hepatocyte-specific contrast agents. Radiographics. 2011;31(6):1547–68.
50. Hama Y, Tate E. Superparamagnetic iron oxide-enhanced MRI-guided stereotactic ablative radiation therapy for liver metastasis. Rep Pract Oncol Radiother. 2021;26(3):470–4.
51. Namasivayam S, Martin DR, Saini S. Imaging of liver metastases: MRI. Cancer Imaging. 2007;7(1):2.
52. Witt JS, Rosenberg SA, Bassetti MF. MRI-guided adaptive radiotherapy for liver tumours: visualising the future. Lancet Oncol. 2020;21(2):e74–82.
53. Hassanzadeh C, Rudra S, Bommireddy A, Hawkins WG, Wang-Gillam A, Fields RC, et al. Ablative five-fraction stereotactic body radiation therapy for inoperable pancreatic cancer using online MR-guided adaptation. Adv Radiat Oncol. 2021;6(1):100506.
54. Rudra S, Jiang N, Rosenberg SA, Olsen JR, Roach MC, Wan L, et al. Using adaptive magnetic resonance image-guided radiation therapy for treatment of inoperable pancreatic cancer. Cancer Med. 2019;8(5):2123–32.
55. Palacios MA, Bohoudi O, Bruynzeel AM, de Koste JRVS, Cobussen P, Slotman BJ, et al. Role of daily plan adaptation in MR-guided stereotactic ablative radiation therapy for adrenal metastases. Int J Radiat Oncol Biol Phys. 2018;102(2):426–33.
56. Rudra S, Fischer-Valuck B, Pachynski R, Daly M, Green O. Magnetic resonance image guided stereotactic body radiation therapy to the primary renal mass in metastatic renal cell carcinoma. Adv Radiat Oncol. 2019;4(4):566.
57. Tetar SU, Bohoudi O, Senan S, Palacios MA, Oei SS, Wel AM, et al. The role of daily adaptive stereotactic MR-guided radiotherapy for renal cell cancer. Cancers. 2020;12(10):2763.
58. Kutuk T, McCulloch J, Mittauer KE, Romaguera T, Alvarez D, Gutierrez AN, et al. Daily online adaptive magnetic resonance image (MRI)-guided stereotactic body radiation therapy for primary renal cell cancer. Med Dosim. 2021;46(3):289–94.
59. Bruynzeel AM, Tetar SU, Oei SS, Senan S, Haasbeek CJ, Spoelstra FO, et al. A prospective single-arm phase 2 study of stereotactic magnetic resonance guided adaptive radiation therapy for prostate cancer: early toxicity results. Int J Radiat Oncol Biol Phys. 2019;105(5):1086–94.
60. Tetar SU, Bruynzeel AM, Oei SS, Senan S, Fraikin T, Slotman BJ, et al. Magnetic resonance-guided stereotactic radiotherapy for localized prostate cancer: final results on patient-reported outcomes of a prospective phase 2 study. Eur Urol Oncol. 2021;4(4):628–34.

61. Tetar SU, Bruynzeel AM, Lagerwaard FJ, Slotman BJ, Bohoudi O, Palacios MA. Clinical implementation of magnetic resonance imaging guided adaptive radiotherapy for localized prostate cancer. Phys Imaging Radiat Oncol. 2019;9:69–76.
62. Mazzola R, Cuccia F, Figlia V, Rigo M, Nicosia L, Giaj-Levra N, et al. Stereotactic body radiotherapy for oligometastatic castration sensitive prostate cancer using 1.5 T MRI-Linac: preliminary data on feasibility and acute patient-reported outcomes. La radiologia medica. 2021;126(7):1–9.
63. Cuccia F, Corradini S, Mazzola R, Spiazzi L, Rigo M, Bonù ML, et al. MR-guided Hypofractionated radiotherapy: current emerging data and promising perspectives for localized prostate cancer. Cancers. 2021;13(8):1791.
64. Alongi F, Rigo M, Figlia V, Cuccia F, Giaj-Levra N, Nicosia L, et al. 1.5 T MR-guided and daily adapted SBRT for prostate cancer: feasibility, preliminary clinical tolerability, quality of life and patient-reported outcomes during treatment. Radiat Oncol. 2020;15(1):1–9.
65. Cuccia F, Mazzola R, Nicosia L, Figlia V, Giaj-Levra N, Ricchetti F, et al. Impact of hydrogel peri-rectal spacer insertion on prostate gland intra-fraction motion during 1.5 T MR-guided stereotactic body radiotherapy. Radiat Oncol. 2020;15(1):1–9.
66. Nicosia L, Sicignano G, Rigo M, Figlia V, Cuccia F, De Simone A, et al. Daily dosimetric variation between image-guided volumetric modulated arc radiotherapy and MR-guided daily adaptive radiotherapy for prostate cancer stereotactic body radiotherapy. Acta Oncol. 2021;60(2):215–21.
67. Sahin B, Mustafayev TZ, Gungor G, Aydin G, Yapici B, Atalar B, Ozyar E. First 500 fractions delivered with a magnetic resonance-guided radiotherapy system: initial experience. Cureus. 2019;11(12):e6457.
68. Ugurluer G, Atalar B, Zoto Mustafayev T, Gungor G, Aydin G, Sengoz M, et al. Magnetic resonance image-guided adaptive stereotactic body radiotherapy for prostate cancer: preliminary results of outcome and toxicity. Br J Radiol. 2021;94(1117):20200696.
69. Boldrini L, Piras A, Chiloiro G, Autorino R, Cellini F, Cusumano D, et al. Low Tesla magnetic resonance-guided radiotherapy for locally advanced cervical cancer: first clinical experience. Tumori J. 2020;106(6):497–505.
70. Henke LE, Stanley JA, Robinson C, Srivastava A, Contreras JA, Curcuru A, et al. Phase I trial of stereotactic MRI-guided online adaptive radiation therapy (SMART) for the treatment of oligometastatic ovarian cancer. Int J Radiat Oncol Biol Phys. 2021;112(2):379–89.
71. Chiloiro G, Boldrini L, Meldolesi E, Re A, Cellini F, Cusumano D, et al. MR-guided radiotherapy in rectal cancer: first clinical experience of an innovative technology. Clin Translat Radiat Oncol. 2019;18:80–6.
72. Hijab A, Tocco B, Hanson I, Meijer H, Nyborg CJ, Bertelsen AS, et al. MR-guided adaptive radiotherapy for bladder cancer. Front Oncol. 2021;11:637591.

8 Image-Guided Adaptive Brachytherapy

Bradley Pieters and Taran Paulsen-Hellebust

8.1 Introduction

The developments in imaging and particularly its integration in the workflow of radiotherapy have had a major impact in the way modern radiotherapy is advancing. Highly conformal radiation treatment planning became possible since the introduction of the computed tomography (CT)-scan.

In 1960, Egan and Johnson [1] described a multisection transverse tomography technique for head and neck implants. With this technique, they were able to reconstruct an implant in three dimensions. Especially for large implants, this technique gave more 3-dimensional (3D) insight and improved dosimetry. Munzenrider et al. [2] published on the use of the CT-scan for radiotherapy and also the potential application and benefits for contouring and brachytherapy dosimetry. In 1980, Lee et al. [3] reported on a method to use a CT-scan after an intrauterine-vaginal application in 20 patients. The CT images clearly showed the position of the applicator in relation to the pelvic organs. The authors also mentioned misplacement of the intrauterine tandem. Besides anatomical and topographical information obtained from the CT-scan, it was also possible to show isodose plots superimposed on the CT-scan. Since then, more and more publications on the use of CT-scan for brachytherapy became available, later on followed by other imaging modalities.

B. Pieters (✉)
Department of Radiation Oncology, Amsterdam University Medical Centers, University of Amsterdam, Amsterdam, The Netherlands

Cancer Center Amsterdam, Imaging and Biomarkers, Amsterdam, The Netherlands
e-mail: b.r.pieters@amsterdamumc.nl

T. Paulsen-Hellebust
Department of Medical Physics, The Radium Hospital, Oslo University Hospital, Oslo, Norway

Department of Physics, University of Oslo, Oslo, Norway
e-mail: tph@ous-hf.no

E. G. C. Troost (ed.), *Image-Guided High-Precision Radiotherapy*,
https://doi.org/10.1007/978-3-031-08601-4_8

Imaging for brachytherapy is used at several time points [4]. These are grossly divided in: (1) before the implantation, (2) during the implantation, (3) for treatment planning, and (4) connected to dose delivery and its quality assurance.

1. Before the implantation, imaging is used to prepare for the intervention. Preparation consists of the choice of the applicator to be used and the desired position of the applicator. This preparation is necessary to decide on the implantation technique and procedure to be used.
2. During the implantation, imaging can guide the brachytherapist with the procedure. It is of high importance to have the applicator placed in the correct position for optimal dosimetry. Because of its flexibility to bring it to every operating theater, ultrasound (US) is the most commonly used modality, although other imaging modalities are also useful.
3. For treatment planning, to cover target volumes with the prescribed dose as well as possible and to avoid dose to organs at risk (OAR) as much as possible, imaging is essential in this respect. On the images, volumes of interest are contoured and used in the treatment planning process. Several dose constraints can be applied to (sub)volumes, which are used for calculation of dose distribution.
4. The last aspect of imaging is its use for quality assurance. After treatment planning, changes may occur that will influence the dose distribution and as such the calculated doses on the different volumes of interest. These changes are caused by applicator movement, tumor regression, and organ motion. By imaging just prior to and during the course of brachytherapy (BT), the delivered dose can be estimated much more accurately.

Nowadays modern brachytherapy is performed as image-guided adaptive brachytherapy. Imaging is essential for optimal placement of the applicator and conformal treatment planning. Because of continuous changes that happen during the treatment course, adapting to these anatomical variations is necessary. This is where imaging plays an important role. Although imaging is applied to nearly all indications for brachytherapy, this chapter will restrict itself mainly to cervix and prostate cancer.

8.2 Clinical Aspects in Imaging for Cervix Brachytherapy

Traditionally, BT dosimetry for cancer of the uterine cervix was based on standard 2D plans. Prescription of dose was done on the so-called point A, which was a fixed point related to the applicator used [5, 6]. This point A is easily identified on two orthogonal pelvic X-ray radiographs. However, on the radiograph there is neither visualization of the cervix and tumor, nor of the adjacent organs at risk such as bladder, rectum, and sigmoid. Fiducial structures, such as a Foley-balloon and rectum tube can identify the position of these organs such that the dose to these organs can be roughly estimated. Even so, a drawback of this approach is that there is no possibility to create conformal treatment plans and as a result, underdosage in tumor subvolumes can occur or overdosage to healthy organs. As a consequence, underdosage in parts of the tumor will lead to higher probability of tumor relapse, while high dose to healthy organs is related to increased toxicity.

With the introduction of 3D treatment planning in BT, the possibility arose to create conformal treatment plans, preventing the above problems of 2D planning drawbacks as much as possible. With CT as imaging modality, it became possible to contour whole organs and, in that way, calculate dose volume parameters. It was evident that dose point values calculated on 2D radiographs did not correspond with the maximum dose to CT-planning and point A dose being a poor surrogate for the high-risk clinical target volume dose [7, 8]. Also, apart from the traditional dose calculation on the bladder and rectum, with a CT-scan also estimation of dose to the sigmoid and small bowel became possible.

An important development for the concept of image-guided BT was the introduction of magnetic resonance imaging (MRI) in this radiation treatment modality. With MRI, a new target concept for the treatment of cervix cancer was developed with clear definitions of gross tumor volume (GTV) and clinical target volume (CTV) [9, 10]. With MRI, in particular the GTV can be better identified than with any other imaging modality. This element of the image-guided treatment approach, together with necessary clinical information obtained from inspection and palpation is the basis for the high local control rates achieved nowadays [11–14].

8.2.1 Ultrasound

US is ideal to use for guidance of the correct applicator positioning. The applicator for cervix BT consists of two parts. The first part is an intrauterine tandem, which is placed in the uterine cavity. The second part consists of two ovoids or one ring, which are/is placed in the top of the vagina just touching the cervix. Placing the intrauterine tandem into the uterine cavity using the intrauterine canal seems to be a straight-forward procedure. However, in cases in which the external cervix ostium cannot be recognized due to the presence of tumor or in which the tumor is blocking the intrauterine canal, misplacement of the intrauterine tandem can happen. The tandem may be placed in the uterus wall (myometrium) or even perforate the uterus at the anterior or posterior wall. The incidence rate of uterine perforation during applicator positioning is about 15% [15]. In such cases, no optimal dosimetry of the BT application can be guaranteed, since the intrauterine tandem is not positioned centrally of the tumor. In order to cover the whole tumor with the prescribed dose, unacceptably high doses would need to be approved in the OARs, usually sigmoid, bladder or small bowel. A method to prevent such misplacement of the intrauterine tandem is by inserting the intrauterine tandem under abdominal US-guidance [16, 17]. With abdominal US, the cervix and the body of the uterus can be easily recognized. Placement in the correct position in the uterine fundus is facilitated by guidance in both sagittal and transversal view.

An important aspect of the BT procedure is the treatment planning for BT dose distribution. For treatment planning, it is necessary to the contour target volumes and OARs, and to perform a reconstruction of the inserted applicator on the image data set. The golden standard is to perform the contouring on MRI (see below). However, ongoing studies aim to investigate the possibility of using US in the contouring process. The high-risk CTV (CTV_{HR}) on US appears to be similar to MRI and within the interobserver variability of MRI [18]. In practice, the CTV_{HR}, as contoured on transrectal US (TRUS), and a 3D library model of the applicator are registered onto a CT image data set. Subsequently, the contoured target volume on US is transferred to CT for the final treatment planning [19]. However, this workflow still has many imperfections that need to be resolved before it can be introduced in clinical practice. This TRUS/CT-based approach can be a solution for institutes with low access to MRI. A prospective study reported on high agreement between MRI contouring and CT-based with TRUS-aided contouring [20].

8.2.2 MRI

A major break-through in image-guided adaptive BT for cervical cancer was the introduction of MRI in the workflow. In 2005, the *Groupe Européen de Curiethérapie* – European Society for Radiotherapy and Oncology (GEC-ESTRO) introduced a target concept mainly based on MR images [9]. The concept has been further developed in the ICRU report number 89 [10]. For target volume contouring, both MRIs, the one at diagnosis and the other at time of BT, are considered.

On MRI, the GTV can be easily identified as a high intensity mass on fast spin echo T2-weighted sequences. During radiotherapy, the regression of the GTV is apparent, and these changes are used for an adaptive approach of the treatment [9].

Another volume to consider according to this target concept is the CTV_{HR}. This volume represents the whole cervix including the presumed extracervical tumor extension at the time of BT. The extracervical extension is assessed by clinical examination, ideally performed at the initial staging and at the time of BT. On T2-weighted MRI, this volume is recognized by so-called residual "gray"-zones in parametria, uterine corpus, vagina, rectum, or bladder, and also includes any other residual pathologic tissue on MRI.

The last volume to consider is the intermediate-risk clinical target volume (CTV_{IR}), which carries a significant microscopic tumor load. This volume encompasses a margin of 5–10 mm beyond the CTV_{HR} and covers at least the tumor extension at initial clinical investigation and staging of the disease before start of radiotherapy.

The definition of this target concept made it possible to also develop a dosimetry system based on dose to the respective target volume, independent of the type of BT applicator used. This dosimetry system based on volumes substantially differs from the traditional systems based on dose points [21]. Besides defining doses to a volume and using this for dose prescription, also dose-volume parameters are defined for OARs. These OAR parameters are used to guide in calculating an optimal treatment plan. The OARs in the pelvic area can be either contoured on CT or MRI. There is hardly any difference in dose values of the OAR when contoured on either of these two modalities.

The value of imaging and especially MRI is evident in the outcome of the retroEMBRACE and EMBRACE studies. A five-year local control rate of 89% is reported in the retroEMBRACE study, with also high rates for stage IIIB tumors (75%) [14]. Not surprisingly, the better local outcome is seen in case of an intracavitary application combined with interstitial needle insertions [12]. This improvement in local control was primarily enabled by the use of imaging techniques to better depict the target volumes and to place of applicators in the correct position. Late toxicity was found to be acceptably low, despite the high doses prescribed to the CTV_{HR}; 5-year grade 3–5 toxicity of 5% for bladder, 7% for gastrointestinal tract, and 5% for vagina has been reported [14]. Further investigations in the successive EMBRACE study show a strong association between dose-volume-histogram (DVH) parameters and both local control and toxicity, emphasizing the importance of adjustments of therapy based on information from imaging [22].

8.2.3 Image-Guided Adaptive Brachytherapy

With the introduction of imaging techniques, radiotherapy in general has evolved to a high-tech treatment taking into account changes occurring during treatment. This development is not different for BT. Adaptive BT considers tumor shrinkage and organ changes, facilitating the adaptation of the given dose to different subvolumes whenever necessary.

In the EMBRACE study, different patterns of parametrial invasion were recognized; (1) expansive with spiculae, (2) expansive with spiculae and infiltrating parts, (3) infiltrative into the inner third of the parametrial space, (4) infiltrative into the middle third of the parametrial space, (5) infiltrative into the outer third of the parametrial space. Residual tumor after external beam and prior to BT was more often present in patterns 3–5 compared to 1 and 2 [23]. As a consequence, patients with patterns 3–5 resulted in having a larger CTV_{HR} leading to high doses to larger volumes. Conversely, if the response to external beam radio(chemo)therapy is good, the target volumes can be reduced significantly.

To safely encompass large volumes, care should be taken to use appropriate applicators in order to reach the periphery of the target volume, i.e., CTV_{HR} and CTV_{IR}. With the advent of 3D imaging in BT, new applicators have been developed allowing the insertion of additional interstitial needles next to the standard intracavitary component of the applicators [24, 25]. The interstitial needles can be directed to the outer surface of the tumor volume to guarantee an optimal dose coverage of these parts. The use of interstitial needles is more common for infiltrative tumors than for expansive tumors [26].

Not only tumor shrinkage during external beam radio(chemo)therapy is of importance to recognize, but also further shrinkage in between BT applications. In BT, the OARs show the largest variations in dose to a certain volume of interest. These variations are due to changes in shape and size because of filling and motion of these organs, e.g., bladder, small bowel, sigmoid, and rectum. Larger variation in dose occurs between applications (interapplication variation) than during one application (intra-application variation), with larger variations for sigmoid compared to bladder and rectum. Mean dose differences of 7% between applications can be expected for sigmoid with large variations between individuals [27]. No general value for dose variation to OAR can be given, because this variation is not only dependent on the specific OAR, but also on the treatment approach, e.g., number of fractions or the use of a BT treatment plan for one or several applications [28]. This expected variation on OAR dose between, but also during applications emphasizes the importance of repeated imaging as part of quality assurance. For OAR assessment, CT is as useful and accurate as MRI as opposed to the assessment of the GTV as already mentioned above.

Next to calculation of the dose for every BT application, the total dose is given by summing up the dose of the whole treatment, i.e., the entire course of EBRT and all BT applications. For rectum and bladder, the most reliable method is by adding up the DVH parameters of each fraction, which is a good approximation of the given dose [29]. For organs that show larger motion, such as sigmoid and small bowel, this method overestimates the dose. For these organs, deformable image registration (DIR) may improve dose assessment, provided better models for DIR are developed [30, 31].

8.3 Clinical Aspects in Imaging for Prostate Brachytherapy

8.3.1 US-Guided Applications

Prostate BT became successful after the introduction of image-guided implantation using US in 1983 by Holm et al. [32]. The technique, which has been the standard approach for more than three decades, combines transrectal US with transperineal implantations.

Two main prostate BT methods are regularly performed; low-dose rate (LDR) and high-dose rate (HDR) BT. With LDR-BT, low activity-encapsulated sources of about 5-mm long are placed in the prostate. These sources are introduced with hollow, open-end needles in the correct position. Treatment planning indicates the position of the sources. By combining axial and sagittal US views of the prostate, both the radial as the depth of source insertion can be assessed.

HDR-BT implantations are performed in similar way as LDR implantation in lithotomy position. Instead of using the needles to insert radioactive sources, these needles stay in place to be connected to an afterloading BT machine. Via the needles, a stepping-source remains on several positions in the prostate for dose delivery.

Developments in the field of prostate BT resulted in dedicated hard- and software to aid with implantations. Systems allow for the import of US images into a BT planning system for intraoperative treatment planning (see Fig. 8.1a). The template mounted on the US probe, to guide needle placement, is calibrated with the coordinate system of the US machine [33]. This enables planned virtual needle positions to be exactly placed in the prostate via the template.

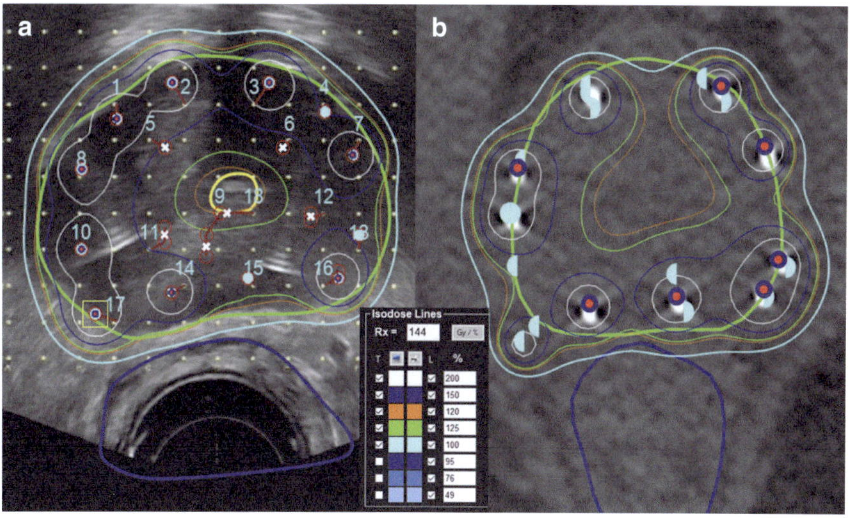

Fig. 8.1 Images of a LDR prostate implant of the same patient. Panel A represents the preplan with virtual positions of the needles (sequentially numbered) on ultrasound and the isodose distribution. Panel B represents the postoperative dosimetry on CT-scan done 30 days after the implantation. The actual position of the sources with isodose distribution is illustrated. The outer aqua blue isodose line is the reference 100% isodose (144 Gy) line

One of the greatest advantages of real-time US imaging is the possibility of dynamic dose calculation. Actual source placement for LDR-BT is recorded and real-time dosimetry is provided. Also, prostate shape and size variations are considered. This methodology also allows for extra placement of sources if underdosed areas are detected. The main drawback of only US-based dynamic dose calculation is that not all sources can be detected with high accuracy. To resolve this drawback, combined fluoroscopy and US systems have been developed and employed. X-rays, from a C-arm fluoroscopy device, have much more accuracy in detecting source positions than US [34]. Several multidirectional fluoroscopy images can be taken to construct a 3D seed position distribution. As a next step, fluoroscopy-US registration is done to allow the calculated dose distribution be projected on the US-contoured prostate gland. This technique showed dosimetric values of registered fluoroscopy-US to be closer to postop dosimetry on CT or MRI than by US alone [35].

Ultrasound gives the opportunity for interactive treatment planning during prostate HDR-BT. The first step in such procedure is to image the prostate gland. Then a preplan is elaborated, including delineation of the gland and positioning of the needles (see Fig. 8.2a) [36, 37]. When all the needles are inserted, using US guidance, another image acquisition is performed and the treatment planning will be performed using this image set. At this stage, there is still possibility to modify the position of a needle or even place additional needles. A major challenge is that the presence of the needles will preclude the image quality. Therefore, treatment planning systems usually allow transferring the initial gland delineation into the image

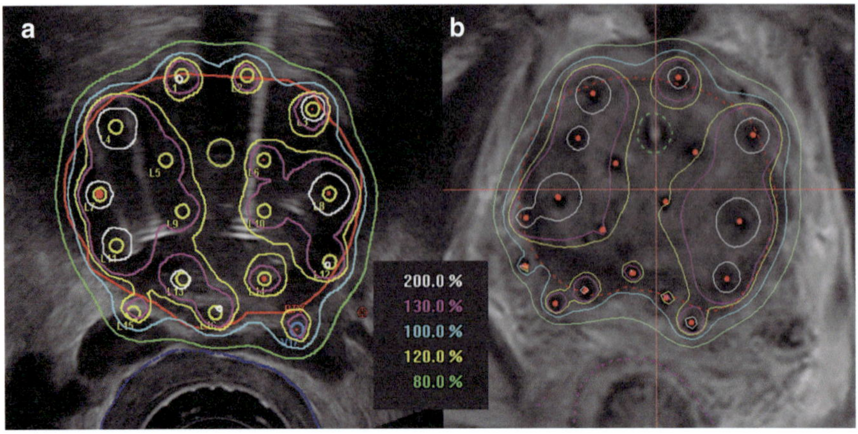

Fig. 8.2 Images of a temporary prostate implant for HDR of the same patient. Panel A represents the preplan with virtual positions of the needles on ultrasound and the isodose distribution. Panel B represents the definitive treatment plan on MRI. The actual position of the flexible catheters with isodose distribution is illustrated. The outer aqua blue isodose line is the reference 100% isodose (15 Gy) line

set with the needles to guide the definition of the prostate in this second image set. For HDR-BT, inverse optimization will usually give a good result in shorter time than traditional forward planning using for example graphical optimization [38].

All these techniques allow the possibility to improve the dose distribution, by either extra source placement or re-optimization of stepping source dose distribution, before the patient leaves the operation room.

8.3.2 CT during Implantation and CT Postplanning

When performing LDR-BT, a C-arm for fluoroscopy purposes can also be used to make images of cone-beam-CT (CBCT) quality, as developed by Westendorp et al. [39]. Both increase of D_{90} as V_{100} (i.e., the minimal dose D to 90% of the target and the target volume V encompassed by the 100% isodose) was observed on day 30 postimplantation dosimetry by placing remedial sources because of foreseen underdosage during the implantation [39]. A 13% difference in biochemical recurrence-free survival was found between patients having only US compared to patients evaluated by CBCT with even an overall survival benefit for high-risk profile patients [40].

For LDR-BT, immediate postimplant dosimetry can be obtained by dynamic dose calculation. However, because of edema of the prostate occurring during the implantation, calculated dose-volume (DV) parameters are not representative for the whole treatment lasting several weeks. Prostate volume after implant can be 36% larger compared to the preimplant volume. Because of resolution of edema, an increase of V_{100} and D_{90} is expected in the following 30 days, with a largest effect for initial “low” coverage implants [41]. In the recommendations of the European

Society for Radiotherapy and Oncology (ESTRO) and the American Brachytherapy Society (ABS), CT-scan postoperative dosimetry is recommended for dosimetric analysis (see Fig. 8.1b) [42, 43]. Another reason besides recording of accurate DV parameters is that postoperative dosimetry is also used for quality assurance. In this way, the operator can evaluate his/her own achievements and use this knowledge for quality improvements. Possible established low-coverage areas in the prostate can be still corrected for by placing extra sources in this specific area. A third reason to perform CT dosimetry after 4 weeks is to check if sources have migrated, causing "cold spots" that can be corrected for [44]. On average, seed displacement of up to 3–5 mm has been reported dependent on the area of interest [45].

8.3.3 CT- and MRI-Based Treatment Planning

When performing implantation for HDR-BT, catheters/needles will stay in situ. One option for treatment planning is to perform it based on US images. Further explanation about this method is described in Sect. 8.4. After the implantation, these catheters will be connected to the afterloader BT machine for the treatment itself.

A second option is to use CT or MR for treatment planning. In contrast to US-based treatment planning, the patient needs to be transferred to a CT- or MRI-scanner for imaging. The image dataset is imported to the treatment planning computer and can be processed for treatment planning purposes (see Fig. 8.2b).

One reason to choose for CT- or MRI-based treatment planning is that catheters can be better identified on CT and MRI compared to US. This will decrease the catheter reconstruction uncertainty (see Sect. 8.4). However, it has been shown that prostate gland delineation on CT is less accurate than on US resulting in a volume of approx. 10% larger [46–48]. This is caused by a decreased visibility of the prostate gland after implantation, thus leading to a delineation of the outer catheters rather than of the prostate gland itself. In contrast, MRI identifies the outer contour of the prostate much better than CT [49]. Also, the concordance of prostate volume between MRI and US is better than between CT and US [50]. Dinkla et al. evaluated CT-based treatment plans re-planned on MRI contours [51]. It appeared that the new plans based on MR-contoured prostate resulted in 3% less V100, particularly because of missing part of the prostate gland at the base, which was confirmed by others [52]. This study showed also a 6–10% higher tumor control probability for MR-based treatment plans compared to CT-based.

8.3.4 Focused Boost

The biggest advantage of MRI above all other imaging modalities is the ability to visualize intraprostatic lesions (IL) [53]. By identifying IL, targeted dose deposition can be accomplished within the prostate gland. This highly accurate and precise dose deposition facilitates possibilities for focused and focal BT. *Focused* BT is thereby defined as a higher dose given on an IL as part of treatment of the entire prostate gland, whereas *focal* BT is treatment of the dominant intraprostatic lesion

(DIL) as part of a partial gland treatment. For both techniques, it is of eminent importance to visualize the IL.

In a proof-of-principle study, Pieters et al. [54] showed the value of identifying ILs for dosimetry using contrast-enhanced ultrasound. The $V_{140\%}$ on the IL increased by as much as 45%, in case the localization of the IL on imaging was considered during planning. Although the technique of using contrast-enhanced US for BT has never been used clinically, it shows the importance of accurately locating IL for high dose to these lesions.

Also MRI is routinely used for diagnosis and identification of the ILs. With multiparametric MRI (mpMRI), in which T1- and T2-weighted images are combined with dynamic contrast-enhancement and diffusion-weighted imaging, accurate localization of IL can be obtained. In a systematic review, a sensitivity of 58–96% was reported, although the positive predicted value was only 34–68%, emphasizing the need for histologic confirmation [55]. Magnetic resonance spectroscopy can be added for better identification of visible lesions.

As a next step, MR images are registered to the planning transrectal US images. The identified ILs are transposed to the US images. For treatment planning, a standard single-dose of 10–15 Gy is prescribed to the prostate volume with an HDR-focused boost on the DIL [56]. This procedure allows for further dose-escalation within the visible ILs. A mean biologically equivalent dose of 140 Gy is reachable on the DIL when combining external beam radiotherapy with HDR-BT [57].

Functional MR sequences offer a unique possibility to increase the dose to areas with biological characteristics indicating radioresistance, not only in prostate MR-based BT, but also in gynecological BT. This concept was explored by Rylander et al. [58] for prostate BT and by Li et al. [59] for cervical cancer BT. In focal BT, multiparametric MR imaging is a tool that can assist in defining the target volume for such treatment [60].

A different approach to the use of focused boost is to de-escalate the dose to the whole prostate gland, while maintaining or increasing the dose to the ILs. Preliminary research has been performed to investigate this treatment approach [61]. The rationale of this approach is to maintain high dose to the tumor lesions itself while reducing toxicity by decreasing the dose to nonaffected parts of the prostate and the surrounding structures and organs, such as nerves, bladder, and rectum.

When performing MR imaging after needle insertion into the prostate, there are certain aspects of tumor visualization to consider. In case of treatment planning on MR-images, it is still useful to have a preoperative mpMRI for identification of ILs. Since trauma and edema effect the visibility, ILs are vanished on postoperative MR images obstructing identification of these structures. In these cases, registration to a preoperative MRI can be useful.

8.3.5 Focal and Partial Prostate Brachytherapy

Focal and partial prostate BT is a new treatment approach for patients with low-risk disease or recurrent prostate cancer after previous radiotherapy [62, 63]. Some studies are already published and several trials are ongoing [64–69]. The introduction of mpMRI in the diagnostic workup of prostate cancer enables the identification of the ILs with high accuracy, particularly if the tumor is more than 5 mm in size and if it belongs to ISUP (International Society of Urological Pathology) grade group 4–5 [53, 70]. To increase the diagnostic accuracy and to avoid missing low-grade small size tumor lesions, biopsies mapping the prostate are part of the work-up [71, 72].

LDR as well as HDR are useful techniques for focal BT. The margin to be applied around the visible ILs in order to achieve adequate dose coverage is subject of current research. A margin of 5 mm has been found to be sufficient for this purpose [73]. The use of MRI to US registration techniques is a prerequisite to perform for treatment planning [74]. In that respect, there is no difference in the approach of focal or focused boost technique. However, since focal BT does not include treatment of the entire gland, the definition of the safety margin is more critical.

8.4 Physics Imaging Aspects for Brachytherapy

8.4.1 Applicator Reconstruction Using MR and/or CT

As elaborated on above, modern imaging has enabled accurate and precise definition of the target volumes and OAR, and due to the steep dose gradients in BT, highly tailored dose distribution can therefore be generated. However, to be able to produce such optimized dose distribution, not only the anatomy should be visualized, but also it is equally important to localize the applicator(s) or sources in the images [75]. The choice of the imaging modality has even its implication on the applicator to be used [76]. CT- and MR-compatible applicators have been developed to be used in image-guided BT. A wrongly positioned source path can lead to considerably under- or over-dosage [77]. This means that the optimal image modality should visualize the patient's anatomy *as well as* the applicator(s)/sources. Often, the most optimal modality for depicting the anatomy is not optimal for applicators or source localization and vice versa. For example, radiographic films (x-ray imaging) visualize the applicator(s) or sources very well, but do not provide any soft tissue contrast. Also, in CT imaging, the applicator(s)/sources or the lumen of a rigid applicator used for gynecological BT is clearly visible (Fig. 8.3a). The lumen of the applicator represents the source channel, and CT imaging will therefore be excellent to localize the possible source dwell positions in an applicator. However, CT imaging is of limited use, for example, to assess the boundaries of the tumor versus the cervix/uterus and of parametrial invasion [75]. In contrast to CT, MR is superior for defining the target volume for several BT sites [78, 79]. MRI could, however, be prone to geometrical distortion and since there are large dose gradients in BT, it is important to be aware of the magnitude of these distortions. The spatial accuracy decreases with the distance from the isocenter of the magnet [80]. This means that in prostate and gynecology BT, the distortions are smallest in the area of

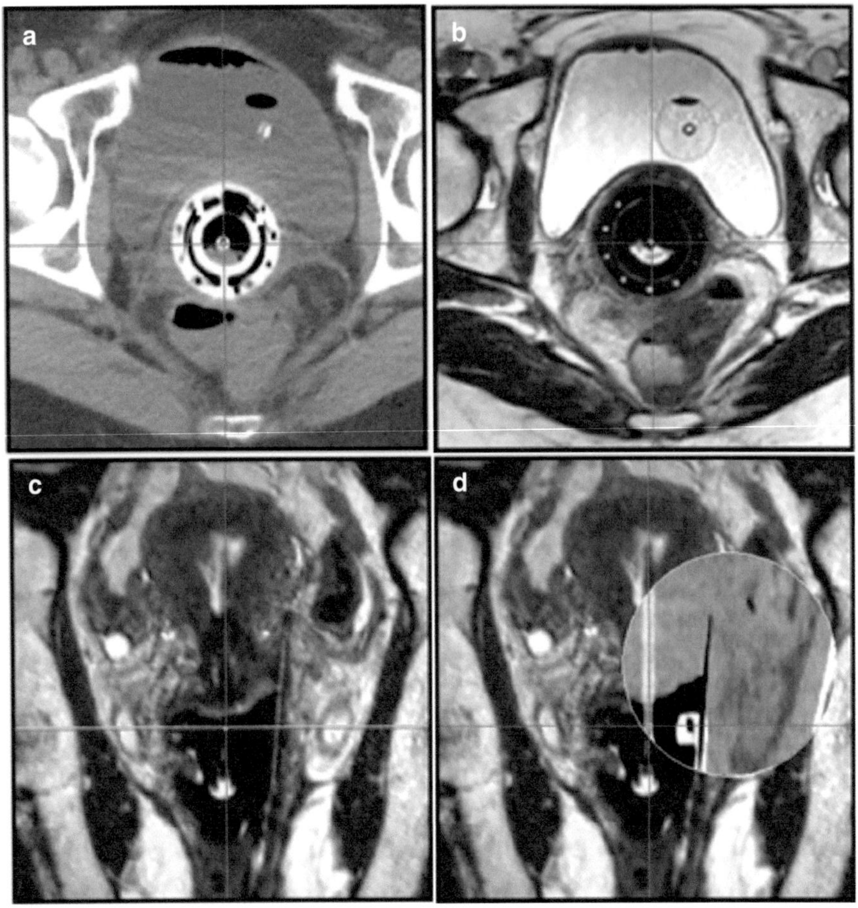

Fig. 8.3 Images from a patient with a ring/tandem applicator with three needles: (**a**) CT image through the ring, (**b**) T2-weighted MR image through the ring, (**c**) T2-weighted MR image in a para-coronal plan showing one of the needles, and (**d**) the same image with a spyglass function with CT information. During CT imaging, an x-ray marker string is used in the ring applicator, while a marker tube filled with copper sulfate is used in the ring during the MR imaging

the implant. Wills et al. [81] showed that if appropriate sequences are used for a field strength of 1.5 T together with distortion correction algorithms provided by the manufacturers, the geometrical distortion is considered to be small (<2 mm) in the region of interest in pelvic BT.

A major challenge in the use of MRI is the ability to reconstruct the applicator [77]. Some applicators (e.g., steel applicators or shielded applicators) are not even MR compatible and should not be used in combination with MR imaging. Plastic/carbon fiber and titanium applicators are MR compatible and can be safely used. In CT imaging, the source channel is readily visible, while this is not the case for MR imaging. This means that some kind of marker is needed to visualize the source

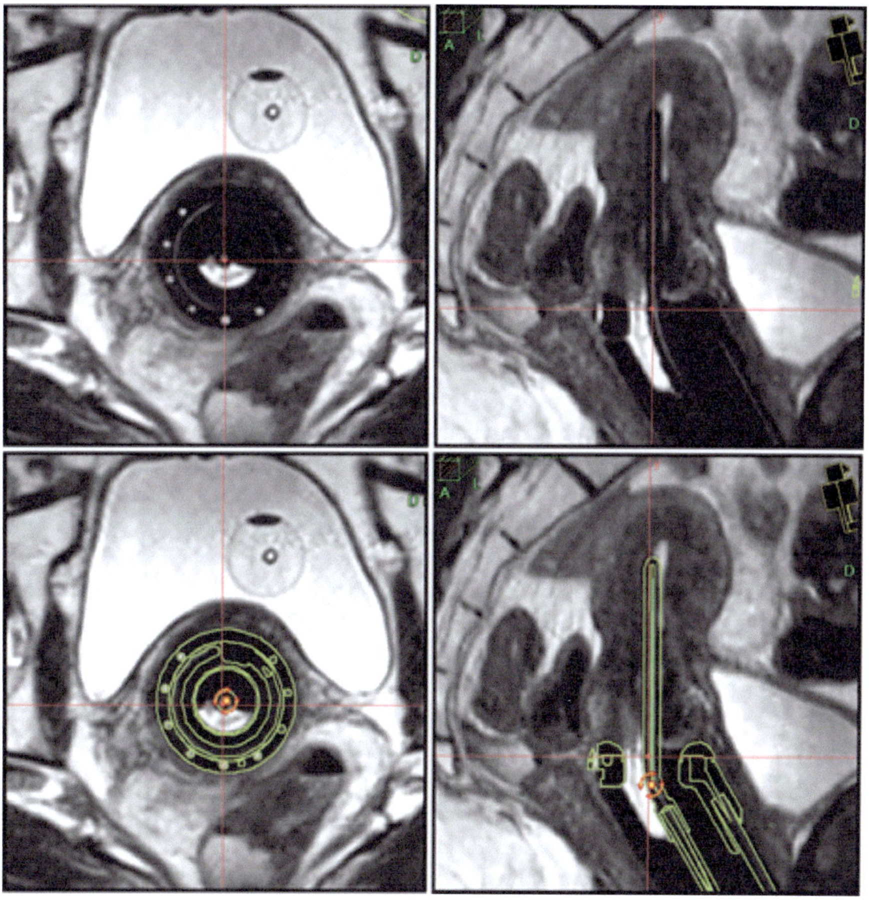

Fig. 8.4 T2-weighted MR images from a patient with a ring/tandem applicator with three needles in para-transversal (left panels) and para-sagittal (right panels) planes. In the lower panels, the library applicator is imported and positioned in the MR images

channel, as shown in Fig. 8.3b [77, 82]. However, in most modern treatment planning systems, so-called library applicator files may be used to easily and accurately reconstruct rigid applicators (e.g., plastic tandem-ring-applicator). The applicator file includes information about the applicator surface dimensions and the source path, can be imported into the MR images, and rotated and translated until it matches the images. This technique is illustrated in Fig. 8.4.

Because of superior soft-tissue resolution of MRI, postoperative dosimetry with MR images results in more reliable assessment of postplanning dosimetry. With CT, the contouring of the prostate tends to follow the seeds, while on MRI better distinction of the prostate toward surrounding tissues is visible. CT is the most frequently used image modality for postimplant dosimetry of permanent prostate seed implants, but MR can also be used as suggested by Moerland et al. [83] in 1997.

With CT the seeds can be easily identified, often with a computerized algorithm. Using MR, however, such procedure is challenging. De Brabandere et al. [79] analyzed data from seven observers that reconstructed the seed positions on CT and MRI images from three patients and found that the interobserver variability in seed detection resulted in a standard deviation for the D_{90} of 1.5% and 6.6% for CT and MRI, respectively.

Even though TRUS is considered to be the gold standard for HDR prostate BT, several groups have started to use MRI as a part of such procedure, either intraoperatively [84] or for treatment planning after TRUS-guided implantation [51, 85].

8.4.2 CT-MR Registration

As described above, it is in many situations not the same modality that fulfills the two criteria of reproducing the anatomy and localization of the applicator(s)/sources with high precision; CT could be the most optimal modality for reconstruction of the applicator, while MRI could be better for target delineation. Additionally, the availability of the image modalities is often different. Most centers do have easy access to CT, while the capacity for MRI is often limited. This means that combination of CT and MR imaging could be the optimal solution in some situations, either during the same session or for different fractions. For example, for centers with limited access to MRI, Nesvacil et al. [86] described a technique using MRI for the first BT fractions and CT for the subsequent fractions for adaptive treatment of cervical cancer. For prostate cancer BT, a combinations of CT and MRI have been suggested by De Brabandere et al. [79] and by Brown et al. [52]. When two image modalities are combined, so-called image registration procedures are used and it is important to understand the principles and limitations of such procedures. In a newly published review, Swamidas et al. [30] explain the principle of image registration for gynecological BT and give an overview of studies addressing this topic. If MR imaging modality is used for target delineation and CT imaging for applicator reconstruction/source localization, it is important to evaluate the uncertainties that are introduced by combining these image modalities compared to the uncertainties that are present by using only one modality. If the applicator shifts it position relative to the bony anatomy between the two image acquisitions, the target volume and even parts of the OARs will move together with the applicator. It is therefore recommended to use rigid registration with the applicator as the reference system and not the bony anatomy to perform the registration between the MR and CT images [77]. In rigid registration, minimum three points should be localized in both image sets. Since the applicator appears differently in CT and MR images, it could sometimes be difficult to define such points, often referred to as landmarks. However, if a combined intracavitary/interstitial applicator is used, the unused needles' holes will be filled by fluid and can be used as landmarks (see Fig. 8.3b).

Using MR imaging for applicator reconstruction during interstitial BT is usually feasible with modern treatment planning system and well-designed MR acquisition.

However, occasionally, it could be challenging to identify the tip of the needles accurately. In such situation, a CT acquisition could be helpful to guide the needle reconstruction, as shown in Fig. 8.3c, d.

8.4.3 Ultrasound and Brachytherapy

Accurately identification of the needles during US prostate BT could be challenging. CT imaging is the gold standard for optimal geometrical precision in reconstruction of needle positions. Schmid et al. [87] compared needle reconstruction in a phantom using CT and US. They identified two sources of errors using US. Firstly, using the bright echoes in the transversal US images for localizing the needles will result in a systematic error that has to be corrected for. Secondly, they observed challenges in identifying the needle tip and errors up to 5.8 mm were observed. This latter challenge can be solved by measuring the residuals needle length, as described by Zheng et al. [88]. Moreover, a biplane US transducer can be used and Batchelar et al. [89] found discrepancies of more than 3 mm for only 3% of the needles when needle reconstruction utilizing such transducer was compared with needle reconstruction using CBCT. However, a biplane US transducer can potentially introduce systematic shifts during the axial- to sagittal image registration step. Hrinivich et al. [90] explored a yet another TRUS-imaging technique where the probe was rotated using a motor and simultaneously captured the images in order to create a 3D image set. For 12 patients, this method was compared with the method described by Batchelar et al. [91] and found statistically significantly smaller insertion depth errors.

Since US is a rather inexpensive modality, widely available, and offers fast image acquisition, it is interesting to use US for other body sites than the prostate. In cervical cancer BT, transabdominal ultrasound (TAUS) is primarily used to ensure a safe applicator placement [16, 17]. A study on 192 cervical cancer BT patients where the patients were imaged with both MRI and transabdominal US found that the differences between these two image modalities were within clinical acceptable limits [92]. Mahanshetty et al. [93] also found an excellent correlation between TAUS and MRI, but with limitations in the posterior uterine wall and in the highly relevant areas of the parametrial space. Schmid et al. [18, 94] therefore explored the use of 3D TRUS for cervical cancer BT and demonstrated 3D TRUS to be noninferior to T2-weighted MRI for defining the dimensions of the CTV_{HR}. A full workflow, including 3D TRUS, was tested in an in-house developed system by the same group [19]. They found superior image quality by rotating the probe during image acquisition compared to a pulling back procedure. They also found that the applicator reconstruction was challenging. In a test series, they were able to reconstruct the applicator with acceptable precision only for 20% of the patients [95]. Thus, for the time being it is not feasible to perform the whole procedure with 3D TRUS. Further development of hardware, software, and operation procedures is required to increase image quality to be able to delineate the target and to reconstruct the applicator with sufficient precision.

8.4.4 Treatment Planning

In external beam radiotherapy (EBRT), the median dose to the target volumes is usually used for normalization and reporting. Due to the very steep dose gradients in BT, such procedure will not work since this will lead to very low minimum dose to the target. Therefore, the minimal dose to 90% of the target volume, referred to as D_{90}, is usually used for evaluation and reporting in BT. Moreover, evaluation and reporting of dose to OARs are different in BT compared to EBRT. In BT, the dose to the most exposed part of the organ is used, for example the dose to the 2 cm^3 most exposed volume, referred to as D_{2cm^3}.

Traditionally, the prescribed dose is referred to as the dose the patients should receive and it is determined before the treatment, typically by specifying the fractionation schedule. Usually similar patients (same diagnosis, stage, type of treatment, etc.) will be treated with similar fractionation schedule. However, during 3D image-based BT planning, an individualized optimization will be performed resulting in different dose distribution from patient to patient and reflects the dose the patients receive. Therefore, for 3D image-based BT, the goal for the treatment planning is now referred to as the planning-aim dose and the prescribed dose is achievable dose to a specific volume of the target (e.g., D_{90}) [10]. The prescribed dose could be equal to the planning-aim dose, but is often not.

What you are able to achieve during the optimization is closely related to your implant and to the applicator(s) that is used. For example, to have an acceptable D_{90} for a large CTV_{HR} in cervical cancer implants without increasing the dose to the organs at risk, it is usually necessary to use a combined intracavitary/interstitial (IC/IS) applicator [96, 97]. To use such technique, 3D imaging is required. Data from an EMBRACE cohort showed a better dose conformity for intermediate and large CTV_{HR} volumes when IC/IS applicators were used, compared to only IC [98]. Furthermore, the retroEMBRACE data showed the 3-year local control rate was 10% higher for IC/IS patient compared to IC patients with no increase in the treatment-related morbidity for patients with $CTV_{HR} \geq 30\ cm^3$ [12].

The dose to the recto-vaginal-point [ICRU 89] correlates with vaginal stenosis according to an analysis performed by Kirchheiner et al. on 630 patients from the EMBRACE study [99]. They suggested to keep the dose to this point ≤65 GY EQD2 (EBRT + BT). This can be achieved by de-escalating the dose in the vaginal part of the implant. Such procedure can only be performed with 3D image-based treatment planning.

8.5 Conclusion

Imaging in brachytherapy is used on subsequent time points. Before the implantation of an applicator, imaging will help in the decision of how to perform the invasive procedure and where to exactly place the applicators.

Image-guided insertion of applicators have resulted in an improvement of well-placed applicators and as a consequence better dosimetry and treatment outcome.

Imaging is essential as part of treatment planning. Traditional dose prescription, recording, and reporting on dose points have been replaced by volumes. Target volume concepts are necessary to design conformal treatment plans with specific doses on subvolumes. The optimal image modality should reproduce both the anatomy and localization of the applicator(s)/sources with high precision, but in many situations it is not the same modality that fulfills these two criteria. Eventually a compromise is necessary or the different imaging modalities need to be registered to each other.

Imaging lastly serves quality assurance purposes. It provides information on the actual dose that occurs because of applicator movement, tumor regression, and organ motion. This information is not only important to register, but also to take measures for adapting the treatment.

References

1. Egan R, Johnson GC. Multisection transverse tomography in radium implant calculations. Radiology. 1960;74:407–13.
2. Munzenrider JE, Pilepich M, Rene-Ferrero JB, Tchakarova I, Carter BL. Use of body scanner in radiotherapy treatment planning. Cancer. 1977;40:170–9.
3. Lee KR, Mansfield CM, Dwyer SJ III, Cox HL, Levine E, Templeton AW. CT for intracavitary radiotherapy planning. Am J Radiol. 1980;135:809–13.
4. Pötter R. Modern imaging in brachytherapy. In: The GEC-ESTRO handbook of brachytherapy. Leuven: ESTRO; 2002.
5. Tod M, Meredith WJ. Treatment of cancer of the cervix uteri, a revised Manchester method. Br J Radiol. 1953;26:252–7.
6. ICRU. International Commission on Radiation Units and Measurements. Dose and volume specification for reporting intracavitary therapy in gynaecology, ICRU report 38, Oxford University Press, Oxford, United Kingdom. 1985.
7. Jamema SV, Saju S, Mahantshetty U, Palad S, Deshpande DD, Shrivastava SK, et al. Dosimetric evaluation of rectum and bladder using image-based CT planning and orthogonal radiographs with ICRU 38 recommendations in intracavitary brachytherapy. J Med Phys. 2008;33:3–8.
8. Tanderup K, Nielsen SK, Nyvang G-B, Pedersen EM, Røhl L, Aagaard T, et al. From point a to the sculpted pear: MR image guidance significantly improves tumour dose and sparing of organs at risk in brachytherapy of cervical cancer. Radiother Oncol. 2010;94(2):173–80.
9. Haie-Meder C, Pötter R, van Limbergen E, Briot E, De Brabandere M, Dimopoulos J, et al. Recommendations from Gynaecological (GYN) GEC-ESTRO Working Group I: concepts and terms in 3D image-based 3D treatment planning in cervix cancer brachytherapy with emphasis on MRI assessment of GTV and CTV. Radiother Oncol. 2005;74:235–45.
10. Pötter R, Kirisits C, Erickson B, Haie-Meder C, Van Limbergen E, Lindegaard JC, et al. Prescribing, recording, and reporting brachytherapy for cancer of the cervix, ICRU report 89. Oxford: Oxford University Press; 2016.
11. Mazeron R, Castelnau-Marchand P, Dumas I, del Campo ER, Kom LK, Martinetti F, et al. Impact of treatment time and dose escalation on local control in locally advanced cervical cancer treated by chemoradiation and image-guided pulsed-dose rate adaptive brachytherapy. Radiother Oncol. 2015;114(2):257–63.
12. Fokdal L, Sturdza A, Mazeron R, Haie-Meder C, Tan LT, Gillham C, et al. Image-guided adaptive brachytherapy with combined intracavitary and interstitial technique improves the therapeutic ratio in locally advanced cervical cancer: analysis from the retroEMBRACE study. Radiother Oncol. 2016;120(3):434–40.
13. Pötter R, Georg P, Dimopoulos J, Grimm M, Berger D, Nesvacil N, et al. Clinical outcome of protocol-based image (MRI)-guided adaptive brachytherapy combined with 3D conformal

radiotherapy with or without chemotherapy in patients with locally advanced cervical cancer. Radiother Oncol. 2011;100(1):116–23.
14. Sturdza A, Potter R, Fokdal LU, Haie-Meder C, Tan LT, Mazeron R, et al. Image-guided brachytherapy in locally advanced cervical cancer: improved pelvic control and survival in RetroEMBRACE, a multicenter cohort study. Radiother Oncol. 2016;120(3):428–33.
15. Barnes EA, Thomas G, Ackerman I, Barbera L, Letourneau D, Lam KL, et al. Prospective comparison of clinical and computed tomography assessment in detecting uterine perforation with intracavitary brachytherapy for carcinoma of the cervix. Int J Gynecol Cancer. 2007;17:821–6.
16. Mayr NA, Montebello JF, Sorosky JI, Daugherty JS, Nguyen DL, Mardirossian G, et al. Brachytherapy management of the retroverted uterus using ultrasound-guided implant applicator placement. Brachytherapy. 2005;4(1):24–9.
17. Davidson MT, Yuen J, D'Souza DP, Radwan JS, Hammond JA, Batchelar DL. Optimization of high-dose-rate cervix brachytherapy applicator placement: the benefits of intraoperative ultrasound guidance. Brachytherapy. 2008;7(3):248–53.
18. Schmid MP, Nesvacil N, Potter R, Kronreif G, Kirisits C. Transrectal ultrasound for image-guided adaptive brachytherapy in cervix cancer - an alternative to MRI for target definition? Radiother Oncol. 2016;120(3):467–72.
19. Nesvacil N, Schmid MP, Potter R, Kronreif G, Kirisits C. Combining transrectal ultrasound and CT for image-guided adaptive brachytherapy of cervical cancer: proof of concept. Brachytherapy. 2016;15(6):839–44.
20. Mahantshetty U, Naga CP, Khadanga CR, Gudi S, Chopra S, Gurram L, et al. A prospective comparison of computed tomography with transrectal ultrasonography assistance and magnetic resonance imaging-based target-volume definition during image- guided adaptive brachytherapy for cervical cancers. Int J Radiat Oncol Biol Phys. 2018;102(5):1448–56.
21. Pötter R, Haie-Meder C, van Limbergen E, Barillot I, De Brabandere M, Dimopoulos J, et al. Recomendations from gynaecological (GYN) GEC ESTRO working group (II): concepts and terms in 3D image-based treatment planning in cervix cancer brachytherapy - 3D dose volume parameters and aspects of 3D image-based anatomy, radiation physics, radiobiology. Radiother Oncol. 2006;78:67–77.
22. Mazeron R, Fokdal LU, Kirchheiner K, Georg P, Jastaniyah N, Segedin B, et al. Dose-volume effect relationships for late rectal morbidity in patients treated with chemoradiation and MRI-guided adaptive brachytherapy for locally advanced cervical cancer: results from the prospective multicenter EMBRACE study. Radiother Oncol. 2016;120(3):412–9.
23. Schmid MP, Fidarova E, Pötter R, Petric P, Bauer V, Woehs V, et al. Magnetic resonance imaging for assessment of parametrial tumour spread and regression patterns in adaptive cervix cancer radiotherapy. Acta Oncol. 2013;52:1384–90.
24. Nomden CN, de Leeuw AA, Moerland MA, Roesink JM, Tersteeg RJ, Jurgenliemk-Schulz IM. Clinical use of the Utrecht applicator for combined intracavitary/interstitial brachytherapy treatment in locally advanced cervical cancer. Int J Radiat Oncol Biol Phys. 2012;82(4):1424–30.
25. Dimopoulos JCA, Kirisits C, Petric P, Georg P, Lang S, Berger D, et al. The Vienna applicator for combined intracavitary and interstitial brachytherapy of cervical cancer: clinical feasibility and preliminary results. Int J Radiat Oncol Biol Phys. 2006;66(1):83–90.
26. Yoshida K, Jastaniyah N, Sturdza A, Lindegaard J, Segedin B, Mahantshetty U, et al. Assessment of parametrial response by growth pattern in patients with International Federation of Gynecology and Obstetrics Stage IIB and IIIB cervical cancer: analysis of patients from a prospective, multicenter trial (EMBRACE). Int J Radiat Oncol Biol Phys. 2015;93(4):788–96.
27. Nesvacil N, Tanderup K, Hellebust TP, De Leeuw A, Lang S, Mohamed S, et al. A multicentre comparison of the dosimetric impact of inter- and intra-fractional anatomical variations in fractionated cervix cancer brachytherapy. Radiother Oncol. 2013;107(1):20–5.
28. Kirisits C, Rivard MJ, Baltas D, Ballester F, De Brabandere M, van der Laarse R, et al. Review of clinical brachytherapy uncertainties: analysis guidelines of GEC-ESTRO and the AAPM. Radiother Oncol. 2014;110(1):199–212.
29. van Heerden LE, Houweling AC, Koedooder K, van Kesteren Z, van Wieringen N, Rasch CRN, et al. Structure-based deformable image registration: added value for dose accumula-

tion of external beam radiotherapy and brachytherapy in cervical cancer. Radiother Oncol. 2017;123(2):319–24.
30. Swamidas J, Kirisits C, De Brabandere M, Hellebust TP, Siebert FA, Tanderup K. Image registration, contour propagation and dose accumulation of external beam and brachytherapy in gynecological radiotherapy. Radiother Oncol. 2020;143:1–11.
31. van Heerden LE, van Wieringen N, Koedooder K, Rasch CRN, Pieters BR, Bel A. Dose warping uncertainties for the accumulated rectal wall dose in cervical cancer brachytherapy. Brachytherapy. 2018;17(2):449–55.
32. Holm HH, Juul N, Pedersen JF, Hansen H, Strøyer I. Transperineal 125iodine seed implantation in prostatic cancer guided by transrectal ultrasonography. J Urol. 1983;130(2):283–6.
33. Siebert FA, Kirisits C, Hellebust TP, Baltas D, Verhaegen F, Camps S, et al. GEC-ESTRO/ACROP recommendations for quality assurance of ultrasound imaging in brachytherapy. Radiother Oncol. 2020;148:51–6.
34. Orio PF 3rd, Tutar IB, Narayanan S, Arthurs S, Cho PS, Kim Y, et al. Intraoperative ultrasound-fluoroscopy fusion can enhance prostate brachytherapy quality. Int J Radiat Oncol Biol Phys. 2007;69(1):302–7.
35. Lee J, Mian OY, Le Y, Bae HJ, Burdette EC, DeWeese TL, et al. Intraoperative registered ultrasound and fluoroscopy (iRUF) for dose calculation during prostate brachytherapy: improved accuracy compared to standard ultrasound-based dosimetry. Radiother Oncol. 2017;124(1):61–7.
36. Kovács G, Pötter R, Loch T, Hammer J, Kolkman-Deurloo I, de la Rosette JJMCH, et al. GEC/ESTRO-EAU recommendations on temporary brachytherapy using stepping sources for localised prostate cancer. Radiother Oncol. 2005;74:137–48.
37. Hoskin PJ, Colombo A, Henry A, Niehoff P, Paulsen Hellebust T, Siebert F, et al. GEC/ESTRO recommendations on high-dose-rate afterloading brachytherapy for localised prostate cancer: an update. Radiother Oncol. 2013;107(3):325–32.
38. Dinkla AM, van der Laarse R, Kaljouw E, Pieters BR, Koedooder K, van Wieringen N, et al. A comparison of inverse optimization algorithms for HDR/PDR prostate brachytherapy treatment planning. Brachytherapy. 2015;14(2):279–88.
39. Westendorp H, Nuver TT, Moerland MA, Minken AW. An automated, fast and accurate registration method to link stranded seeds in permanent prostate implants. Phys Med Biol. 2015;60(20):N391–403.
40. Peters M, Smit Duijzentkunst DA, Westendorp H, van de Pol SMG, Kattevilder R, Schellekens A, et al. Adaptive cone-beam CT planning improves long-term biochemical disease-free survival for 125 I prostate brachytherapy. Brachytherapy. 2017;16(2):282–90.
41. Tanaka O, Hayashi S, Matsuo M, Nakano M, Uno H, Ohtakara K, et al. Effect of edema on postimplant dosimetry in prostate brachytherapy using CT/MRI fusion. Int J Radiat Oncol Biol Phys. 2007;69(2):614–8.
42. Ash D, Flynn A, Battermann J, de Reijke T, Lavagnini P, Blank L. ESTRO/EAU/EORTC recommendations on permanent seed implantation for localized prostate cancer. Radiother Oncol. 2000;57:315–21.
43. Bittner NHJ, Orio PF, Merrick GS, Prestidge BR, Hartford AC, Rosenthal SA. The American College of Radiology and the American brachytherapy society practice parameter for transperineal permanent brachytherapy of prostate cancer. Brachytherapy. 2017;16(1):59–67.
44. Fuller DB, Koziol JA, Feng AC. Prostate brachytherapy seed migration and dosimetry: analysis of stranded sources and other potential predictive factors. Brachytherapy. 2004;3(1):10–9.
45. Westendorp H, Nuver TT, Hoekstra CJ, Moerland MA, Minken AW. Edema and seed displacements affect intraoperative permanent prostate brachytherapy dosimetry. Int J Radiat Oncol Biol Phys. 2016;96(1):197–205.
46. Ohashi T, Yorozu A, Toya K, Saito S, Momma T, Nagata H, et al. Comparison of intraoperative ultrasound with postimplant computed tomography--dosimetric values at Day 1 and Day 30 after prostate brachytherapy. Brachytherapy. 2007;6(4):246–53.
47. Stone NN, Hong S, Lo Y-C, Howard V, Stock RG. Comparison of intraoperative dosimetric implant representation with postimplant dosimetry in patients receiving prostate brachytherapy. Brachytherapy. 2003;2(1):17–25.

48. Chauveinc L, Flam T, Solignac S, Thiounn N, Firmin F, Debre B, et al. Prostate cancer brachytherapy: is real-time ultrasound-based dosimetry predictive of subsequent CT-based dose distribution calculation? A study of 450 patients by the Institut curie/hospital Cochin (Paris) group. Int J Radiat Oncol Biol Phys. 2004;59(3):691–5.
49. Petrik D, Araujo C, Kim D, Halperin R, Crook JM. Implications of CT imaging for postplan quality assessment in prostate brachytherapy. Brachytherapy. 2012;11(6):435–40.
50. Bowes D, Crook JM, Araujo C, Batchelar D. Ultrasound–CT fusion compared with MR–CT fusion for postimplant dosimetry in permanent prostate brachytherapy. Brachytherapy. 2013;12(1):38–43.
51. Dinkla A, Pieters BR, Koedooder K, van Wieringen N, van der Laarse R, van der Grient JN, et al. Improved tumor control probability with MRI-based prostate brachytherapy treatment planning. Ann Oncol. 2013;52(3):658–65.
52. Brown AP, Pugh TJ, Swanson DA, Kudchadker RJ, Bruno TL, Christensen EN, et al. Improving prostate brachytherapy quality assurance with MRI-CT fusion-based sector analysis in a phase II prospective trial of men with intermediate-risk prostate cancer. Brachytherapy. 2013;12(5):401–7.
53. Anderson ES, Margolis DJ, Mesko S, Banerjee R, Wang PC, Demanes DJ, et al. Multiparametric MRI identifies and stratifies prostate cancer lesions: implications for targeting intraprostatic targets. Brachytherapy. 2014;13(3):292–8.
54. Pieters BR, Wijkstra H, van Herk M, Kuipers R, Kaljouw E, de la Rosette J, et al. Contrast-enhanced ultrasound as support for prostate brachytherapy treatment planning. J Contemp Brachyther. 2012;4(2):67–74.
55. Futterer JJ, Briganti A, De Visschere P, Emberton M, Giannarini G, Kirkham A, et al. Can clinically significant prostate cancer be detected with multiparametric magnetic resonance imaging? A systematic review of the literature. Eur Urol. 2015;68(6):1045–53.
56. Crook J, Ots A, Gaztanaga M, Schmid M, Araujo C, Hilts M, et al. Ultrasound-planned high-dose-rate prostate brachytherapy: dose painting to the dominant intraprostatic lesion. Brachytherapy. 2014;13(5):433–41.
57. von Eyben FE, Kiljunen T, Kangasmaki A, Kairemo K, von Eyben R, Joensuu T. Radiotherapy boost for the dominant intraprostatic cancer lesion-a systematic review and meta-analysis. Clin Genitourin Cancer. 2016;14(3):189–97.
58. Rylander S, Polders D, Steggerda MJ, Moonen LM, Tanderup K, Van der Heide UA. Re-distribution of brachytherapy dose using a differential dose prescription adapted to risk of local failure in low-risk prostate cancer patients. Radiother Oncol. 2015;115(3):308–13.
59. Li A, Andersen E, Lervåg C, Julin CH, Lyng H, Hellebust TP, et al. Dynamic contrast- enhanced magnetic resonance imaging for hypoxia mapping and potential for brachytherapy targeting. Phys Imaging Radiat Oncol. 2017;2:1–6.
60. Mason J, Al-Qaisieh B, Bownes P, Wilson D, Buckley DL, Thwaites D, et al. Multi-parametric MRI-guided focal tumor boost using HDR prostate brachytherapy: a feasibility study. Brachytherapy. 2014;13(2):137–45.
61. Ennis RD, Quinn SA, Trichter F, Ryemon S, Jain A, Saigal K, et al. Phase I/II prospective trial of cancer-specific imaging using ultrasound spectrum analysis tissue-type imaging to guide dose-painting prostate brachytherapy. Brachytherapy. 2015;14(6):801–8.
62. Kovacs G, Cosset JM, Carey B. Focal radiotherapy as focal therapy of prostate cancer. Curr Opin Urol. 2014;24(3):231–5.
63. Duijzentkunst DA, Peters M, van der Voort van Zyp JR, Moerland MA, van Vulpen M. Focal salvage therapy for local prostate cancer recurrences after primary radiotherapy: a comprehensive review. World J Urol. 2016;34(11):1521–31.
64. Cosset JM, Cathelineau X, Wakil G, Pierrat N, Quenzer O, Prapotnich D, et al. Focal brachytherapy for selected low-risk prostate cancers: a pilot study. Brachytherapy. 2013;12(4):331–7.
65. Nguyen PL, Chen MH, Zhang Y, Tempany CM, Cormack RA, Beard CJ, et al. Updated results of magnetic resonance imaging-guided partial prostate brachytherapy for favorable risk prostate cancer: implications for focal therapy. J Urol. 2012;188(4):1151–6.

66. Maenhout M, Peters M, van Vulpen M, Moerland MA, Meijer RP, van den Bosch M, et al. Focal MRI-guided salvage high-dose-rate brachytherapy in patients with Radiorecurrent prostate cancer. Technol Cancer Res Treat. 2017;16(6):1194–201.
67. Maenhout M, Peters M, Moerland MA, Meijer RP, van den Bosch M, Frank SJ, et al. MRI-guided focal HDR brachytherapy for localized prostate cancer: toxicity, biochemical outcome and quality of life. Radiother Oncol. 2018;129(3):554–60.
68. Murgic J, Morton G, Loblaw A, D'Alimonte L, Ravi A, Wronski M, et al. Focal salvage high-dose-rate brachytherapy for locally recurrent prostate cancer after primary radiation therapy failure: results from a prospective clinical trial. Int J Radiat Oncol Biol Phys. 2018;102(3):561–7.
69. Brun T, Bachaud JM, Graff-Cailleaud P, Malavaud B, Portalez D, Popotte C, et al. New approach of ultra-focal brachytherapy for low- and intermediate-risk prostate cancer with custom-linked I-125 seeds: a feasibility study of optimal dose coverage. Brachytherapy. 2018;17(3):544–55.
70. Turkbey B, Mani H, Shah V, Rastinehad AR, Bernardo M, Pohida T, et al. Multiparametric 3T prostate magnetic resonance imaging to detect cancer: histopathological correlation using prostatectomy specimens processed in customized magnetic resonance imaging-based molds. J Urol. 2011;186(5):1818–24.
71. Ahmed HU, Hu Y, Carter T, Arumainayagam N, Lecornet E, Freeman A, et al. Characterizing clinically significant prostate cancer using template prostate mapping biopsy. J Urol. 2011;186(2):458–64.
72. Langley S, Ahmed HU, Al-Qaisieh B, Bostwick D, Dickinson L, Gomez Veiga F, et al. Report of a consensus meeting on focal low-dose rate brachytherapy for prostate cancer. BJU Int. 2012;109(Supl 1):7–16.
73. Polders DL, Steggerda M, van Herk M, Nichol K, Witteveen T, Moonen L, et al. Establishing implantation uncertainties for focal brachytherapy with I-125 seeds for the treatment of localized prostate cancer. Acta Oncol. 2015;54(6):839–46.
74. Mayer A, Zholkover A, Portnoy O, Raviv G, Konen E, Symon Z. Deformable registration of trans-rectal ultrasound (TRUS) and magnetic resonance imaging (MRI) for focal prostate brachytherapy. Int J Comput Assist Radiol Surg. 2016;11(6):1015–23.
75. Hellebust TP. Place of modern imaging in brachytherapy planning. Cancer Radiother. 2018;22(4):326–33.
76. Steggerda. An analysis of the effect of ovoid shields in a selectron-LDR cervical applicator on dose distributions in rectum and bladder. Int J Radiat Oncol Biol Phys. 1997;39:237–45.
77. Hellebust TP, Kirisits C, Berger D, Perez-Calatayud J, De Brabandere M, De Leeuw A, et al. Recommendations from gynaecological (GYN) GEC-ESTRO working group: considerations and pitfalls in commissioning and applicator reconstruction in 3D image-based treatment planning of cervix cancer brachytherapy. Radiother Oncol. 2010;96(2):153–60.
78. Viswanathan AN, Dimopoulos J, Kirisits C, Berger D, Pötter R. Computed tomography versus magnetic resonance imaging-based contouring in cervical cancer brachytherapy: results of a prospective trial and preliminary guidelines for standardized contours. Int J Radiat Oncol Biol Phys. 2007;68(2):491–8.
79. De Brabandere M, Hoskin P, Haustermans K, Van den Heuvel F, Siebert FA. Prostate post-implant dosimetry: interobserver variability in seed localisation, contouring and fusion. Radiother Oncol. 2012;104(2):192–8.
80. Fransson A, Andreo P, Pötter R. Aspects of MR image distortions in radiotherapy treatment planning. Strahlenther Onkol. 2001;177:59–73.
81. Wills R, Lowe G, Inchley D, Anderson C, Beenstock V, Hoskin P. Applicator reconstruction for HDR cervix treatment planning using images from 0.35T open MR scanner. Radiother Oncol. 2010;94(3):346–52.
82. Perez-Calatayud J, Kuipers F, Ballester F, Granero D, Richart J, Rodriguez S, et al. Exclusive MRI-based tandem and colpostats reconstruction in gynaecological brachytherapy treatment planning. Radiother Oncol. 2009;91(2):181–6.

83. Moerland MA, Wijrdeman HK, Beersma R, Bakker CJG, Battermann JJ. Evaluation of permanent I-125 prostate implants using radiography and magnetic resonance imaging. Int J Radiat Oncol Biol Phys. 1997;37:927–33.
84. Ménard C, Susil RC, Choyke P, Gustafson GS, Kammerer W, Ning H, et al. MRI-guided HDR prostate brachytherapy in standard 1.5T scanner. Int J Radiat Oncol Biol Phys. 2004;59(5):1414–23.
85. Rylander S, Buus S, Pedersen EM, Bentzen L, Tanderup K. Dosimetric impact of contouring and needle reconstruction uncertainties in US-, CT- and MRI-based high-dose-rate prostate brachytherapy treatment planning. Radiother Oncol. 2017;123(1):125–32.
86. Nesvacil N, Pötter R, Sturdza A, Hegazy N, Federico M, Kirisits C. Adaptive image- guided brachytherapy for cervical cancer: a combined MRI-/CT-planning technique with MRI only at first fraction. Radiother Oncol. 2013;107(1):75–81.
87. Schmid M, Crook JM, Batchelar D, Araujo C, Petrik D, Kim D, et al. A phantom study to assess accuracy of needle identification in real-time planning of ultrasound-guided high-dose-rate prostate implants. Brachytherapy. 2013;12(1):56–64.
88. Zheng D, Todor DA. A novel method for accurate needle-tip identification in trans-rectal ultrasound-based high-dose-rate prostate brachytherapy. Brachytherapy. 2011;10(6):466–73.
89. Batchelar D, Gaztanaga M, Schmid M, Araujo C, Bachand F, Crook J. Validation study of ultrasound-based high-dose-rate prostate brachytherapy planning compared with CT-based planning. Brachytherapy. 2014;13(1):75–9.
90. Hrinivich WT, Hoover DA, Surry K, Edirisinghe C, Montreuil J, D'Souza D, et al. Three-dimensional transrectal ultrasound-guided high-dose-rate prostate brachytherapy: a comparison of needle segmentation accuracy with two-dimensional image guidance. Brachytherapy. 2016;15(2):231–9.
91. Hrinivich WT, Hoover DA, Surry K, Edirisinghe C, Velker V, Bauman G, et al. Accuracy and variability of high-dose-rate prostate brachytherapy needle tip localization using live two-dimensional and sagittally reconstructed three-dimensional ultrasound. Brachytherapy. 2017;16(5):1035–43.
92. van Dyk S, Kondalsamy-Chennakesavan S, Schneider M, Bernshaw D, Narayan K. Comparison of measurements of the uterus and cervix obtained by magnetic resonance and transabdominal ultrasound imaging to identify the brachytherapy target in patients with cervix cancer. Int J Radiat Oncol Biol Phys. 2014;88(4):860–5.
93. Mahantshetty U, Khanna N, Swamidas J, Engineer R, Thakur MH, Merchant NH, et al. Trans-abdominal ultrasound (US) and magnetic resonance imaging (MRI) correlation for conformal intracavitary brachytherapy in carcinoma of the uterine cervix. Radiother Oncol. 2012;102(1):130–4.
94. Schmid MP, Potter R, Brader P, Kratochwil A, Goldner G, Kirchheiner K, et al. Feasibility of transrectal ultrasonography for assessment of cervical cancer. Strahlenther Onkol. 2013;189(2):123–8.
95. Schmid MP, Beaulieu L, Nesvacil N, Pieters BR, Postema AW, Schalk SG, et al. Ultrasound. In: Song WY, Tanderup K, Pieters BR, editors. Emerging technologies in brachytherapy. Medical physics and biomedical engineering. Boca Raton: CRC Press; 2017.
96. Berger D, Pötter R, Dimopoulos JA, Kirisits C. New Vienna applicator design for distal parametrial disease in cervical cancer. Brachytherapy. 2010;9:S51–S2.
97. Kirisits C, Lang S, Dimopoulos J, Berger D, Georg D, Pötter R. The Vienna applicator for combined intracavitary and interstitial brachytherapy of cervical cancer: design, application, treatment planning, and dosimetric results. Int J Radiat Oncol Biol Phys. 2006;65(2):624–30.
98. Serban M, Kirisits C, de Leeuw A, Potter R, Jurgenliemk-Schulz I, Nesvacil N, et al. Ring versus Ovoids and Intracavitary versus Intracavitary-interstitial applicators in cervical cancer brachytherapy: results from the EMBRACE I study. Int J Radiat Oncol Biol Phys. 2020;106(5):1052–62.
99. Kirchheiner K, Nout RA, Lindegaard JC, Haie-Meder C, Mahantshetty U, Segedin B, et al. Dose-effect relationship and risk factors for vaginal stenosis after definitive radio(chemo)therapy with image-guided brachytherapy for locally advanced cervical cancer in the EMBRACE study. Radiother Oncol. 2016;118(1):160–6.

Ultrasonography in Image-Guided Radiotherapy: Current Status and Future Challenges

9

Davide Fontanarosa, Emma Harris, Alex Grimwood, Saskia Camps, Maria Antico, Erika Cavanagh, and Chris Edwards

9.1 Ultrasound-Guided Radiotherapy

Ultrasound (US) is an imaging modality, which has been known mainly for its applications in radiology: for example, foetal scanning, cardiac diagnostics, sports injuries evaluation or breast cancer investigations. But its popularity has grown in recent years also for quantitative applications, such as localisation, definition and tracking of structures or tools [1, 2]. It is cost-effective, radiation-free, portable and with excellent imaging characteristics, among which virtually unlimited resolution and high soft tissue contrast. Moreover, the image creation process (see Sect. 9.2) is

D. Fontanarosa (✉) · E. Cavanagh · C. Edwards
Centre for Biomedical Technologies (CBT), Queensland University of Technology, Brisbane, QLD, Australia

School of Clinical Sciences, Queensland University of Technology, Brisbane, QLD, Australia
e-mail: d3.fontanarosa@qut.edu.au; ej1.robinson@hdr.qut.edu.au; c8.edwards@qut.edu.au

E. Harris
Joint Department of Physics, Institute of Cancer Research, London, UK
e-mail: Emma.Harris@icr.ac.uk

A. Grimwood
Division of Radiotherapy and Imaging, Institute of Cancer Research, London, UK
e-mail: Alex.Grimwood@icr.ac.uk

S. Camps
EBAMed SA, Geneva, Switzerland
e-mail: saskia.camps@eba-med.com

M. Antico
Centre for Biomedical Technologies (CBT), Queensland University of Technology, Brisbane, QLD, Australia

School of Mechanical, Medical and Process Engineering, Queensland University of Technology, Brisbane, QLD, Australia
e-mail: maria.antico@hdr.qut.edu.au

E. G. C. Troost (ed.), *Image-Guided High-Precision Radiotherapy*,
https://doi.org/10.1007/978-3-031-08601-4_9

inherently real-time and, in advanced systems, volumetric. This combination of properties makes US the only 4D modality currently suitable for applications in radiotherapy (RT) bunkers or in operating theatres.

In the RT workflow, US is clinically used to help contour the target and the clinical structures, to set up the patient prior to treatment fractions, and to monitor the position of the tumour during treatment delivery [2, 3]. The advantages over other more established modalities for inter-fraction patient setup, such as films [4], electronic portal imaging (EPI) [5] or Cone-Beam CT (CBCT) [6], are that US can use soft tissue for alignment, while the others typically rely on bony structures. This approach is more effective when relative changes happen between the target and the bony structures between the simulation and the treatment stages. Other modalities, which allow (to various degrees) soft tissue tracking, such as implanted markers or MRI, are invasive (the former) or are extremely more expensive (the latter). For intra-fraction monitoring, instead, the main competitors are the global positioning system (GPS) for body localisation [7, 8], which is also invasive and is potentially prone to migration of the beacons; fluoroscopy, which only provides projected planar information [7] and optical surface guidance [9], which only tracks the surface of the body of the patient, which does not necessarily always show reliable spatial correlation with the internal structures for which it acts as surrogate.

Traditionally, US has been regarded as an operator-dependent modality because, especially in its diagnostic aspect, it relies heavily on user's skills and expertise. In literature, studies have shown significant inter-operator variability when quantitative applications are considered [10, 11]. Other challenges introduced by the use of this modality include, among others, possible probe-induced tissue displacement [12, 13], interference with the treatment beam [14], loss of acoustic coupling during the treatment, localisation errors produced by aberrations [15] and limited field of view. In recent years, though, several improvements have been introduced and, most importantly, innovative approaches have been envisioned, to minimise these limitations. These include new scanning protocols, aberration correction algorithms [16], advanced transducer technologies, improved image formation methods, robotic probe holders [17], viscous coupling gels, automatic image interpretation [18] and automatic probe positioning [19].

Historically, the first US systems started to appear in mid-90s [20] and were mainly focussed on post-surgery breast seroma localisation for electron boost treatments. The first commercial product, the B-mode Acquisition and Targeting (BAT) system (Best NOMOS, Pittsburgh, PA) using a 2D probe and a mechanical arm to track the transducer, was initially developed for prostate localisation [21]. Other systems introduced later replaced the arm with optical or infrared cameras for probe tracking, an approach that also allowed the acquisition of manually swept 3D volumes. These included the Sonarray system (Varian Medical Systems, Palo Alto, CA), the Restitu System (Resonant Medical, Montreal, Canada; now Clarity system Elekta AB, Stockholm, Sweden) and the Exactrac US Module (Brainlab AG, Munich, Germany). Also the BAT system has eventually implemented infrared camera tracking and is currently marketed as the BATCAM. Together with the Clarity system (Fig. 9.1), it is the only commercial product clinically available at the

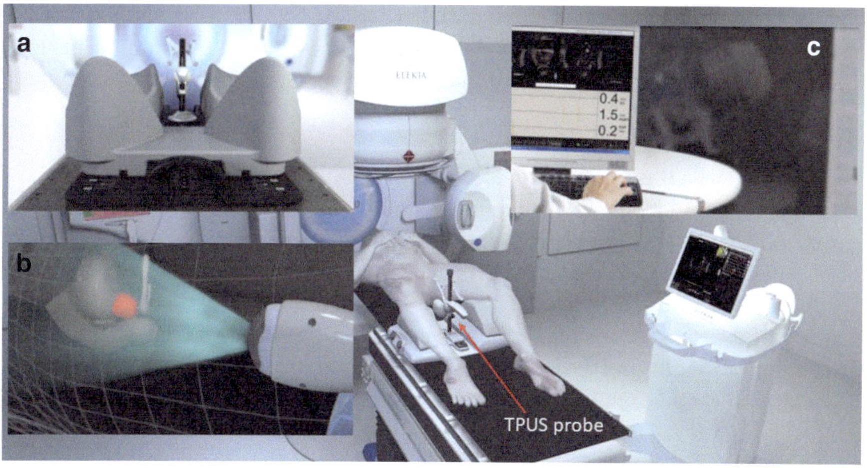

Fig. 9.1 Clarity autoscan system (images courtesy of Elekta AB, Stockholm, Sweden): the transperineal US (TPUS) probe is positioned against the perineum of the patient to scan the prostate. (**a**) US probe holder and patient support. (**b**) US beam volumetrically scanning the target and the organs at risk. (**c**) Setup and monitoring software in the control room

time of writing this book chapter. Besides the two main clinical sites of interest for US guidance, as mentioned, i.e. prostate [22] and breast [23], several other body regions have been investigated and clinical applications are already available for some of them, including liver [24], uterine cervix [25], upper abdomen [26], pancreas [27], gallbladder [28], head and neck lymph nodes [29] and bladder [30].

In this chapter, after this initial introduction to the topic, in Sect. 9.2, the main concepts of US imaging are introduced, from the basic principles to image formation; then the contribution of quantitative US in the RT workflow is discussed in Sect. 9.3, with particular attention to the most advanced applications and future vision, besides what is currently already available clinically. The following Sect. 9.4, presents the applications of US for guidance prior (inter-fraction) or during (intra-fraction) each treatment fraction, reporting the main works in literature for each clinical site. In Sect. 9.5, automatic applications are investigated from the most traditional image processing tools to the most innovative machine learning-based techniques. Finally, in the last Sect. 9.6, future directions are explored, with particular attention to new treatment techniques and innovative applications.

9.2 Ultrasound Imaging Technology

9.2.1 Basic Principles of Ultrasound Imaging

US in medical imaging uses high frequency sound waves transmitted into the body to create an image of a person's internal anatomy. Short ultrasonic pulses (at a frequency higher than the human ear can detect) can be imparted into the human body, and the echoes of these pulses can be captured to form an image of the internal tissue. Differentiation between the types of tissues shown on the resulting image is made by the strength (amplitude) of the returning echoes, and is demonstrated as a grey-scale image.

Sound waves are generated and returning echoes are detected by a device called a transducer, which is typically made from tiny piezoelectric crystals. These allow the conversion of electrical signals into sound waves (for transmission) and sound waves into an electrical signal (for detection). The crystals transmit sound in a very short pulse and then listen and wait for the structures in the path of the ultrasound beam to reflect returning echoes. The transmission of sound waves accounts for less than 1% of the transducer's total functioning time, with 99% of operating time spent detecting and amplifying the returning echoes.

Returning echoes, which have been detected, amplified and digitally processed, are displayed on the US monitor using a grey-scale (from black to white). Tissues, which produce a stronger reflection, are displayed in lighter shades of grey or even white, while black pertains to an absence of returning echoes, meaning that the sound waves transmit directly through that structure without any reflection. Grey-scale US images may therefore be described as B-mode (brightness modulation) images, because the amplitude of the echoes returning to the transducer is used to modulate the brightness of the image.

9.2.2 Attenuation of Ultrasound

When an US beam is propagated through soft tissues, it reduces in amplitude and intensity by losing energy. This is called attenuation. Different types of tissue attenuate the US beam at different rates; for example, US attenuation in bone is much greater than the attenuation in the liver. The rate of attenuation of the US beam is also dependent on the frequency of the sound waves being generated by the transducer. Low-amplitude returning echoes will have insufficient effect on the crystal to generate a signal, therefore there is a practical limit to the tissue depth capable of generating an image. There is a trade-off between image resolution and penetration inherent in all US imaging. In general, higher frequency sound waves give a greater spatial resolution image, but they are much more readily attenuated, thus limiting the tissue penetration. Lower frequency sound waves allow for a greater possible depth penetration, but spatial resolution is compromised.

The strength of the returning echo also depends on the difference in tissue density and compressibility between the various body organs. The greater the difference between two organs, the stronger the echoes from the interface defining the margins between the two organs will be. Thus, organs of vastly different acoustic impedance (for example, the liver and gallbladder) will be much more readily differentiated on an US image than organs with similar acoustic impedance (for example, the liver and kidney).

In US imaging, the beam can be attenuated in four main different ways: reflection, refraction, scattering and absorption (Fig. 9.2). Reflection refers to the

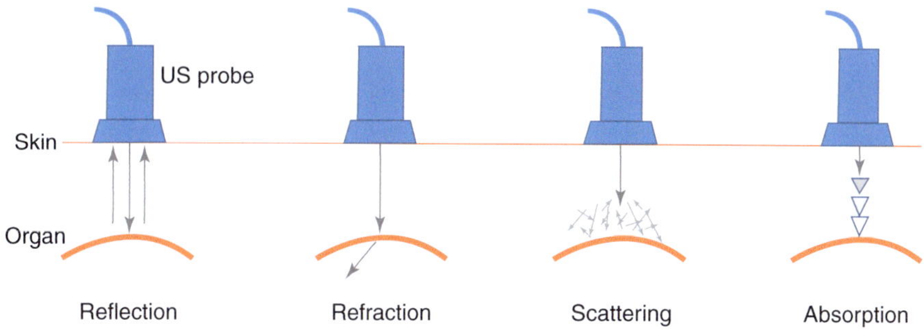

Fig. 9.2 Four different types of attenuation: from the left, reflection, refraction, scattering and absorption effects on the US beam from the US probe (transducer) through the tissues

interaction between the US beam and the interface between two structures of different acoustic impedances. At this point, some of the US beams are reflected back to the transducer as an echo, and the remainder of the US beam is transmitted into the deeper structure. The amount of energy reflected at the interface depends on the angle that the US beam is propagated onto the interface and the degree difference in acoustic impedance between the two structures. Where the angle of incidence of the US beam to the interface is 90°, the greatest amount of energy is reflected back to the transducer, creating a very bright signal called 'specular reflection'. As the angle of incidence of the US beam moves away from 90°, the amplitude of the returning echoes gradually decreases. Refraction is the deviation in the path of the US beam, caused by the beam passing through an interface between tissues with different speeds of sound, and by the interface between the tissues being not perpendicular. The degree of refraction and the angle of the refraction depend on the relative speeds of sound in the two different tissues. The resulting image may be displayed as a duplication or ghosting appearance of the structures, and may mislead the observer. US beam refraction is often referred to as an acoustic artefact in US (an appearance that does not accurately correspond to the anatomical characteristics being imaged) and is usually an undesirable degradation to the image. Scattering occurs when the US beam interacts with an acoustic interface, and results in attenuation of the US beam. Scattering at an angle perpendicular to the US beam is reflection. Scattered echoes of tiny interfaces within the tissue that are propagated back to the transducer, allow an image of the tissue to be formed. Thus, the strength of the returning echoes in tissue is not determined by the tissue density, but rather by the scatter of the US beam. Absorption refers to the transfer of the US beam energy. Absorption of sound produces a thermal effect on tissues, and accounts for the majority of US beam attenuation in diagnostic US.

The total beam attenuation in any given circumstance can be attributed to multiple processes, for example, an US beam transmitted through a kidney may be subject to absorption, scattering and reflection, whereas an US beam transmitted through lung tissue may be almost entirely attenuated by reflection.

9.2.3 Speed of Sound

US machines rely on the assumption that the speed of sound in soft tissue is always 1540 m/s. This assumption is incorrect, but because the US beam always travels through several types of body tissue in any one image, an average value must be taken to allow the machine to calculate the depth at which to display each returning echo [31]. In actual fact, the propagation speed varies subtly from 1540 m/s with each different tissue type, and can vary greatly with tissues such as bone and lung. This difference in propagation speed often leads to depth artefacts in the US image, where the displayed image does not accurately correspond to the tissue encountered in the US scan plane.

9.2.4 Ultrasound Transducers

An US transducer is a bidirectional piezoelectric device used to generate a sound wave and to receive returning echoes. The piezoelectric crystal component of the transducer converts the electrical pulse into acoustic energy (sound wave) in transmission, and acoustic energy to an electrical signal on reception of the echo. The US transducer is the most critical component of the US system because of its role in influencing image quality, dependent on the transducer's spatial and contrast resolution.

The main type of transducers used in real-time diagnostic US is an array transducer, where the piezoelectric crystals are arranged in separate parallel segments known as crystal elements. Diagnostic US transducers typically operate between 2 and 18 MHz (around 1000 times higher frequency than audible sound). US transducers are usually named according to the frequency of the US that they operate at, for example, a linear array transducer operating over a range of 9–5 MHz may be referred to as 'L9–5'.

9.2.5 Image Formation and Different Types of Imaging

The basis for image formation in diagnostic US is the 'pulse-echo' principle. Short pulses of sound are generated by the transducer and transmitted into the patient. The echoes generated by the US beam attenuation are received by the transducer and then processed and displayed in a grey-scale format. The amplitude of the returning sound waves determines the brightness of each element in the displayed image. This echo information can be displayed in several different forms or modes. A-mode (amplitude modulation) is a one-dimensional display of echoes as a series of peaks on the display. The amplitude of the echo is represented on the Y-axis and the distance or depth is represented on the X-axis. The main application of A-mode US is in ophthalmology to accurately calculate ocular dimensions. B-mode produces a two-dimensional image, and is the most common mode of US display. The US beam is 'tracked' for the duration of the scan, allowing the transmitted US beam position and orientation to accurately determine the origin and strength of the returning echoes in two dimensions. M-mode (motion mode) is a continuously updated B-mode display from a single line of sight, mostly used in echocardiography. The US beam is kept in a fixed position and transmits and receives along this single axis. The echo display is swept along the X-axis (time) on the monitor, and any vertical movement along the axis of the US beam is recorded along the Y-axis of the display. M-mode thus provides information about the movement (speed and acceleration) of an individual structure.

US imaging allows for visualisation of anatomical structures that are difficult to visualise with other image modalities. For example, the urethra is difficult to identify on a CT scan [32], while it is typically clearly visible in a US volume. In addition to B-mode imaging, there are several other imaging techniques currently clinically available or being investigated that fall under the US imaging umbrella. The most known one is probably Doppler [33], which allows for imaging of blood flow in the vasculature. As tumours typically have a different vasculature than the surrounding normal tissue, this approach has been used to assist in target identification. US elastography allows visualisation of the shear elastic moduli of different tissues [34], in other words, the stiffness of the tissues. Also in this case, tumour tissues typically have different stiffness characteristics than normal tissue. Combining these additional tissue-typing modalities with a B-mode US image and the simulation CT scan could potentially result in more accurate treatment planning [35].

9.3 Ultrasound in the Radiotherapy Workflow

US imaging can be of use during several phases of the RT workflow (see Fig. 9.3). This image modality allows for visualisation of certain anatomical structures or tissue properties that cannot or only poorly visualised with other image modalities.

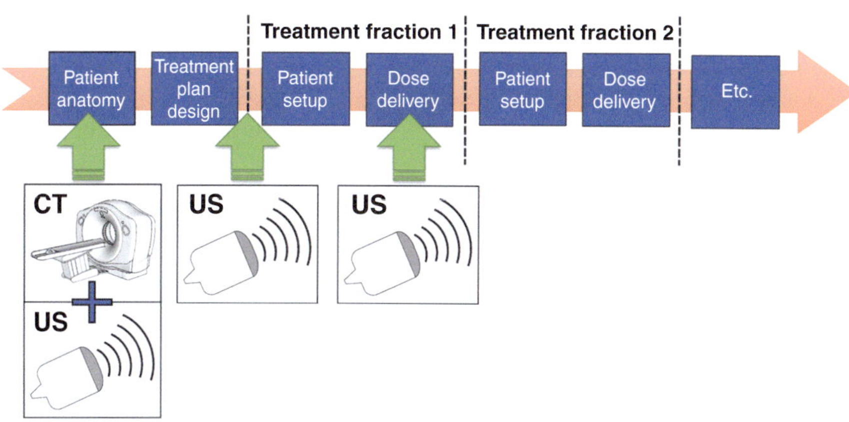

Fig. 9.3 Typical RT workflow with US imaging included for both inter-fraction and intra-fraction motion monitoring during one treatment fraction

For this reason, information from the US images could be used to help identify the target and/or organs at risk for treatment planning purposes [36]. In addition, it can also be used for both inter- and intra-fraction motion monitoring of a variety of anatomical structures, such as prostate, uterine cervix, liver and pancreas [2, 3, 22]. The motion monitoring possibilities are covered in more detail in Sect. 9.4, while US imaging for treatment planning purposes can be found in this section.

Despite the several roles that US imaging can fulfil in RT workflows, its use in these workflows is not yet widespread. This can be partially attributed to the need for a skilled operator to acquire and interpret the US images. This operator needs to position the US probe on the body of the patient and, while moving it around, interprets the live images to understand if the correct anatomical structures are visualised with sufficient quality. Typically, the technicians who are responsible for patient setup and monitoring during both simulation and treatment stage are not trained to acquire US images. For this reason, it is paramount to introduce automation into the ultrasound-guided radiotherapy (USgRT) workflows to allow for, for example, US probe setup guidance [19], image quality assessment [18] and automatic segmentation [25]. Section 9.5 dives deeper into automatic US image processing.

To allow for treatment planning and/or accurate motion management using US imaging, the US images need to be registered to the CT-scan coordinate system, as this is the coordinate system, in which the treatment plan was prepared. As introduced in Sect. 9.1, the newest USgRT systems have US probe tracking functionality, which, after calibration, allows for this registration. Ideally, the US images at the simulation stage would not only be registered to the CT coordinates, but also acquired simultaneously with the CT scan. In this way, anatomical structure shifts in between both image acquisitions due to, for example, probe pressure effects [17, 37, 38] can be avoided.

Currently, this simultaneous US-CT acquisition is not performed in clinical practice for a number of reasons. First, probe tracking systems typically do not allow tracking inside the bore of the CT. Secondly, the US probe contains metal components and if these components are present in the beam path of the CT scanner, they may create aberrations in the CT scan [39]. This could significantly deteriorate the resulting CT scan and so affect the quality of the RT treatment plan that can be prepared based on this scan. Schlosser and Hristov [39] have developed a translucent US probe that allows for 4D US imaging while causing minimal interference with the CT scan, specifically intended for use during RT workflows. This US probe is, however, not clinically available yet. For this reason, at the simulation stage of the RT workflow, the US image is typically acquired right before or after the CT scan.

To allow for intra-fraction motion monitoring (see Sect. 9.4), US images have to be acquired continuously while the radiation dose is being delivered. This raises a similar issue as with the simulation CT scan: the presence of the probe in the path of the radiation beam could potentially result in dose delivery errors. In literature, several solutions have been proposed for this issue, including the earlier mentioned translucent US probe [39]. Other solutions are the complete avoidance of the US probe during radiation delivery [17] or irradiation through the probe while possible dose deviations have already been taken into account during treatment planning [40].

The possible interventions that can be performed when inter- or intra-fraction motions are detected primarily allow for the correction of rigid motion, for example, by moving the treatment couch or by gating the radiation beam. In order to also correct for tissue deformations, a change of the treatment plan is often necessary. For this reason, adaptive RT strategies have been introduced by Yan et al. [41]. In adaptive RT, there are two main approaches followed: the first approach focusses on correction of systematic anatomical changes that have occurred between simulation and treatment stage. This so-called 'triggered replanning' can be performed at specific time slots in the treatment trajectory, for example, after delivery of a certain amount of dose; half-way during the treatment; or when under-dosage of the target is likely [42–44]. The second approach does not focus on systematic changes, but instead it corrects for daily changes in the patient's anatomy. To enable this correction, a library of treatment plans can be prepared prior to treatment commencement. Subsequently, some type of imaging has to be performed at every fraction to understand which treatment plan from the library will be used as the plan of the day (POTD) [45, 46]. It is also possible to generate the plan of the day prior to the treatment fraction during online replanning instead of selecting it from a library.

US imaging could provide the anatomical information required for both adaptive RT strategies, especially because right now it is the only volumetric imaging modality that allows for real-time image acquisition in a RT environment. For both strategies, it is important to understand how the anatomical structures have shifted and deformed over time. This implies that the segmentation and tracking of these anatomical structures on US images are critical. These topics are both extensively covered in Sect. 9.5.

At the time of writing this chapter, there are three publications available in literature that look into solutions for adaptive RT based on US imaging. Two of them focus on the generation of pseudo-CT scans based on deformable registration of US volumes [47, 48]. These pseudo-CT scans could potentially be used for (online) replanning purposes without the need to acquire an additional CT scan. The other publication compares the use of US imaging and CBCT specifically for the terms of adaptive RT of patients with cancer of the uterine cervix [49]. More research is necessary to further explore these promising directions.

9.4 Inter-Fractional and Intra-Fractional Organ Motion Estimation Using Ultrasound

This section summarises the main clinical applications of USgRT. State-of-the-art image-guided radiotherapy increasingly relies upon direct imaging of the tumour and surrounding soft tissues [50]. In turn, new imaging technologies are contributing to the development of high-precision delivery methods, such as stereotactic body radiotherapy (SBRT) and ultrahypofractionation [51–53]. As mentioned previously, US as one such technology, is characterised by excellent soft tissue contrast, an ability to scan in real time and to produce both volumetric and 4D images.

NOMOS BATCAM and Elekta Clarity, introduced in Sect. 9.1, are the only commercially available USgRT systems. Both are capable of inter-fraction image guidance and have been used for a variety of applications. Clarity, specifically, has been approved for monitoring intra-fraction prostate motion during RT delivery [54]. Early clinical applications are extensively summarised in two review papers by Fontanarosa et al. [2] and O'shea et al. [3]. More recent studies are discussed in this section. No recent reports of BATCAM have been identified, so this section will focus primarily on applications involving Elekta Clarity [22].

Two types of probe are available for use with Clarity: transabdominal (TAUS) and transperineal (TPUS). TAUS probes are used for freehand scanning of the abdomen during patient setup, which can lead to significant tissue motion and increased geometric uncertainties as a result of probe pressure. Even so, TAUS patient studies have demonstrated improvements to uterus localisation and segmentation in RT planning and adaptation [55, 56].

A TPUS probe affixed to the treatment couch is used for patient setup and intra-fraction monitoring during prostate radiotherapy. The fixation device mitigates variations in probe pressure, enables remote scanning during beam delivery and transperineal imaging ensures the probe remains outside the treatment beam field during therapy. Elekta Clarity is approved for prostate and post-prostatectomy (prostate bed) RT, hence a majority of studies address this clinical application. During treatment, prostate displacement is characterised by a slow anterioposterior drift caused by muscle relaxation, punctuated with abrupt shifts associated with muscle clenching and gas passing through the rectum [57, 58]. Intra-fraction motion ranges from <2 mm to shifts >10 mm across acquisition times spanning 100–600 s, with displacement magnitude correlated to fraction duration [54, 59–62]. Subsequently, margin size estimates increase during the first 15 min of monitoring up to maximal values of 4.29 mm superior-inferior, 1.84 mm left-right and 4.63 mm anteroposterior [63].

USgRT accuracy is typically quantified through comparisons against other well-established image guidance technologies. The current gold standard is cone-beam CT in combination with implanted fiducial markers, which are clearly visible in the resulting images. TPUS intra-fraction prostate motion monitoring was validated against both CBCT/electronic portal imaging (EPI) and implanted electromagnetic (EM) transponders (RayPilot: Micropos AB, Sweden). The different techniques were found to be comparable, with 95% limits of agreement <3 mm ([59, 60, 64]. Both EM and Clarity struggle to estimate prostate rotation, although Clarity errors were typically larger at 6.9 mm for 15° rotations compared to 3.8 mm for RayPilot.

Inter-fraction 3D TAUS guidance was reported as comparable to CBCT [65]. Moreover, improved concordance with CBCT for prostate and prostate bed matching was reported when using TPUS [66]. The improvement was attributed to reduced probe pressure and increased image quality. Guidance published in 2011 from AAPM Task Group 154 identified localisation uncertainties between US and CBCT of 3–5 mm; however, these early studies were performed using TAUS probes [67].

Average setup differences between CBCT and US of 6 mm have been recorded [68]. As CBCT with markers is the current gold standard for patient setup, it was concluded that this guidance method should be combined with US intra-fraction monitoring to capitalise on both techniques' strengths.

Motion estimation is still an ongoing challenge in USgRT. Elekta Clarity incorporates a 3D registration algorithm for tracking rigid prostate motion across six degrees of freedom during intra-fraction monitoring; however, it is susceptible to large rotations (>15°) [59]. Furthermore, real-time deformable registration algorithms are yet to be clinically implemented and manual registration is still used for daily inter-fraction matching. To realise the advantages associated with US imaging, improvements in automating registration are required to ensure the next generation of adaptive RTs can be delivered. Numerous methods have been reported, including template matching, feature-based approaches and hybrid B-spline registration [69–71], all showing potential in USgRT.

In addition to prostate applications, daily positioning and intra-fraction monitoring during breath hold for liver SBRT have been studied [72]. The liver is susceptible to respiratory motion and multiple breath holds are required during treatment, so image guidance is particularly desirable [73, 74]. A mean error of 5.4 ± 3.3 mm was reported between CBCT and TAUS for inter-fraction positioning, while intra-fraction motion >10 mm was identified in 0.8% of cases, underscoring the need for real-time motion monitoring. The same study reported monitoring diaphragm motion as a surrogate for abdominal lesions that could not be directly imaged with TAUS [75]. Other applications explored include: Intra-fraction monitoring of the diaphragm combined with intermittent kV imaging in lung cancer patients undergoing RT [76]; monitoring of the pancreatic head and surrogate structures in pancreatic RT patients [77] and monitoring of lumpectomy cavity motion during breast RT—where treatment margin reductions of 1–2 mm were reported [78].

For all applications, it is of utmost importance to adequately train the staff to achieve the desired efficacy of US image guidance, e.g. during RT of the prostate or prostate bed [79].

9.5 Automatic Image Processing Applications

As described in Sect. 9.3, US imaging in external-beam RT is not used at its full potential, yet, mostly due to the inherent complexity of US image acquisition and interpretation. To make the use of US imaging more widespread, automatic image analysis needs to be enabled to extract the useful information from the US images. This could produce enormous benefits if implemented in clinical practice. Automation will allow for: fast and precise patient setup; reduced clinician training-time; minimised inter–/intra-operator variability; inter-/intra-fraction dose re-calculation; facilitated offline and online adaptive strategies and possibly enabled real-time treatment adaptations. Section 9.4 reports on the commercially available systems and the current use of US in RT, which has applications for prostate, liver, uterine cervix, pancreas and breast cancer. In this section, the existing US-based automatic image processing techniques are covered, which were implemented for these body regions and could be applied at different stages of the EBRT workflow.

In the literature, many studies investigated prostate automatic segmentation on TRUS images [80]. TRUS is not typically utilised for USgRT since it is invasive and the US probe would interfere with the treatment beam path. However, this type of scan could be used in RT for planning purposes to complement the information provided by the simulation CT scan. The segmentation methods developed can be categorised in contour- and shape-based; region-based; supervised and unsupervised techniques and hybrid methods. The first category includes automatic deformable model-based approaches, which consist of active contours models using either external energies (balloon force [81] and gradient vector flow [82]) or Gabor filters to guide the deformable segmentation [83]. Several works have been reported on supervised and unsupervised techniques, which make use of image features to discriminate between the background and target (e.g. prostate) pixels. These image features can be learned through a labelled training dataset for supervised methods or by identifying clusters of similar objects for unsupervised methods [80, 84, 85]. Among the supervised methods, two types of algorithms have been developed: traditional machine learning approaches, using support vector machines or random forest algorithms [86–89] and deep learning methods, among which the most popular are convolutional neural networks (CNN) [90, 91]. Automatic hybrid approaches have also been reported, combining in different ways different flavours of contour- and shape-, region-based and supervised methods. Compared to the other types, these methods have been proven to be typically more robust to artefacts and noise [80].

Several studies investigated automatic image processing techniques for TPUS imaging, which is the scan type currently clinically used for prostate USgRT (see Sect. 9.4). The aim of these works was primarily to assess TPUS image quality and to ensure optimal probe positioning prior to treatment delivery.

Image quality evaluation has been implemented training a CNN combined with Gaussian Processes to automatically distinguish between good and poor quality TPUS images, where good quality were the images on which an experienced operator could identify the prostate boundaries [18]. The results were very promising as they showed that the algorithm could perform comparably to the experts involved in the study.

Two different approaches have been developed for optimal probe positioning. The first was to enable a patient-specific probe setup for RT using the patient's TPUS 3D volume, the simulation CT scan and the corresponding segmented structures to propose an optimal TPUS probe position for treatment [19]. The setups proposed in this study proved to be successful in including all the anatomical structures required for prostate RT and enabled the visualisation of 94% of the overall structures. The second approach assumed instead that TPUS imaging would be used at simulation stage and prior to the treatment and proposed a CNN to automatically register the US scans acquired at the different times [92]. The results reported an error smaller than 5 mm in about 80% of the cases analysed and showed a performance higher than manual and intensity-based registrations. This type of algorithm could be potentially used also for US intra-fraction motion estimation if used to register the US volumes acquired intra-fraction.

As mentioned in Sect. 9.4, intra-fraction monitoring using the commercially available Clarity Autoscan system still represents a challenge. Many other algorithms have been developed and show potential for this purpose. They were tested on phantoms and in vivo to monitor: the prostate, the diaphragm, the liver, the pancreas and lungs surface [3]. Most of these approaches were based on echo pattern matching, which requires selecting a region of interest (ROI) representing the target to be tracked within an US image and computing through a similarity measure the pattern with the best match in the subsequent images. The indirect, or image-based, methods make use instead of additional information supporting target localisation, such as segmentation, pre-calculated motion patterns and models. Deep learning approaches have also been developed involving CNNs able to track landmarks on an image patch by automatically extracting the relevant image features to be compared to the candidate image patches [93, 94]. The localisation accuracy achieved by the different methods was in the range of a few millimetres when phantoms were considered and slightly worse for in vivo studies.

9.6 Future Directions

In our opinion, the future of USgRT relies on continued progress in automation. Automation will not only serve to reduce, or even eliminate, operator and observer errors, it will speed-up acquisition times and potentially improve image quality. On-going efforts to employ robotic US within the RT workflow have begun to make this a reality [95, 96]. Although this workflow has focussed specifically on the integration of robotic US with the CyberKnife platform (Accuray Inc.,Sunnyvale, CA), this technology is translatable to any photon or particle treatment delivery system. Robotic-guided surgery already has public acceptance, indeed the CyberKnife itself is described as a robotic linear accelerator (LINAC); however, regulatory approval of fully automated robotic technologies, which, for example, find the best US imaging plane, may still be a significant hurdle to overcome. The use of sophisticated commercially available robots, already CE-marked and FDA-approved for use in humans, although costly, is key to accelerating translation of robotics into the clinic. We have reviewed a number of methods for the automated processing of images (see above). Automated image processing and interpretation of US images will be required to automatically select optimal imaging parameters or to determine the patient inter- or intra-fraction motion. The recent rapid development of new Deep Learning technologies, and their application to image processing and interpretation [97], presents numerous opportunities to explore these tools for the automation of USgRT [18].

Few publications have explored USgRT for particle therapies [98]. There is, however, growing interest in the use of US to localise the Bragg peak for the purpose of verification of ion beam therapies [99]. The use of US in this context may pave the way for US guidance to be used to also estimate tissue motion during particle therapy delivery. US remains the only modality that can rapidly capture volumetric images in real-time with volume rates of up to tens of Hz, opening up the possibility of capturing motion of the organs at risk as well as the target tissues. This may be especially useful for the guidance of protons, for which the deformation of overlying tissues may significantly affect the delivered dose distribution. Moving into an era of wider use of proton therapy and particularly with a focus on paediatrics [100], US also presents advantages because it is a non-ionising imaging modality and children tend to have anatomy favourable for US.

The invention of the magnetic resonance (MR) LINAC [101] has further stimulated research into adaptive on-line RT and MR-only RT workflows with significant research efforts being made in the area of automated ultrafast replanning [102] and image segmentation on MR images. The possibility of using 3D US in the context of adaptive RT has yet to be fully explored; however, preliminary work, which developed a method for the generation of pseudo-CT from US images prostate RT replanning [48], and the combination of 3D US and CBCT to visualise the uterine boundary [49] have shown US to be a promising technology. Furthermore, limitations on the volumetric imaging rates of MR have driven the investigation of combining US's real-time 3D imaging capability with MR cross-sectional imaging for the assessment of motion [103], including the exciting new development of a MR-compatible 2D matrix array [104].

Finally, US is not only an anatomical imaging modality. Using functional US imaging, closer examination of the tumour microenvironment may be a useful tool to assess the response of tumours to RT. Using power Doppler, colour Doppler and dynamic contrast-enhanced (DCE) modes of operation, US may be used to characterise the tumour vasculature, using metrics of flow and perfusion, which have been shown to change post-RT. Evidence from both preclinical [105] and clinical studies [106–108] have shown that these metrics have the potential to be used as early (<4 weeks) biomarkers of tumour response to therapy. In addition to interrogation of the tumour vasculature, changes in tumour stiffness in response to radiation have been observed in clinical studies using US strain elastography to measure the response of cervical cancer to radiation [109, 110] and quantitative shear wave elastography to measure the radiation response of rectal cancer [111]. As shown in this chapter, US image guidance technology has already been successfully integrated into the RT clinic for prostate RT, and research in cervical and liver cancer has demonstrated to have significant promise. Extending the use of this technology to monitor tumour response to RT may not only further improve the cost-effectiveness of US, but it opens up exciting new avenues for more personalised RT in which patient's treatments can be adapted according to their response to radiation.

References

1. Antico M, Sasazawa F, Wu L, et al. Ultrasound guidance in minimally invasive robotic procedures. Med Image Anal. 2019;54:149–67.
2. Fontanarosa D, van der Meer S, Bamber J, Harris E, O'Shea T, Verhaegen F. Review of ultrasound image guidance in external beam radiotherapy: I. treatment planning and inter-fraction motion management. Phys Med Biol. 2015;60(3):R77–114.
3. O'Shea T, Bamber J, Fontanarosa D, van der Meer S, Verhaegen F, Harris E. Review of ultrasound image guidance in external beam radiotherapy part II: intra-fraction motion management and novel applications. Phys Med Biol. 2016;61(8):R90–137.

4. Schewe JE, Balter JM, Lam KL, ten Haken RK. Measurement of patient setup errors using port films and a computer-aided graphical alignment tool. Med Dosim. 1996;21(2):97–104.
5. Bel A, Vos PH, Rodrigus PT, et al. High-precision prostate cancer irradiation by clinical application of an offline patient setup verification procedure, using portal imaging. Int J Radiat Oncol Biol Phys. 1996;35(2):321–32.
6. Srinivasan K, Mohammadi M, Shepherd J. Applications of linac-mounted kilovoltage cone-beam computed tomography in modern radiation therapy: a review. Pol J Rad. 2014;79:181–93.
7. Shirato H, Shimizu S, Kitamura K, et al. Four-dimensional treatment planning and fluoroscopic real-time tumor tracking radiotherapy for moving tumor. Int J Radiat Oncol Biol Phys. 2000;48(2):435–42.
8. Willoughby TR, Kupelian PA, Pouliot J, et al. Target localization and real-time tracking using the calypso 4D localization system in patients with localized prostate cancer. Int J Radiat Oncol Biol Phys. 2006;65(2):528–34.
9. Covington EL, Fiveash JB, Wu X, et al. Optical surface guidance for submillimeter monitoring of patient position during frameless stereotactic radiotherapy. J Appl Clin Med Phys/Am Coll Med Phys. 2019;20(6):91–8.
10. Enke C, Ayyangar K, Saw CB, Zhen W, Thompson RB, Raman NV. Inter-observer variation in prostate localization utilizing BAT. Int J Radiat Oncol Biol Phys. 2002;54(2):269.
11. Langen KM, Pouliot J, Anezinos C, et al. Evaluation of ultrasound-based prostate localization for image-guided radiotherapy. Int J Radiat Oncol Biol Phys. 2003;57(3):635–44.
12. Artignan X, Smitsmans MHP, Lebesque JV, Jaffray DA, van Her M, Bartelink H. Online ultrasound image guidance for radiotherapy of prostate cancer: impact of image acquisition on prostate displacement. Int J Radiat Oncol Biol Phys. 2004;59(2):595–601.
13. van der Meer S, Bloemen-van Gurp E, Hermans J, et al. Critical assessment of intramodality 3D ultrasound imaging for prostate IGRT compared to fiducial markers. Med Phys. 2013;40(7):071707.
14. Martyn M, O'Shea TP, Harris E, Bamber J, Gilroy S, Foley MJ. A Monte Carlo study of the effect of an ultrasound transducer on surface dose during intrafraction motion imaging for external beam radiation therapy. Med Phys. 2017;44(10):5020–33.
15. Fontanarosa D, van der Meer S, Bloemen-van Gurp E, Stroian G, Verhaegen F. Magnitude of speed of sound aberration corrections for ultrasound image-guided radiotherapy for prostate and other anatomical sites. Med Phys. 2012;39(8):5286–92.
16. Fontanarosa D, van der Meer S, Harris E, Verhaegen F. A CT-based correction method for speed of sound aberration for ultrasound-based image-guided radiotherapy. Med Phys. 2011;38(5):2665–73.
17. Schlosser J, Salisbury K, Hristov D. Telerobotic system concept for real-time soft-tissue imaging during radiotherapy beam delivery. Med Phys. 2010;37(12):6357–67.
18. Camps SM, Houben T, Carneiro G, et al. Automatic quality assessment of transperineal ultrasound images of the male pelvic region, using deep learning. Ultrasound Med Biol. 2020;46(2):445–54.
19. Camps SM, Verhaegen F, Vanneste BGL, de With PHN, Fontanarosa D. Automated patient-specific transperineal ultrasound probe setups for prostate cancer patients undergoing radiotherapy. Med Phys. 2018b;45(7):3185–95.
20. Troccaz J, Laieb N, Vassal P, et al. Patient setup optimization for external conformal radiotherapy. J Image Guid Surg. 1995;1(2):113–20.
21. Lattanzi J, McNeeley S, Donnelly S, et al. Ultrasound-based stereotactic guidance in prostate cancer--quantification of organ motion and set-up errors in external beam radiation therapy. Comput Aided Surg. 2000;5(4):289–95.
22. Camps SM, Fontanarosa D, de With PHN, Verhaegen F, Vanneste BGL. The use of ultrasound imaging in the external beam radiotherapy workflow of prostate cancer patients. Biomed Res Int. 2018a;2018:7569590.
23. Fraser DJ, Wong P, Sultanem K, Verhaegen F. Dosimetric evolution of the breast electron boost target using 3D ultrasound imaging. Radiother Oncol. 2010;96(2):185–91.

24. Bloemen-van Gurp E, van der Meer S, Hendry J, et al. Active breathing control in combination with ultrasound imaging: a feasibility study of image guidance in stereotactic body radiation therapy of liver lesions. Int J Radiat Oncol Biol Phys. 2013;85(4):1096–102.
25. Mason SA, O'Shea TP, White IM, et al. Towards ultrasound-guided adaptive radiotherapy for cervical cancer: evaluation of Elekta's semiautomated uterine segmentation method on 3D ultrasound images. Med Phys. 2017;44(7):3630–8.
26. Fuss M, Salter BJ, Cavanaugh SX, et al. Daily ultrasound-based image-guided targeting for radiotherapy of upper abdominal malignancies. Int J Radiat Oncol Biol Phys. 2004;59(4):1245–56.
27. Fuss M, Wong A, Fuller CD, Salter BJ, Fuss C, Thomas CR. Image-guided intensity-modulated radiotherapy for pancreatic carcinoma. Gastrointest Cancer Res. 2007;1(1):2–11.
28. Fuller CD, Thomas CR, Wong A, et al. Image-guided intensity-modulated radiation therapy for gallbladder carcinoma. Radiother Oncol. 2006;81(1):65–72.
29. Fraser D, Fava P, Cury F, Vuong T, Falco T, Verhaegen F. Evaluation of a prototype 3D ultrasound system for multimodality imaging of cervical nodes for adaptive radiation therapy. In: Cleary KR, Miga MI, editors. Medical Imaging 2007: Visualization and Image-Guided Procedures. SPIE Proceedings. Bellingham: SPIE; 2007. p. 65090Y.
30. McBain CA, Green MM, Stratford J, et al. Ultrasound imaging to assess inter- and intra-fraction motion during bladder radiotherapy and its potential as a verification tool. Clin Oncol (R Coll Radiol). 2009;21(5):385–93.
31. Gill R. The physics and technology of diagnostic ultrasound: a practitioner's guide. High Frequency Publishing; Sydney, Australia. 2012.
32. Kataria T, Gupta D, Goyal S, et al. Simple diagrammatic method to delineate male urethra in prostate cancer radiotherapy: an MRI-based approach. Br J Radiol. 2016;89(1068):20160348.
33. Merritt CR. Doppler color flow imaging. J Clin Ultrasound. 1987;15(9):591–7.
34. Bamber J, Cosgrove D, Dietrich CF, et al. EFSUMB guidelines and recommendations on the clinical use of ultrasound elastography. Part 1: basic principles and technology. Ultraschall in der Medizin (Stuttgart, Germany : 1980). 2013;34(2):169–84.
35. Zhang P, Osterman KS, Liu T, et al. How does performance of ultrasound tissue typing affect design of prostate IMRT dose-painting protocols? Int J Radiat Oncol Biol Phys. 2007;67(2):362–8.
36. Wein W, Röper B, Navab N. Integrating diagnostic B-mode ultrasonography into CT-based radiation treatment planning. IEEE Trans Med Imaging. 2007;26(6):866–79.
37. Fargier-Voiron M, Presles B, Pommier P, et al. Impact of probe pressure variability on prostate localization for ultrasound-based image-guided radiotherapy. Radiother Oncol. 2014;111(1):132–7.
38. Li M, Hegemann N-S, Manapov F, et al. Prefraction displacement and intrafraction drift of the prostate due to perineal ultrasound probe pressure. Strahlenther Onkol. 2017b;193(6):459–65.
39. Schlosser J, Hristov D. Radiolucent 4D ultrasound imaging: system design and application to radiotherapy guidance. IEEE Trans Med Imaging. 2016;35(10):2292–300.
40. Bazalova-Carter M, Schlosser J, Chen J, Hristov D. Monte Carlo modeling of ultrasound probes for image-guided radiotherapy. Med Phys. 2015;42(10):5745–56.
41. Yan D, Vicini F, Wong J, Martinez A. Adaptive radiation therapy. Phys Med Biol. 1997;42(1):123–32.
42. Birkner M, Yan D, Alber M, Liang J, Nüsslin F. Adapting inverse planning to patient and organ geometrical variation: algorithm and implementation. Med Phys. 2003;30(10):2822–31.
43. Lim K, Stewart J, Kelly V, et al. Dosimetrically triggered adaptive intensity modulated radiation therapy for cervical cancer. Int J Radiat Oncol Biol Phys. 2014;90(1):147–54.
44. Li T, Thongphiew D, Zhu X, et al. Adaptive prostate IGRT combining online re-optimization and re-positioning: a feasibility study. Phys Med Biol. 2011;56(5):1243–58.
45. Gill S, Pham D, Dang K, et al. Plan of the day selection for online image-guided adaptive post-prostatectomy radiotherapy. Radiother Oncol. 2013;107(2):165–70.
46. Sharfo AWM, Breedveld S, Voet PWJ, et al. Validation of fully automated VMAT plan generation for library-based plan-of-the-day cervical cancer radiotherapy. PLoS One. 2016;11(12):e0169202.

47. Camps S, van der Meer S, Verhaegen F, Fontanarosa D. Various approaches for pseudo-CT scan creation based on ultrasound to ultrasound deformable image registration between different treatment time points for radiotherapy treatment plan adaptation in prostate cancer patients. Biomed Phys Eng Exp. 2016;2(3):035018.
48. van der Meer S, Camps SM, van Elmpt WJC, et al. Simulation of pseudo-CT images based on deformable image registration of ultrasound images: a proof of concept for transabdominal ultrasound imaging of the prostate during radiotherapy. Med Phys. 2016;43(4):1913.
49. Mason SA, White IM, O'Shea, T, et al. Combined ultrasound and cone-beam CT improves target segmentation for image-guided radiation therapy in uterine cervix cancer. Int J Radiat Oncol Biol Phys. 2019;104(3):685–93.
50. Bertholet J, Knopf A, Eiben B, et al. Real-time intrafraction motion monitoring in external beam radiotherapy. Phys Med Biol. 2019;64(15):15TR01.
51. Loblaw A. Ultrahypofractionation should be a standard of care option for intermediate-risk prostate cancer. Clin Oncol (R Coll Radiol). 2020;32(3):170–4.
52. Tree A, Ostler P, van As N. New horizons and hurdles for UK radiotherapy: can prostate stereotactic body radiotherapy show the way? Clin Oncol (R Coll Radiol). 2014;26(1):1–3.
53. Wang H, Jin C, Fang L, Sun H, Cheng W, Hu S. Health economic evaluation of stereotactic body radiotherapy (SBRT) for hepatocellular carcinoma: a systematic review. Cost Eff Res Alloc. 2020;18:1.
54. Richter A, Exner F, Weick S, et al. Evaluation of intrafraction prostate motion tracking using the clarity autoscan system for safety margin validation. Z Med Phys. 2020;30(2):135–41.
55. Baker M, Cooper DT, Behrens CF. Evaluation of uterine ultrasound imaging in cervical radiotherapy; a comparison of autoscan and conventional probe. Br J Radiol. 2016;89(1066):20160510.
56. Mason SA, White IM, Lalondrelle S, Bamber JC, Harris EJ. The stacked-ellipse algorithm: an ultrasound-based 3-D uterine segmentation tool for enabling adaptive radiotherapy for uterine cervix cancer. Ultrasound Med Biol. 2020;46(4):1040–52.
57. Ballhausen H, Li M, Hegemann NS, Ganswindt U, Belka C. Intra-fraction motion of the prostate is a random walk. Phys Med Biol. 2015;60(2):549–63.
58. Pommer T, Oh JH, Munck AF, Rosenschöld P, Deasy JO. Simulating intrafraction prostate motion with a random walk model. Adv Radiat Oncol. 2017;2(3):429–36.
59. Biston M-C, Zaragori T, Delcoudert L, et al. Comparison of electromagnetic transmitter and ultrasound imaging for intrafraction monitoring of prostate radiotherapy. Radiother Oncol. 2019;136:1–8.
60. Han B, Najafi M, Cooper DT, et al. Evaluation of transperineal ultrasound imaging as a potential solution for target tracking during hypofractionated radiotherapy for prostate cancer. Radiat Oncol. 2018;13(1):151.
61. Richardson AK, Jacobs P. Intrafraction monitoring of prostate motion during radiotherapy using the clarity® autoscan Transperineal ultrasound (TPUS) system. Radiography (London, England : 1995). 2017;23(4):310–3.
62. Sihono DSK, Ehmann M, Heitmann S, et al. Determination of Intrafraction prostate motion during external beam radiation therapy With a Transperineal 4-dimensional ultrasound real-time tracking system. Int J Radiat Oncol Biol Phys. 2018;101(1):136–43.
63. Pang EPP, Knight K, Park SY, et al. Duration-dependent margins for prostate radiotherapy-a practical motion mitigation strategy. Strahlenther Onkol. 2020;196(7):657–63.
64. Grimwood A, McNair HA, O'Shea TP, et al. In vivo validation of Elekta's clarity autoscan for ultrasound-based Intrafraction motion estimation of the prostate during radiation therapy. Int J Radiat Oncol Biol Phys. 2018;102(4):912–21.
65. Li M, Ballhausen H, Hegemann N-S, et al. Comparison of prostate positioning guided by three-dimensional transperineal ultrasound and cone-beam CT. Strahlenther Onkol. 2017a;193(3):221–8.
66. Fargier-Voiron M, Presles B, Pommier P, et al. Evaluation of a new transperineal ultrasound probe for inter-fraction image-guidance for definitive and post-operative prostate cancer radiotherapy. Phys Med. 2016;32(3):499–505.

67. Molloy JA, Chan G, Markovic A, et al. Quality assurance of U.S.-guided external beam radiotherapy for prostate cancer: report of AAPM task group 154. Med Phys. 2011;38(2):857–71.
68. Richter A, Polat B, Lawrenz I, et al. Initial results for patient setup verification using transperineal ultrasound and cone-beam CT in external beam radiation therapy of prostate cancer. Radiat Oncol. 2016;11(1):147.
69. De Luca V, Banerjee J, Hallack A, et al. Evaluation of 2D and 3D ultrasound tracking algorithms and impact on ultrasound-guided liver radiotherapy margins. Med Phys. 2018;45(11):4986–5003.
70. Rivaz H, Collins DL. Near real-time robust non-rigid registration of volumetric ultrasound images for neurosurgery. Ultrasound Med Biol. 2015;41(2):574–87.
71. Wulff D, Kuhlemann I, Ernst F, Schweikard A, Ipsen S. Robust motion tracking of deformable targets in the liver using binary feature libraries in 4D ultrasound. Curr Direct Biomed Eng. 2019;5(1):601–4.
72. Boda-Heggemann J, Sihono DSK, Streb L, et al. Ultrasound-based repositioning and real-time monitoring for abdominal SBRT in DIBH. Phys Med. 2019;65:46–52.
73. Betgen A, Alderliesten T, Sonke J-J, van Vliet-Vroegindeweij C, Bartelink H, Remeijer P. Assessment of set-up variability during deep inspiration breath hold radiotherapy for breast cancer patients by 3D-surface imaging. Radiother Oncol. 2013;106(2):225–30.
74. Dhont J, Vandemeulebroucke J, Burghelea M, et al. The long- and short-term variability of breathing-induced tumor motion in lung and liver over the course of a radiotherapy treatment. Radiother Oncol. 2018;126(2):339–46.
75. Vogel L, Sihono DSK, Weiss C, et al. Intra-breath-hold residual motion of image-guided DIBH liver-SBRT: an estimation by ultrasound-based monitoring correlated with diaphragm position in CBCT. Radiother Oncol. 2018;129(3):441–8.
76. Mostafaei F, Tai A, Gore E, et al. Feasibility of real-time lung tumor motion monitoring using intrafractional ultrasound and kV cone-beam projection images. Med Phys. 2018;45(10):4619–26.
77. Omari EA, Erickson B, Ehlers C, et al. Preliminary results on the feasibility of using ultrasound to monitor intrafractional motion during radiation therapy for pancreatic cancer. Med Phys. 2016;43(9):5252.
78. Heimann R, Hard D. A comparison of three dimensional ultrasound, clips and CT for measuring interfractional breast lumpectomy cavity motion. J Nucl Med Radiat Ther. 2016;07(02)
79. Hilman S, Smith R, Masson S, et al. Implementation of a daily transperineal ultrasound system as image-guided radiotherapy for prostate cancer. Clin Oncol (R Coll Radiol). 2017;29(1):e49.
80. Ghose S, Oliver A, Martí R, et al. A survey of prostate segmentation methodologies in ultrasound, magnetic resonance and computed tomography images. Comput Methods Prog Biomed. 2012b;108(1):262–87.
81. Knoll C, Alcañiz M, Grau V, Monserrat C, Carmen Juan M. Outlining of the prostate using snakes with shape restrictions based on the wavelet transform (doctoral thesis: dissertation). Pattern Recogn. 1999;32(10):1767–81.
82. Zaim A, Jankun J. 2007. An energy-based segmentation of prostate from ultrasound images using dot-pattern select cells. In: *2007 IEEE International Conference on Acoustics, Speech and Signal Processing - ICASSP '07*. IEEE, pp. I-297-I–300.
83. Shen D, Zhan Y, Davatzikos C. Segmentation of prostate boundaries from ultrasound images using statistical shape model. IEEE Trans Med Imaging. 2003;22(4):539–51.
84. Richard WD, Keen CG. Automated texture-based segmentation of ultrasound images of the prostate. Comput Med Imaging Graph. 1996;20(3):131–40.
85. Zaim A. Automatic segmentation of the prostate from ultrasound data using feature-based self organizing map. In: Kalviainen H, Parkkinen J, Kaarna A, editors. Image analysis. Lecture notes in computer science. Berlin, Heidelberg: Springer Berlin Heidelberg; 2005. p. 1259–65.
86. Akbari H, Yang X, Halig LV, Fei B. 3D segmentation of prostate ultrasound images using wavelet transform. Proc SPIE. 2011;7962:79622K.

87. Ghose S, Mitra J, Oliver A, et al. A supervised learning framework for automatic prostate segmentation in trans rectal ultrasound images. In: Blanc-Talon J, Philips W, Popescu D, Scheunders P, Zemčík P, editors. Advanced concepts for intelligent vision systems. Lecture notes in computer science. Berlin, Heidelberg: Springer Berlin Heidelberg; 2012a. p. 190–200.
88. Nouranian S, Ramezani M, Spadinger I, Morris WJ, Salcudean SE, Abolmaesumi P. Learning-based multi-label segmentation of Transrectal ultrasound images for prostate brachytherapy. IEEE Trans Med Imaging. 2016;35(3):921–32.
89. Zaim A, Yi T, Keck R. 2007. Feature-based classification of prostate ultrasound images using multiwavelet and kernel support vector machines. In: *2007 International Joint Conference on Neural Networks*. IEEE, pp. 278–281.
90. Ghavami N, Hu Y, Bonmati E, et al. Automatic slice segmentation of intraoperative transrectal ultrasound images using convolutional neural networks. In: Webster RJ, Fei B, editors. Medical imaging 2018: image-guided procedures, robotic interventions, and modeling. Bellingham: SPIE; 2018. p. 2.
91. Lei Y, Tian S, He X, et al. Ultrasound prostate segmentation based on multidirectional deeply supervised V-net. Med Phys. 2019;46(7):3194–206.
92. Zhu N, Najafi M, Han B, Hancock S, Hristov D. Feasibility of image registration for ultrasound-guided prostate radiotherapy based on similarity measurement by a convolutional neural network. Technol Cancer Res Treat. 2019;18:1533033818821964.
93. De Luca V, Benz T, Kondo S, et al. The 2014 liver ultrasound tracking benchmark. Phys Med Biol. 2015;60(14):5571–99.
94. Gomariz A, Li W, Ozkan E, Tanner C, Goksel O. 2019. Siamese networks with location prior for landmark tracking in liver ultrasound sequences. In: *2019 IEEE 16th International Symposium on Biomedical Imaging (ISBI 2019)*. IEEE, pp. 1757–1760.
95. Gerlach S, Kuhlemann I, Jauer P, et al. Robotic ultrasound-guided SBRT of the prostate: feasibility with respect to plan quality. Int J Comput Assist Radiol Surg. 2017;12(1):149–59.
96. Ipsen S, Bruder R, Kuhlemann I, et al. 2018. A visual probe positioning tool for 4D ultrasound-guided radiotherapy *Conference Proceedings: Annual International Conference of the IEEE Engineering in Medicine and Biology Society* 2018, pp. 883–886.
97. Brattain LJ, Telfer BA, Dhyani M, Grajo JR, Samir AE. Machine learning for medical ultrasound: status, methods, and future opportunities. Abdom Radiol (New York). 2018;43(4):786–99.
98. Schwaab J, Prall M, Sarti C, et al. Ultrasound tracking for intra-fractional motion compensation in radiation therapy. Phys Med. 2014;30(5):578–82.
99. Kellnberger S, Assmann W, Lehrack S, et al. Ionoacoustic tomography of the proton Bragg peak in combination with ultrasound and optoacoustic imaging. Sci Rep. 2016;6:29305.
100. Journy N, Indelicato DJ, Withrow DR, et al. Patterns of proton therapy use in pediatric cancer management in 2016: an international survey. Radiother Oncol. 2019;132:155–61.
101. Lagendijk JJW, Raaymakers BW, van Vulpen M. The magnetic resonance imaging-linac system. Semin Radiat Oncol. 2014;24(3):207–9.
102. Ziegenhein P, Kamerling CP, Fast MF, Oelfke U. Real-time energy/mass transfer mapping for online 4D dose reconstruction. Sci Rep. 2018;8(1):3662.
103. Giger A, Stadelmann M, Preiswerk F, et al. Ultrasound-driven 4D MRI. Phys Med Biol. 2018;63(14):145015.
104. Lee W, Chan H, Chan P, et al. A magnetic resonance compatible E4D ultrasound probe for motion management of radiation therapy. IEEE Netw. 2017;2017
105. Arteaga-Marrero N, Mainou-Gomez JF, Brekke Rygh C, et al. Radiation treatment monitoring with DCE-US in CWR22 prostate tumor xenografts. Acta Radiologica (Stockholm, Sweden : 1987). 2019;60(6):788–97.
106. Detsky JS, Milot L, Ko Y-J, et al. Perfusion imaging of colorectal liver metastases treated with bevacizumab and stereotactic body radiotherapy. Phys Imaging Radiat Oncol. 2018;5:9–12.
107. Li H, Liu J, Chen M, Li H, Long L. Therapeutic evaluation of radiotherapy with contrast-enhanced ultrasound in non-Resectable hepatocellular carcinoma patients with portal vein tumor thrombosis. Med Sci Monit. 2018;24:8183–9.

108. Shiozawa K, Watanabe M, Ikehara T, et al. Evaluation of contrast-enhanced ultrasonography for hepatocellular carcinoma prior to and following stereotactic body radiation therapy using the CyberKnife® system: a preliminary report. Oncol Lett. 2016;11(1):208–12.
109. Mabuchi S, Sasano T, Kuroda H, Takahashi R, Nakagawa S, Kimura T. Real-time tissue sonoelastography for early response monitoring in cervical cancer patients treated with definitive chemoradiotherapy: preliminary results. J Med Ultrason (2001). 2015;42(3):379–85.
110. Xu Y, Zhu L, Liu B, et al. Strain elastography imaging for early detection and prediction of tumor response to concurrent chemo-radiotherapy in locally advanced cervical cancer: feasibility study. BMC Cancer. 2017;17(1):427.
111. Rafaelsen SR, Vagn-Hansen C, Sørensen T, Lindebjerg J, Pløen J, Jakobsen A. Ultrasound elastography in patients with rectal cancer treated with chemoradiation. Eur J Radiol. 2013;82(6):913–7.

10 Means for Target Volume Delineation and Stabilisation: Fiducial Markers, Balloons and Others

Ben G. L. Vanneste, Oleksandr Boychak, Marianne Nordsmark, and Lone Hoffmann

Abbreviations

3D-CRT	3D Conventional RadioTherapy
ARW	Ano-Rectal Wall
CBCT	Cone-Beam Computed Tomography
CT	Computed Tomography
EDD	Endo-rectal Displacement Device
EPIC	Expanded Prostate Cancer Index Composite
ERB	Endo-Rectal Balloons
ERD	Endo-Rectal Devices
HA	Hyaluronic Acid
IMRT	Intensity-Modulated RadioTherapy
IRS	Implanted Rectum Spacers
MRI	Magnetic Resonance Imaging
PEG	PolyEthylene-Glycol

B. G. L. Vanneste (✉)
Department of Radiation Oncology (MAASTRO), GROW—School for Oncology and Developmental Biology, Maastricht University Medical Centre, Maastricht, The Netherlands

Department of Radiation Oncology, Ghent University Hospital, Ghent, Belgium

Department of Human Structure and Repair, Ghent University, Ghent, Belgium
e-mail: ben.vanneste@uzgent.be

O. Boychak
Department of Radiation Oncology, St Luke's Radiation Oncology Network, Dublin, Republic of Ireland
e-mail: Oleksandr.Boychak@slh.ie

M. Nordsmark · L. Hoffmann
Department of Oncology, Aarhus University Hospital, Aarhus, Denmark
e-mail: marianne@oncology.au.dk; lone.hoffmann@aarhus.rm.dk

E. G. C. Troost (ed.), *Image-Guided High-Precision Radiotherapy*,
https://doi.org/10.1007/978-3-031-08601-4_10

PTV	Planning Target Volume
QALY	Quality-Adjusted Life Year
RBI	Rectal Balloon Implant
RT	RadioTherapy
TRUS	TransRectal UltraSonography

10.1 Introduction

In general, solid tumours originate from soft tissues and are therefore not visible on planar kV- or MV-X-ray-based imaging modalities and only difficult on cone-beam computed tomography (CBCT). In the era of high-precision radiotherapy, an accurate and precise depiction of the tumour, either directly (preferred) or indirectly is mandatory to guarantee the best treatment outcome possible. To illustrate means of target volume demarcation or stabilisation, the following chapter highlights developments for both oesophageal and prostate cancer.

Prostate cancer is the 2nd most common cancer in men worldwide and the 4th most common cancer overall. There were more than 1.4 million new cases of prostate cancer in 2020 [1]. Over the years conducted and published, randomised controlled trials showed that RT dose escalation not only significantly improve local control and biochemical relapse-free survival in prostate cancer patients [2–6] Dose-escalated RT provides a very high cure rate: the 10 years or more survival is approximately 85% in men diagnosed with prostate cancer in the UK (Cancer Statistics for the UK, see cancerresearchuk.org). As survival rates have soured, focus of research has shifted towards improving and maintaining high quality of life. The quality of life can be significantly affected after all treatments due to changes in bowel function, sexual dysfunction and an increased rate of urinary incontinence [7]. The side effects of RT for prostate cancer are mostly related to significant late gastro-intestinal toxicity: increased frequency and diarrhoea, mucus discharge, faecal incontinence, bleeding, urgency and tenesmus [8]. Therefore, many technical advances in clinical practice, recently shifted towards development of safer RT dose escalation. This chapter provides an overview of the improvements of volume delineation and the medical devices used for decreasing rectal dose and reducing rectal toxicities.

Also in other tumour sites, e.g. oesophageal cancer, RT as part of the oncological treatment has successfully attributed to increased survival rates. Oesophageal cancer is the eighth most common cancer worldwide, the sixth most common cause of death from cancer, with >570,000 new cases per year and >500,000 deaths per year [9, 10]. Global cancer statistics 2018: GLOBOCAN estimates of incidence and mortality worldwide for 36 cancers in 185 countries. A high proportion of patients have advanced disease at diagnosis and the survival at 5 years is low, 20%. Patients in good general condition with localised tumours receive treatment with curative intent; either surgery alone, trimodality treatment consisting of surgery combined with neoadjuvant chemoradiotherapy (nCHRT), perioperative chemotherapy, or definitive chemoradiotherapy (dCHRT) [11–21]. Unfortunately, all of these treatments have significant toxicity, reported as high as up to 50–60%. Thus, there is a need for more effective treatments, for reducing toxicity.

10.2 Image Guidance

Previously, patients were positioned on a linear accelerator using surrogate reference points: external reference points such as skin marks or tattoo points, or bony landmarks visualised by conventional plain orthogonal X-ray radiographs (see Chap. 4). However, as it is known that various solid tumours themselves move, shrink, grow or deform during the radiotherapy course and additionally are surrounded by moving organs at risk (OARs), these surrogate reference points may lead to off-target dose delivery, which in turn compromises tumour cure and inflicts higher rates of nearby OARs toxicity [22–24]. This problem is typically compensated for by expanding safety margins used around the target volume, but the disadvantage of this strategy is the irradiation of larger volumes of the surrounding healthy tissues. Different techniques have been developed to handle this problem, and further improved both oncological and toxicity outcomes [25, 26].

The aspects of Cone-beam Computed Tomography (CBCT), magnetic resonance imaging (MRI) and ultrasound are in depth discussed in Chaps. 3, 4, and 9, respectively.

10.2.1 Cone-Beam Computed Tomography

In brief, the use of daily CBCT or in-room CT for patient setup reduces the setup margins [24]. There are different strategies for patient setup, varying from setup using surrogate structures as nearby bony anatomy or high-contrast OARs, as e.g. the carina for mediastinal targets, to soft tissue setup based on the tumour [27]. Low-contrast or motion artefacts in, e.g. the abdomen or thorax may hamper soft tissue matching of the target structure. Implantation of fiducial markers in or in proximity of the tumour may help evaluating the soft tissue match, since the markers are clearly visible on CT/CBCT (see below) [28–30]. Daily setup on the target compared to setup on the bony anatomy reduces margins in oesophageal cancer patients compared to setup on the bony anatomy (Fig. 10.1) [27]. Furthermore, the daily imaging may visualise systematic anatomical changes, which can be mitigated by adaptive radiotherapy (ART) [31]. The concept of ART is to act on anatomical changes by, e.g. rescanning the patient in case of systematic changes [26, 32] or making a variety of treatment plans based on a library of target and OAR positions in case of random changes, e.g. in the pelvic region [33, 34]. The implementation of ART may significantly reduce toxicity, as seen, e.g. in lung cancer patients [35].

Possible disadvantages of CBCT include lower soft-tissue contrast, applied radiation dose and an inter-observer variability in the interpretation of target changes [36]. Therefore, CBCT modality may benefit from being combined with other methods, e.g. fiducial markers acting as surrogates for the tumour.

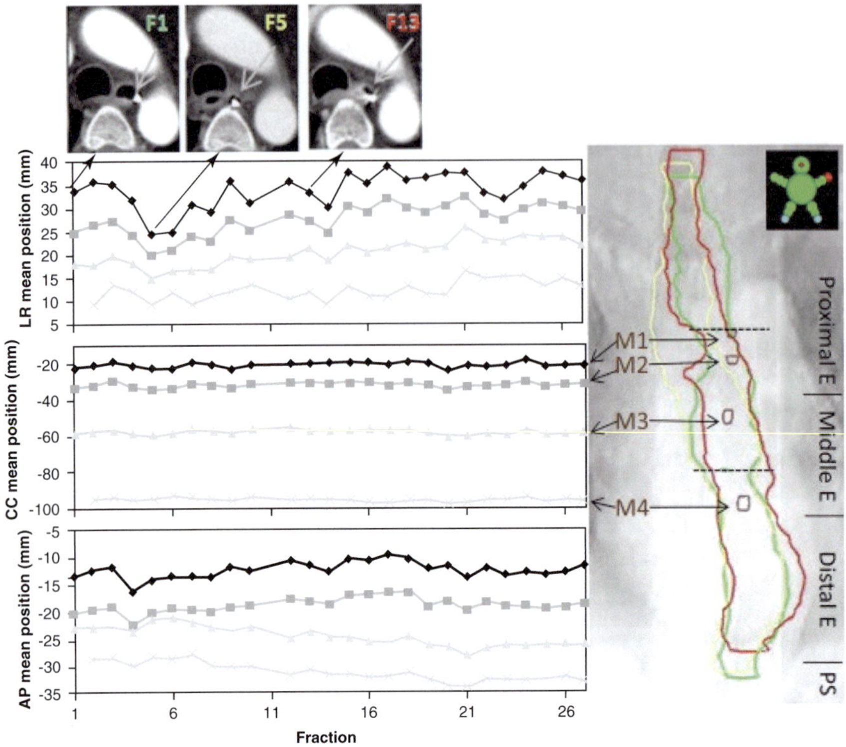

Fig. 10.1 Inter-fractional motion of four markers (M1–M4) during 27 fractions for a patient in the left–right (LR), cranio-caudal (CC) and anterior-posterior (AP) directions. Upper: the position of M1 at fractions 1, 5 and 13. Below-left: All positions are relative to the isocentre after bony anatomy alignment. With permission taken from Hoffmann et al. [27]

10.2.2 Ultrasound

In summary, two ultrasound systems can be used for visualisation of the target volume, i.e. prostate: transperineal and transabdominal ultrasound [37]. Possible advantages are no additional irradiation for the patient, the relatively low price and the possibility for real-time volumetric organ tracking. Some of the limitations of the ultrasound are the inaccessibility of tissues shielded by bone or air, the susceptibility for imaging artefacts and high user dependency, due to its mostly manual operation [38].

10.2.3 MRI

A new on-line imaging tool is the MRI-LINAC providing superior soft-tissue contrast visualisation of the tumour and the surroundings for more accurate and precise radiation delivery [39, 40]. More advantages are the availability of functional and biological information, and real-time image guidance [41]. Furthermore, a workflow entirely based on MRI flow will make the invasive placement of the fiducial markers superfluous [42]. Disadvantages of MRI-LINAC systems include the very high resource demand and complex quality assurance processes [41]. Finally, the long-term clinical benefit and the cost-effectiveness of this pricey treatment modality still need to be proven [43]. Very recently, Hehakaya et al. [44] revealed the cost-effectiveness of MR-LINAC compared to 20–39 fractions external beam radiotherapy. However, to become cost-effective over five fractions, external beam radiotherapy and low-dose rate brachytherapy, it has to reduce complications substantially, in which it has to either reduce grade ≥2 urinary, grade ≥2 bowel and sexual complications (54% and 66%, respectively) or be offered at lower costs. This is further elaborated in detail in Chaps. 6 and 7.

10.3 Medical Devices

10.3.1 Radio-Opaque Fiducial Markers

Radio-opaque fiducial markers are made of metal, e.g. gold or as liquid markers. In order to validate the tumour position during the course of radiotherapy, these markers are placed depending on the target transorally, endoscopically into intra-abdominal organs or transrectally, e.g. into the prostate, into or in proximity of the target volume using a (endoscopic) needle.

In oesophageal cancer, fiducial markers have a high rate of visibility on orthogonal kV and CBCT/CT images and a low migration rate [30, 45]. Conversely, clips placed during surgery, which are often used to mark the position of the tumour, e.g. in oesophageal cancer, show high migration and low stability during the full course of radiotherapy (Hoffmann, unpublished).

The gold markers are typically 1–10-mm long cylinders or coils and have been available for many years [30, 46, 47]. Liquid markers are applied in small volumes, e.g. 0.025–0.1 ml injected into the tissue [28, 29, 48, 49]. After injection, the markers become sticky and gel-like, and stay in the tissue for months or years before decomposition [28, 29]. Liquid markers are compatible with proton therapy as the absorption of radiation dose is low compared to the gold markers [50].

In prostate cancer, three to four radio-opaque markers are inserted into the prostate before acquiring the CT scan for RT treatment planning [51, 52]. In this way, the markers act as a surrogate for the prostate: they are visualised by radiographic imaging (such as CBCT or orthogonal 2D X-ray radiographs). The movement of the prostate can be monitored before and during ('tracking') treatment, and field setups can be adjusted in case of movement of the prostate ensuring correct dose delivery, even with small safety margins. It is the most popular strategy for image guidance because of the easy and quick performance. Disadvantages of this approach is the invasive method (transrectal or transperineal insertion), with consequently risk of infection (lower rates in transperineal insertion), and the lack of information of the movement of the seminal vesicles and the possible rotation angle of the prostate when the fiducials are projected on a small distance [53, 54].

For thoracic and abdominal targets, large intra- and inter-fractional changes are seen in some patients [26, 55, 56]. Oesophageal targets have a large extension with complex shape. The target volume changes in both position and shape due to respiratory and cardiac motions and to other anatomical changes [56–59]. Fiducial markers implanted into or proximal to the target can monitor these changes. Typically, two to four markers are implanted in order to cover all parts of the target [30, 45].

For *radiation treatment planning* in oesophageal cancer, fiducial markers can be implanted at the inferior and superior border of the tumour. This approach, together with oesophagogastroscopy, endoscopic ultrasound (EUS) and ^{18}FDG PET/CT, CT alone and in some cases MRI and ultrasound, aids at defining the primary tumour and metastatic lymph nodes [60–63]. An acceptable correlation between the inferior border marker position and a standardised uptake value (SUV) of 2.5 was reported [45, 64]. For the superior border, larger deviations were described and in 25% of the patients a difference of more than 2 cm was found. Quite large inter-observer variation has been reported for target delineation in oesophageal cancer patients [65]. Implantation of fiducial markers aids the delineation and significantly reduces the inter-observer variation [28, 29]. In particular in the cranio-caudal direction, where variations of 1.4 mm in mean were seen, the implanted markers lead to a reduction in the variability (mean 0.4 cm) [28, 29]. Furthermore, Machiels et al. [28, 29] assessed that a margin of 1–1.5 cm is sufficient to derive the clinical target volume (CTV) from the gross tumour volume (GTV) when employing fiducial markers implanted at the proximal and distal tumour borders.

By segmentation of the setup CBCT scan or orthogonal kV images, both acquired prior to the delivery of the radiation treatment fraction, the motion of the target volume demarcated by fiducial markers can be measured throughout the treatment course [27, 45, 66]. In addition, the motion can be measured intra-fractionally by segmentation of kV images recorded during the actual dose delivery [27, 67]. Noteworthy, the intra-fractional motion is significantly smaller on the 4DCT, taking into account the respiratory motion, than on CBCT scans [27, 67, 68]. This results from the fact that the 4DCT only captures one breathing cycle while many breathing cycles are determined during a full CBCT scan.

In oesophageal cancer patients, the detected *intra-fractional* cardiac motion is small with an average motion of 0.5–2 mm. However, the average respiratory motion can be up to 10 mm and largest in cranio-caudal direction [27, 69]. Large motion is observed in distal tumours especially at the gastro-oesophageal junction and below the diaphragm [27, 70]. Similar intra-fractional motion was found for lung cancer patients. When comparing the average marker position before and after each treatment fraction, a systematic shift of markers in cranial and posterior direction during treatment was found [47, 67, 71]. This shift may result from a change in gravitational forces when the patient lay down on the couch and was small for most patients (on average 1 mm cranial and 2 mm posterior).

Inter-fractional tumour shifts are frequent in the thoracic and abdominal region. The shifts originate from anatomical changes of the target volume and OARs. The shifts may be random or systematic, for instance, the position of the diaphragm may vary randomly between fractions or it may shift systematically between planning and delivery due to different abdominal filling [56, 72]. Differences in the position of the diaphragm may result in target under-dosage, depending on the field directions. For proton therapy, this effect is partly mitigated by choosing beams only from posterior, thus minimizing entrance through the diaphragm [59, 73, 74]. However, for targets localised across the diaphragm, changes in the diaphragm position may extend or compress the target, leading to dosimetric changes for target and OARs. In the abdomen, quite large inter-fractional shifts are observed due to differences in filling and positioning of OARs adjacent to the target. In the thoracic region, especially for lung cancer, large inter-fractional anatomical changes are seen [26, 32]. These changes can be relieved by increasing the margins or by implementing an adaptive strategy, whereby the treatment plan is adapted to the anatomical changes once or more frequently during the treatment course [26, 31, 32, 59, 75]. The margin needed to account for inter-fractional changes depends on the setup strategy. The margins can be determined from imaging of the implanted fiducial markers. For oesophageal cancer, planning target volume (PTV) margins of approximately 10 mm are needed for daily setup when using the bony anatomy as reference. This PTV margin can be reduced to approximately 6–8 mm when applying the daily match on soft tissues [27, 69].

Since the markers are often implanted in the tumour tissue, the markers may not be representative of the full target including the CTV, in case of large tumour growth or shrinkage during the course of treatment [76]. Furthermore, markers may only be implanted at distinct points of the tumour and do not represent the entire tumour volume [27]. Thus, caution should be taken not only to solely rely on the markers' positions at the daily pre-treatment imaging scans for the evaluation of the tumour extension, but also to take into account the information gained by the CBCT or possibly a CT scan on rails in the proton gantry room.

Finally, RT for oesophageal cancer is based on photon treatment. However, proton therapy is an evolving technique with a potential to significantly reduce dose to organs at risk and thus toxicity [59, 77–79]. However, proton therapy is more sensitive to anatomical changes and consequently requires close image guidance [59, 75].

10.3.2 Electromagnetic Transponders

A methodology similar to fiducial markers is the implantation of electromagnetic transponders (Calypso®), which can be monitored by low-frequency radio waves instead of ionizing radiation [36]. Furthermore, the movements of the prostate during treatment can be detected [80–82].

Liver cancer tumours are not directly visible on CBCT scans and thus, visualisation of the tumour position for patient setup and during treatment requires insertion of fiducial markers in or nearby the tumour. For liver tumours, electromagnetic transponders have been implanted near the tumour and used as surrogates to track the position of the target [83, 84]. These patients were treated using respiratory gating in free-breathing patients. The Calypso system was used to track the exhale phase and radiation was only delivered during exhale [84]. Subsequent dose reconstruction showed good agreement between planned dose and delivered dose [85].

Possible disadvantages of the transponders are the interaction of the MRI magnetic and with the transponders. This can induce displacement of Calypso transponders and create a radio-frequency-induced heating of the transponders [86]. In summary, due to the complex setup and workflow, the use of the Calypso system is recommended for specialised centres.

10.3.3 Endo-Rectal Devices

Since the ano-rectal complex is closely located to the prostate, the PTV (at least) partially overlaps with the anterior ano-rectal wall (ARW), such that the latter is included in the high-dose volume. Several investigators have demonstrated that minimizing the radiation dose to the ARW reduces the risk for late rectal bleeding. More precisely, when 20% and 15% of the ano-rectal volume receives a dose of at least 70 and 75 Gray (Gy) (in 2 Gy fractions), the risk of developing Grade 2 and Grade 3 late rectal bleeding is <15% and <10%, respectively [87, 88]. This remains a significant risk despite the ability of modern dose delivery techniques to administer highly conformal dose distributions with very steep dose gradients at the rim of the PTV. Since the overlap of the PTV and the ARW is unavoidable, the only option to prevent rectal volumes from inside the high-radiation doses is to artificially increase the distance between the prostate and the ano-rectal complex. Several devices have been developed to achieve a better sparing of the parts of rectum. These devices can be divided into endo-rectal devices (ERD) or relatively novel implantable rectum spacers (IRS) (Fig. 10.2).

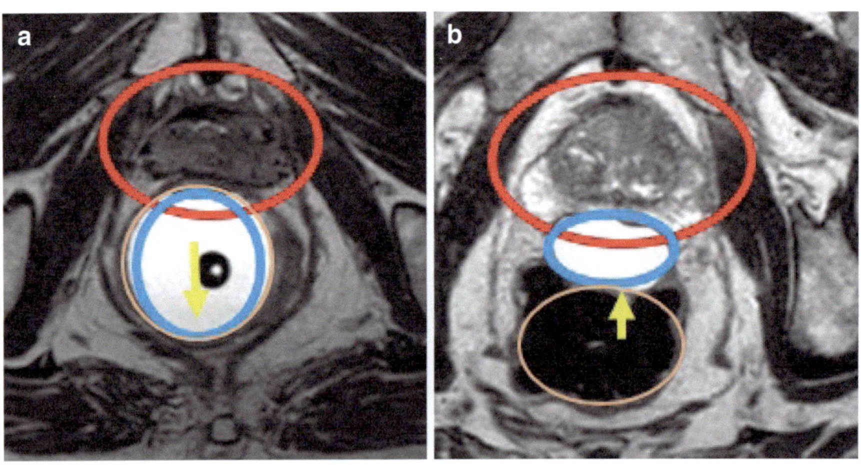

Fig. 10.2 Transversal T2-weighted magnetic resonance images of a prostate cancer patient with an ERB filled with liquid (**a**) and an IRS (**b**) in blue. The PTV-margin (red) around the prostate and rectal wall (brown) are schematically illustrated. The yellow arrow showed the dorsal (**a**) and anterior (**b**) wall of the rectum that is pushed out of the high-dose region in ERB and IRS, respectively. *Abbreviations*: *ERB* endo-rectal balloon; *IRS* implanted rectum spacer; *PTV* planning target volume

10.3.4 Endo-Rectal Balloons

The endo-rectal balloon (ERB) is a silicon or latex device that is filled with either air or water (in case of rectal invasion or its use in proton beam therapy) [89, 90]. An inserted ERB placed prior to each RT fraction can cause discomfort for the patient. The distance from the *dorsal* and *lateral* rectal wall to the PTV is increased (yellow arrow in Fig. 10.2), whereas the *anterior* rectal wall is pushed towards the PTV. Although the ARW is pushed towards the prostate (Fig. 10.2), the overall dosimetric net-effect proved to be beneficial in 3D-CRT and IMRT [91]. Smeenk et al. [92] showed an absolute reduction in the mean dose to the anus of 12 Gy and 7.5 Gy for 3D-CRT and IMRT, respectively.

Another advantage is more prostate immobilisation to reduce inter-fraction (week-to-week) and intra-fraction (pre- and post-treatment) variations. Stool and gas pockets can move the prostate during a treatment fraction: an ERB is able to reduce these intra-fraction motions. Smeenk et al. [91] revealed that an ERB reduces the intra-fraction prostate motion in particular for treatment sessions longer than two and half minutes. Cumulative percentages of prostate deviations of >1, >3, >5 and >7 mm were observed in 57.7, 7.0, 0.7 and 0.3% in the ERB group versus 70.2, 18.1, 4.6 and 1.4% in the no-ERB group after 10 min. The largest reductions in the ERB group were observed in the anterior-posterior direction and no reduction in inter-fraction variation was found.

Furthermore, Jaccard et al. [93] showed an optimal dose sparing of the internal pudendal arteries using an ERB: on average, the dose reduction was 28% ($p = 0.006$) and the median mean dose calculated to be 4.1 Gy versus 5.7 Gy with and without ERB, respectively. The authors' hypothesis that this dose reduction could lead to preservation of the erectile function needs to be confirmed in additional studies.

Clinical outcomes of the use of ERB are listed in Table 10.1. Most published studies have focussed on the dosimetric effects of ERB and are single institution experiences. There are no multi-centre, randomised controlled data on patient- and clinician-reported toxicities of using ERB in RT.

10.3.5 Endo-Rectal Displacement Device

A prostate endo-rectal displacement device (EDD) is a look-alike of an ultrasound probe, and was developed because of the reproducibility of ERB positioning, and additionally, the issue of pushing the anterior part of the rectum into the high-dose region [100]. This EDD is commercially available and developed by Rectafix™ (Scanflex Medical AB, Täby, Sweden). However, the clinical use and proof of clinical benefits are limited, with no large, prospective evidence.

De Leon et al. [101] used the EDD in stereotactic RT and they only observed a small increased intra-fraction stability with the EDD during time of treatment. Nicolae et al. [102] used a similar system in stereotactic RT with the intent of immobilizing the prostate during each treatment fraction. Using the EDD, the authors observed no prostate displacements of more than 3 mm over the course of treatment, but found no statistically significant dosimetric differences for rectum and bladder.

Table 10.1 Clinical outcome after radiotherapy using an endo-rectal balloon

First author	Year	No. of patients + ERB	Study design	ERB (cc)	Radiotherapy technique	Follow-up	Toxicity (no ERB vs. ERB)	Dose-volume histograms(no ERB vs. ERB)
Dubouloz [94]	2018	10	Randomised phase-II trial—dosimetry comparative	Air-filled (100)	SBRT + FMI 36.25Gy/5#	No	NR	Rectal wall: D30%, D40%, D50%, dose median reduced by 50%; D60 rectal wall reduced by 30%
Teh [95]	2018	596	Retrospective	Air-filled (100)	IMRT	62 months	5-year rates of ≥ grade 3 GI toxicity 1.2% GU toxicity 1.1%	NR
Wortel [96]	2017	85	Phase 3 randomised for RT schedule, non-randomised for ERB use	Air-filled (80–100)	IMRT + FMI 64.6Gy/19# vs. 78Gy/39#	4 years	Lower incidences of increased stool frequency (≥4 per day) + mucous loss; incidence of rectal incontinence 23.4% vs. 10.4%	Mean dose of anorectum 30.1 Gy (SD, 7.5 Gy) vs. 25.7 Gy (SD, 3.2 Gy $p < 0.001$) in hypo-fraction arm
Deville [97]	2012	100	Retrospective	Water-filled (100)	IG (IMRT)	3 months	No grade 3 or more toxicities GI toxicity grade 0, 1 and 2: 69, 23 and 8% GU toxicity grade 0, 1 and 2: 17, 41 and 42%	NR
Smeenk	2009	24	Planning study	Air-filled (80)	3D-CRT, IMRT	NR	NR	Absolute reduction of dose mean: 12 Gy (3D-CRT)—7.5 Gy (IMRT)

van Lin [98]	2007	24	Prospective phase 2 randomised	Air-filled (80)	3D-CRT	24	Reduced late GI toxicity: grade ≥1, excess of bowel movements + rectal discharge	Reduced rectal wall volume doses >40 Gy
D'Amico [99]	2006	57	Prospective	Air-filled (60)	3D CRT	1.8 year	Grade 3 rectal bleeding rate 10%	Rectal V70 median 3.7 cc
Bastasch	2006	396	Prospective	Air-filled (100)	3D-CRT, IMRT	8 weeks	No G3–4 toxicity Grade 2 GI toxicities 63.4% anal irritation +36.7% to diarrhoea	NR

Abbreviations: *3D-CRT* 3D- conformal radiotherapy; *ERB* endo-rectal balloon; *FMI* fiducial marker imaging; *GI* gastro-intestinal; *GU* genito-urinary; *IG* image guidance, *IMRT* intensity-modulated radiotherapy; *NR* not reported; *SBRT* stereotactic body radiotherapy

10.3.6 Implanted Rectum Spacers

An implanted rectum spacer (IRS) is inserted as a biodegradable tissue filler between the prostate and the rectum to increase the distance from the anterior rectal wall to the prostate (Fig. 10.3). In contrast to an ERB, where the anterior part of the rectal wall is pushed into the high-dose region of the PTV, while pushing the dorsal and lateral rectal wall away from the prostate, the IRS pushes the complete rectal structure away from the PTV (Figs. 10.2 and 10.4).

Different types of IRS are available and have been applied clinically for external beam RT of prostate cancer: an absorbable hydrogel [104], a hyaluronic acid [105], a saline-filled rectal balloon implant (RBI) [106] and a collagen implant [107]. The main differences between these types of IRS are their chemical composition and the (in)ability to allow for post-implant correction (Table 10.2). Clinical outcomes of the use of IRS are summarised in Table 10.3.

The RBI differs from the other types of IRS, so-called liquid spacers. All types of IRS are implanted through a transperineal approach, which is usually guided by transrectal ultrasound. Vanneste et al. [115] published on the implantation method of an RBI. Implantation can be performed under local, regional or general anaesthesia, with the patient in lithotomy position. All IRS are inserted between the prostate, the Denonvilliers' Fascia and the anterior rectum. Urologists should ideally perform the procedure and/or radiation oncologists experienced in prostate brachytherapy and/or transperineal biopsies: the use of the real-time bi-plane transrectal ultrasonography (TRUS) probe is recommended. A brachytherapy stepper unit is used to stabilise the TRUS probe and allows the operator to use both hands for the implantation. Moreover, fiducial markers are implanted for image-guided external beam prostate irradiation.

Hydrogels are injected as polyethylene-glycol (PEG) liquids and polymerise in situ within a few seconds following the mixture of two liquid hydrogel precursors [104]. The end result is a stable, flexible gel-like structure. This hydrogel is similar to products used in brain surgery, cardiology and ophthalmology [116–118]. The

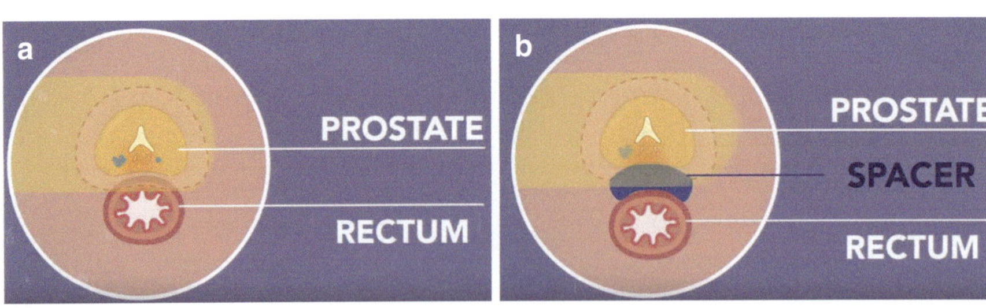

Fig. 10.3 Schematic illustration of prostate irradiation without (**a**) and with (**b**) implanted rectum spacer. In both cases, the dose distribution from a single beam (yellow) conforms to the planning target volume (dashed line). Without spacer, the beam partially overlaps with the rectum, whereas with spacer, the beam does not overlap with the rectum due to the increased distance between the prostate and rectum. (Reproduced as still from movie https://youtu.be/tDlagSXMKqw)

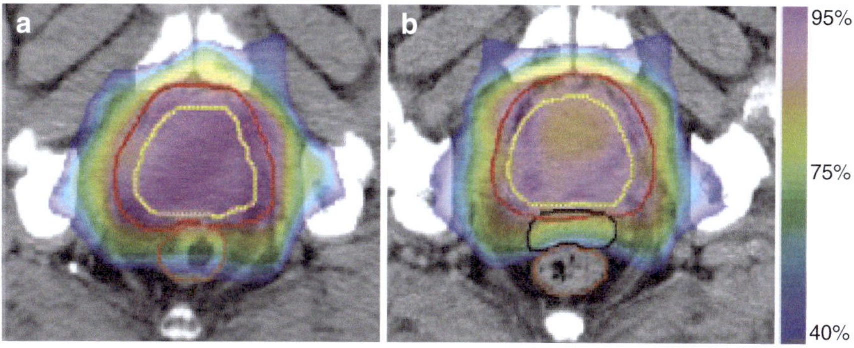

Fig. 10.4 Colour-wash representation of calculated dose distributions superimposed onto an axial computed tomography slice before (**a**) and after (**b**) IRS gel injection in the same patient. Prostate is illustrated in yellow contour, within red contour the PTV margin. Without IRS, the high-dose region >75% (purple) overlaps with the anterior part of the rectum (brown contour), while with IRS in situ the high-dose region spans the IRS (black contour), and not the rectum. The 40% isodose contour (purple) overlaps the entire rectum in (**a**), whereas it overlaps the rectum partially in (**b**). (Reprinted with permission from [103]) *Abbreviation*: *IRS* implantable rectum spacer

commercially developed PEG hydrogel is SpaceOAR (Augmenix, Waktham, MA – Boston Scientific Corporation). Pinkawa et al. [104] proved a relative rectum dose reduction within the 76-Gy isodose of 67% in 3D-CRT, and of 89% in IMRT dose distributions, respectively.

Most reports published with PEG spacers, including a phase 3 multi-centric randomised controlled trial [119, 120]. Mariados et al. [120] published the early results showing a significant reduction in mean volume of the rectum receiving 70 Gy (pre- to post-IRS plans: 12.4% and 3.3%, respectively; $p < 0.0001$). Consequently, they reported on a significant reduction in late (3–15 months) rectal toxicity severity in the IRS group (2.0% and 7.0% in the IRS and control groups, respectively; $p = 0.004$). Hamstra et al. [119] reported the 3-year incidence of grade ≥1 (9.2% vs. 2.0%; $p = 0.028$) and grade ≥2 (5.7% vs. 0%; $p = 0.012$) rectal toxicity favoured the IRS arm. From 6 months onward, bowel quality of life consistently favoured the IRS group ($p = 0.002$), with the difference at 3 years of 5.8 points of the Expanded Prostate Cancer Index Composite (EPIC) ($p < 0.05$). The authors performed a second analysis on this trial to correlate penile bulb dose and sequel quality of life: at 3 years, more men potent at baseline and treated with spacer had 'erections sufficient for intercourse' [control 37.5% vs. spacer 66.7% ($p = 0.046$)] and satisfactory scores in the sexual domain [statistically higher scores on 7 of 13 items [all $p < 0.05$)] [121].

Several other products used in IRS are worthy of being described in detail since their physical properties are very important, mainly in terms of retaining desired form and shape.

Table 10.2 The characteristics of different implantable rectum spacer devices [108]

Characteristic	Hydrogel	Hyaluronic acid	Collagen	Balloon
Material:				
Liquid	+	+	+	–
Biocompatibility	+	+/–	+/–	+
Shape	Variable	Variable	Variable	Constant
Stability	+	+	+	+
Degradation	3–6 months	12 months	6–12 months	3–6 months
Implantation technique:				
Needle	18 G (±1.2 mm)	17G (±1.5 mm)	18 G	2–3 mm
Invasive	+	+	+	+
Corrections	–	–	–	+
High velocity of injection	+	–	–	–
Predictable shape	–	–	–	+
Injected volume	10 cc	3–9 cc	10 cc	Variable, max. ±17 cc
Planning				
CT visibility	–	–	–	+
Prostate-rectum spread	7–15 mm	8–20 mm	13 mm	19 mm
Dose reduction	46–61% (V70Gy)	84% (V70Gy) 74–91% (V90%)	>50% (V40Gy: 40–65%)	50% (V60Gy) 72% (V90%)

Firstly, hyaluronic acid (HA) is a natural polysaccharide (glycosaminoglycan-based polymer) compound found in human tissues as a component of the connective and extracellular matrix [105]. Normally, it is essential in the skin and in the synovial fluid of the joints. This compound is cleaved by the enzyme hyaluronidase to its component subunits, which are predominantly eliminated by hepatic and renal metabolism [122]. When used for treatments in cosmetic skin procedures and osteo-arthritis, the compound is modified, making it stable for a duration close to 1 year before absorption [123]. Several HA-based IRS products are available, each with slight modifications: Barrigel® (Non-Animal Stabilised Hyaluronic Acid, NASHA®, Palette Life sciences, Stockholm, Sweden), Restylane (Q-med, Uppsala, Sweden), Hyalform (Genzyme Corp., Cambridge, MA), Hyalgan (Fidia SPA, Abano Terme, Italy) and Synvisc (Genzyme Corp., Cambridge, MA). Prada et al. [105] published on the use of the HA in combination with brachytherapy. They showed a relative reduction of 28% in the maximum rectum dose averaged over all patients in the cohort.

Secondly, human collagen is the most profuse protein in the human body and is the principle component of connective tissue. It confers stretch resistance to many tissues, such as tendons and ligaments. Collagen is used in ophthalmology, ortho-paedics, dentistry and cosmetics [124]. It is also used to be injected into the perineum for treatment of urinary incontinence [125]. Noyes et al. [107] reported on a mean

Table 10.3 Clinical outcome after radiotherapy using an implantable rectum spacer

First author	Year	No. of patients (+ IRS)	Study design	Radiotherapy technique	Type of spacer (ml injected)	Follow-up	Toxicity (No spacer vs. spacer)	Dose-volume histograms (no spacer vs. spacer)
Quinn [109]	2020	222 (143)	Single-blinded phase 3 randomised	IGRT, IMRT 79.2 Gy, 44#	Hydrogel, SpaceOAR (10)	37 months	Decline in bowel QOL (5-points) 36% vs. 14%	V50 < 26%, V60 < 20%, V65 < 17%, V70 < 13%, V75 < 10%
Karsh [110]	2018					37 months	Sexual QOL: capable of 'erections sufficient for intercourse.' 37.5% vs. 66.7%	Penile bulb: 21.1 Gy vs. 10.8 Gy ($p = 0.036$)
Hamstra	2016					37 months	Grade 1 + GI toxicity 9% vs. 2% ($p < 0.03$) Grade 2 + GI toxicity 6% vs. 0% ($p < 0.015$) Reduction in cumulative grade 1 + GU: 15% vs. 4% ($p = 0.046$)	V50: 21% vs. 10% V70: 10% vs. 2% V80: 4% vs. 0.1% No differences in dosimetry to the bladder/wall
Mariados	2015					3–15 months	GI toxicity: 7.0% vs. 2.0% 10-point declines in bowel quality of life: 21.4% vs. 11.6%	Mean rectal V70: 12.4% vs. 3.3% ($p < 0.0001$) Median rectal V70 dose: 10.5% vs. 2.3 ($p < 0.0001$)

(continued)

Table 10.3 (continued)

First author	Year	No. of patients (+ IRS)	Study design	Radiotherapy technique	Type of spacer (ml injected)	Follow-up	Toxicity (No spacer vs. spacer)	Dose-volume histograms (no spacer vs. spacer)
Uhl [111]	2013	52	Prospective multi-centre phase 2	IMRT 78Gy, 39#	Hydrogel, SpaceOAR (10)	12 months	Grade 1 GI toxicity: 4.3%, no grade 2 + GI toxicity Grade 1—grade 2 GU toxicity: 17.0–2.1%	Mean rectal dose: 8.0 Gy reduction
Pinkawa [112]	2017	114 (54)	Prospective observational	IMRT 76-78Gy, 38–39#	Hydrogel, SpaceOAR (10)	63 months	Bowel urgency: 14% vs. 0% ($p = 0.01$)	NR
Whalley [113]	2016	140 (30)	Phase 1,2 prospective	IMRT 80Gy, 40#	Hydrogel, SpaceOAR (10)	28 months	Acute grade 1 and 2 GI toxicity: 51 vs. 43% - 4.5% vs. 0% Late grade 1 GI: 41.8% vs. 16.6% ($p = 0.04$)	Rectal doses V82 = 1.3% vs. 0.2% V80 = 5.3% vs. 0.8% V75 = 9.5% vs. 2.2% V70 = 12.3% vs. 3.7% V65 = 14.7% vs. 5.4% V40 = 32% vs. 22.9% V30 = 49.4% vs. 42.7%
Chapet [114]	2015	36	Multi-Centre phase 2 study	IMRT 62Gy, 20#	Hyaluronic acid (10)	3 months	Mean pain score of 4.6/10 No grade 2 GI toxicity GU: 11% grade 2 obstruction, 3% hematoma behind the bladder	NA

Prada	2007	27	Multi-Centre phase 2	EBRT 46Gy, 23# + 11.5Gy HDR brachytherapy boost	hyaluronic acid (3–7 mean 6)	–	NR	Median rectal dose 47.1% vs. 39.2% ($p < 0.001$) HDR: Dmax rectum: 7.08 Gy vs. 5.07 Gy ($p < 0.001$) rectum Dmean: 6.08 Gy vs. 4.42 Gy ($p < 0.001$)
Noyes	2012	11	Pilot study	IMRT 75.6 Gy, 42#	Collagen (20)	6.5 years	No GI toxicity	V40Gy: 20–25% vs. 7–15%
Melchert	2013	26	Multi-Centre phase 2	IMRT/3DCRT 74 Gy, 37#	Prospace implantable balloon (17)	NA	NA	Rectal reduction: V70 by 55.3% V80 by 64.0% V90 by 72.0% V100 by 82.3% Rectal D2 cc + D0.1 cc reduced by 15.8 and 3.9%
Vanneste	2017	15	Phase 1, prospective	VMAT, 70 Gy,28#	Prospace implantable balloon (17)	1 year	Mean VAS-score 2/10 Late grade 2 GI toxicity 6% Late grade 1 GI–GU toxicities: 12%	Mean rectal dose 26.2 Gy; V75 Gy: 0.1 cc

Abbreviations: *3D-CRT* 3D- conformal radiotherapy; *FMI* fiducial marker imaging; *GI* gastro-intestinal; *GU* genito-urinary; *HDR* high-dose rate; *IG* image guidance, *IMRT* intensity-modulated radiotherapy; *NR* not reported; *SBRT* stereotactic body radiotherapy; *VAS* visual analogue scale; *VMAT* volumetric-modulated arc radiotherapy reduction in rectal wall of 50% with an IRS: the mean volume of the rectum receiving a radiation dose of 40 Gy decreased from 20–25% to 7–15% in IRS plans.

Thirdly, an inflatable rectal balloon implant is made of poly(L-Lactide-co-caprolactone). This is a co-polymer of polylactide acid and epsilon caprolactone, in a ratio of 70:30. It is a widely used, medically biodegradable material and specifically developed to be used as a tissue spacer [126].

Regarding the stability of RBI, Levy et al. [126] demonstrated the proper functionality of the RBI capability to retain its inflated form during a certain period (e.g. patients' radiation session) in both in vitro and in vivo studies in dogs, guinea pigs and rabbits. In 2013, the first clinical results showed a relative reduction by 82% of the rectal volume receiving 74 Gy [106]. Vanneste et al. [115] published the toxicity data on the implantation: 47% of the patients had no complaints at all, while the other patients had a mild discomfort to slight pain at the perineal region. However, Vanneste et al. [127, 128] observed a significant shrinkage of the RBI volumes: only an average volume of 70.4% compared to that at baseline was detected at the end of the treatment. Although the prostate–rectum separation significantly decreased over time, it remained at least 1 cm. There was no significant increase in ano-rectal volume receiving a dose of 75 Gy. Wolff et al. [129] have also observed the phenomenon of a deflating RBI at an early time point during the course of radiation therapy. They reported on an average volume loss of >50% during a full course of treatment of 37–40 fractions (8 weeks).

Three analyses on the cost-effectiveness of a spacer have been performed [130–132]: an IRS reveals lower toxicities, but also higher costs. Vanneste et al. [132] have calculated an incremental cost-effectiveness ratio of €55,880 per Quality-adjusted life year (QALY) gained. They concluded that for a ceiling ratio of €80,000, an IRS had a 77% probability of being cost-effective. Hutchinson et al. [130] demonstrated the increased cost-effectiveness of SBRT in comparison with conventional RT: an IRS was immediately cost-effective with a savings of $2640 and breakeven risk reduction at 36%. Levy and co-authors calculated an incremental cost-effectiveness ratio of $96,440 per QALY for patients undergoing an IRS implantation in a hospital setting, and $39,286 in an ambulatory facility [131]. This ratio even improved in patients with good baseline erectile dysfunctions: $35,548 per QALY and $9627 per QALY, respectively.

To increase the cost-effectiveness, decision rules based on clinical risk factors have been developed to identify prostate cancer patients with a high risk to develop radiation-induced rectal toxicity prior to IRS implantation [133, 134]. Such clinical rules can be expanded to include patients who have a very high risk to develop rectal toxicity due to, e.g. re-irradiation, inflammatory bowel disease or dosimetric high burden [127, 128]. It is expected that the cost-effectiveness of the IRS will improve because those patients will benefit more from the use of an IRS than others. Finally, a decision support system has been developed to predict the gain in dose and toxicity reduction *prior* to the implantation using a 'virtual' IRS [135, 136]. A 'virtual' IRS (useful for both RBI and hydrogel spacer) is generated using a model that is based on a CT scan without IRS. This model was used to create a deformation field (e.g. virtual IRS) on CT scans of patients without IRS. Predictions of the gain in dose and toxicity reduction can consequently predict if the IRS is cost-effective for the specified patient. This is a very attractive approach because the benefit for an individual patient can be estimated without implanting the IRS. This means no extra discomfort of the operation for the patient and no additional costs of the placement of the IRS.

To conclude, several devices are used to further personalise and individualise radiotherapy to enable high cure rates, with low toxicity rates.

10.4 Summary

Implantation of fiducial markers in the tumour aids delineating the tumour borders at planning CT. Evaluation of fiducial marker positions in the surgical specimen can be used as feedback to the target definition. Furthermore, the markers can be used to aid evaluation of target position for patient setup and during treatment. Hereby, full dose coverage of tumour volume is secured and over dosage of OARs is avoided. Fiducial markers are highly reliable with a low degree of migration and high visibility.

Only the hydrogel spacer is effective proven in a prospective phase 3 trial for prostate cancer. All the other devices are in a non-randomised setting, mostly single centre experiences. However, nowadays, 2 phase 3 trials have been completed to obtain the FDA approval, pending on preliminary results: the ProSpace RBI (NCT03400150) and the Barrigel IRS trial (NCT04189913). The literature is growing on the application of an IRS. In the United States, more than 50,000 men are already treated with spacing devices, and it is commonly used. In Europe, it is used in a single centre, and it is targeted on high risk on rectal toxicity patients. Future clinical studies will determine the definitive role of spacers in that population.

References

1. Sung H, Ferlay J, Siegel RL, Laversanne M, Soerjomataram I, Jemal A, et al. Global Cancer Statistics 2020: GLOBOCAN Estimates of Incidence and Mortality Worldwide for 36 Cancers in 185 Countries. CA Cancer J Clin. 2021;71:209–49.
2. Beckendorf V, Guerif S, Le Prisé E, Cosset JM, Bougnoux A, Chauvet B, Salem N, Chapet O, Bourdain S, Bachaud JM, Maingon P, Hannoun-Levi JM, Malissard L, Simon JM, Pommier P, Hay M, Dubray B, Lagrange JL, Luporsi E, Bey P. 70 Gy versus 80 Gy in localized prostate cancer: 5-year results of GETUG 06 randomized trial. Int J Radiat Oncol Biol Phys. 2011;80(4):1056–63.
3. Dearnaley DP, Jovic G, Syndikus I, Khoo V, Cowan RA, Graham JD, Aird EG, Bottomley D, Huddart RA, Jose CC, Matthews JH, Millar JL, Murphy C, Russell JM, Scrase CD, Parmar MK, Sydes MR. Escalated-dose versus control-dose conformal radiotherapy for prostate cancer: long-term results from the MRC RT01 randomised controlled trial. Lancet Oncol. 2014;15(4):464–73.
4. Heemsbergen WD, Al-Mamgani A, Slot A, Dielwart MF, Lebesque JV. Long-term results of the Dutch randomized prostate cancer trial: impact of dose-escalation on local, biochemical, clinical failure, and survival. Radiother Oncol. 2014;110(1):104–9.

5. Kuban DA, Tucker SL, Dong L, Starkschall G, Huang EH, Cheung MR, et al. Long-term results of the M. D. Anderson randomized dose-escalation trial for prostate cancer. Int J Radiat Oncol Biol Phys. 2008;70:67–74.
6. Michalski JM, Moughan J, Purdy J. A randomized trial of 79.2Gy versus 70.2Gy radiation therapy (RT) for localized prostate cancer. J Clin Oncol. 2015;33. (suppl 7; abstr 4).
7. Lardas M, Liew M, van den Bergh RC, De Santis M, Bellmunt J, Van den Broeck T, Cornford P, Cumberbatch MG, Fossati N, Gross T, Henry AM, Bolla M, Briers E, Joniau S, Lam TB, Mason MD, Mottet N, van der Poel HG, Rouvière O, Schoots IG, Wiegel T, Willemse PM, Yuan CY, Bourke L. Quality of Life Outcomes after Primary Treatment for Clinically Localised Prostate Cancer: A Systematic Review. Eur Urol. 2017;72(6):869–85. https://doi.org/10.1016/j.eururo.2017.06.035. Epub 2017 Jul 27
8. Vanneste BG, Van De Voorde L, de Ridder RJ, Van Limbergen EJ, Lambin P, van Lin EN. Chronic radiation proctitis: tricks to prevent and treat. Int J Colorectal Dis. 2015;30(10):1293–1303. https://doi.org/10.1007/s00384-015-2289-4. Epub 2015 Jul 23
9. Bray F, Ferlay J, Soerjomataram I, Siegel RL, Torre LA, Jemal A. Global cancer statistics 2018: GLOBOCAN estimates of incidence and mortality worldwide for 36 cancers in 185 countries. CA Cancer J Clin. 2018;68(6):394–424. https://doi.org/10.3322/caac.21492. Epub 2018 Sep 12.
10. Global Burden of Disease Cancer Collaboration, Fitzmaurice C, Abate D, Abbasi N, Abbastabar H, Abd-Allah F, Abdel-Rahman O, et al. Global, regional, and national cancer incidence, mortality, years of life lost, years lived with disability, and disability-adjusted life-years for 29 cancer groups, 1990 to 2017: a systematic analysis for the Global Burden of Disease Study. JAMA Oncol. 2019;5(12):1749–68. https://doi.org/10.1001/jamaoncol.2019.2996. Erratum in: JAMA Oncol. 2020;6(3):444. Erratum in: JAMA Oncol. 2020;6(5):789. Erratum in: JAMA Oncol. 2021;7(3):466.
11. Al-Batran S, Homann N, Pauligk C, Goetze T, Meiler J, Kasper S, Kopp H, Mayer F, Haag G, Luley K. FLOT4-AIO investigators perioperative chemotherapy with fluorouracil plus leucovorin, oxaliplatin, and docetaxel versus fluorouracil or capecitabine plus cisplatin and epirubicin for locally advanced, resectable gastric or gastro-oesophageal junction adenocarcinoma (FLOT4) a randomised, phase 2/3 trial. Lancet. 2019;393(10184):1948–57.
12. Chan KKW, et al. Neoadjuvant treatments for locally advanced, resectable esophageal cancer: a network meta-analysis. Int J Cancer. 2018;143:430–7.
13. Conroy T, et al. Definitive chemoradiotherapy with FOLFOX versus fluorouracil and cisplatin in patients with oesophageal cancer (PRODIGE5/ACCORD17): final results of a randomised, phase 2/3 trial. Lancet Oncol. 2014;15(3):305–14.
14. Cooper JS, et al. Chemoradiotherapy of locally advanced esophageal cancer: long-term follow-up of a prospective randomized trial (RTOG 85-01). Radiat Ther Oncol Group JAMA. 1999;281:1623–7.
15. Crosby T, et al. Long-term results and recurrence patterns from SCOPE-1: a phase II/III randomised trial of definitive chemoradiotherapy þ/ cetuximab in oesophageal cancer. Br J Cancer. 2017;116:709–16.
16. Cunningham D, et al. Perioperative chemotherapy versus surgery alone for resectable gastroesophageal cancer. NEJM. 2006;355:11–20.
17. Bartolomeo D. Prognostic and predictive value of microsatellite instability, inflammatory reaction and PD-L1 in gastric cancer patients treated with either adjuvant 5-FU/LV or sequential FOLFIRI followed by Cisplatin and Docetaxel: a translational analysis from the ITACA-S trial. Oncologist. 2020;25:e460–8.
18. Herskovic A, et al. Combined chemotherapy and radiotherapy compared with radiotherapy alone in patients with cancer of the esophagus. NEJM. 1992;326(24):1593–8.
19. Lordick F, et al. Oesophageal cancer: ESMO clinical practice guidelines for diagnosis, treatment and follow-up. Ann Oncol. 2016;27(Suppl 5):v50–7. (Review).
20. Van Hagen P, et al. Preoperative chemoradiotherapy for esophageal or junctional cancer. NEJM. 2012;366:2074–84.

21. Macdonald JS, Smalley SR, Benedetti J, et al. Chemoradiotherapy after surgery com-pared with surgery alone for adenocarcinoma of the stomach or gastroesophageal junction. N Engl J Med. 2001;345:725–30.
22. Liang J, Wu Q, Yan D. The role of seminal vesicle motion in target margin assessment for online image-guided radiotherapy for prostate cancer. Int J Radiat Oncol Biol Phys. 2009;73(3):935–43. https://doi.org/10.1016/j.ijrobp.2008.10.019. Epub 2008 Dec 26.
23. Rijkhorst EJ, Lakeman A, Nijkamp J, de Bois J, van Herk M, Lebesque JV, Sonke JJ. Strategies for online organ motion correction for intensity-modulated radiotherapy of prostate cancer: prostate, rectum, and bladder dose effects. Int J Radiat Oncol Biol Phys. 2009;75(4):1254–60. https://doi.org/10.1016/j.ijrobp.2009.04.034.
24. Knap MM, Hoffmann L, Nordsmark M, Vestergaard A. Daily cone-beam computed tomography used to determine tumour shrinkage and localisation in lung cancer patients. Acta Oncol. 2010;49:1077–84.
25. de Crevoisier R, Bayar MA, Pommier P, Muracciole X, Pêne F, Dudouet P, Latorzeff I, Beckendorf V, Bachaud JM, Laplanche A, Supiot S, Chauvet B, Nguyen TD, Bossi A, Créhange G, Lagrange JL. Daily versus weekly prostate cancer image-guided radiation therapy: phase 3 multicenter randomized trial. Int J Radiat Oncol Biol Phys. 2018;102:1420–9.
26. Møller DS, Holt MI, Alber M, Tvilum M, Khalil AA, Knap MM, Hoffmann L. Adaptive radiotherapy for advanced lung cancer ensures target coverage and decreases lung dose. Radiother Oncol. 2016;121:32–8.
27. Hoffmann L, Poulsen PR, Ravkilde TR, Bertholet J, Kruhlikava I, Helbo BL, Schmidt ML, Nordsmark M. Setup strategies and uncertainties in esophageal radiotherapy based on detailed intra- and interfractional tumor motion mapping. Radiother Oncologia. 2019;136:161–8.
28. Machiels M, Voncken FEM, Jin P, van Dieren JM, Bartels-Rutten A, Alderliesten T, Aleman BMP, van Hooft JE, Hulshof MCCM. A novel liquid fiducial marker in esophageal cancer image-guided radiation therapy: technical feasibility and visibility on imaging. Pract Radiat Oncol. 2019a;9:e506–15.
29. Machiels M, Jin P, van Hooft JE, Gurney-Champion OJ, Jelvehgaran P, Geijsen ED, Jeene PM, Willemijn Kolff M, Oppedijk V, Rasch CRN, van Herk MB, Alderliesten T, Hulshof MCCM. Reduced inter-observer and intra-observer delineation variation in esophageal cancer radiotherapy by use of fiducial markers. Acta Oncol. 2019b;58:943–50.
30. Machiels M, van Hooft J, Jin P, van Berge Henegouwen MI, van Laarhoven HM, Alderliesten T, et al. Endoscopy/EUS-guided fiducial marker placement in patients with esophageal cancer: a comparative analysis of 3 types of markers. Gastrointest Endosc. 2015;82:641–9.
31. Yan D, Vicini F, Wong J, Martinez A. Adaptive radiation therapy. Phys Med Biol. 1997;42:123–32.
32. Kwint M, Walraven I, Burgers S, Hartemink K, Klomp H, Knegjens J, Verheij M, Belderbos J. Outcome of radical local treatment of non-small cell lung cancer patients with synchronous oligometastases. Lung Cancer. 2017;112:134–9. https://doi.org/10.1016/j.lungcan.2017.08.006. Epub 2017 Aug 12
33. Heijkoop ST, Langerak TR, Quint S, Bondar L, Mens JW, Heijmen BJ, Hoogeman MS. Clinical implementation of an online adaptive plan-of-the-day protocol for nonrigid motion management in locally advanced cervical cancer IMRT. Int J Radiat Oncol Biol Phys. 2014;90:673–9.
34. Vestergaard A, Muren LP, Lindberg H, Jakobsen KL, Petersen JB, Elstrøm UV, Agerbæk M, Høyer M. Normal tissue sparing in a phase II trial on daily adaptive plan selection in radiotherapy for urinary bladder cancer. Acta Oncol. 2014;53:997–1004.
35. Tvilum M, Khalil AA, Møller DS, Hoffmann L, Knap MM. Clinical outcome of adaptive radiotherapy in the treatment of lung cancer patients. Acta Oncol. 2015;54:1430–7.
36. Foster RD, Pistenmaa DA, Solberg TD. A comparison of radiographic techniques and electromagnetic transponders for localization of the prostate. Radiat Oncol. 2012;21(7):101. https://doi.org/10.1186/1748-717X-7-101.

37. Camps SM, Fontanarosa D, de With PHN, Verhaegen F, Vanneste BGL. The Use of Ultrasound Imaging in the External Beam Radiotherapy Workflow of Prostate Cancer Patients. Biomed Res Int. 2018;24(2018):7569590. https://doi.org/10.1155/2018/7569590.
38. van der Meer S, Camps S, van Elmpt W, Podesta M, Sanches P, Vanneste BGL, Fontanarosa D, Verhaegen F. Simulation of pseudo-CT images based on deformable image registration of ultrasound images: a proof of concept for transabdominal ultrasound imaging of the prostate during radiotherapy. Med Phys. 2016;43:1913.
39. Raaymakers BW, Jürgenliemk-Schulz IM, Bol GH, Glitzner M, Kotte ANTJ, van Asselen B, de Boer JCJ, Bluemink JJ, Hackett SL, Moerland MA, Woodings SJ, Wolthaus JWH, van Zijp HM, Philippens MEP, Tijssen R, Kok JGM, de Groot-van Breugel EN, Kiekebosch I, Meijers LTC, Nomden CN, Sikkes GG, Doornaert PAH, Eppinga WSC, Kasperts N, Kerkmeijer LGW, Tersteeg JHA, Brown KJ, Pais B, Woodhead P, Lagendijk JJW. First patients treated with a 1.5 T MRI-Linac: clinical proof of concept of a high-precision, high-field MRI-guided radiotherapy treatment. Phys Med Biol 2017;62(23):L41-L50.
40. Raaymakers BW, Lagendijk JJ, Overweg J, Kok JG, Raaijmakers AJ, Kerkhof EM, van der Put RW, Meijsing I, Crijns SP, Benedosso F, van Vulpen M, de Graaff CH, Allen J, Brown KJ. Integrating a 1.5 T MRI scanner with a 6 MV accelerator: proof of concept. Phys Med Biol. 2009;54(12):N229–37.
41. Chen X, Ahunbay E, Paulson ES, Chen G, Li XA. A daily end-to-end quality assurance workflow for MR-guided online adaptive radiation therapy on MR-Linac. J Appl Clin Med Phys. 2020;21(1):205–12.
42. Murray J, Tree AC. Prostate cancer - Advantages and disadvantages of MR-guided RT. Clin Transl Radiat Oncol. 2019;18:68–73. https://doi.org/10.1016/j.ctro.2019.03.006. eCollection 2019 Sep
43. Bruynzeel AME, Tetar SU, Oei SS, Senan S, Haasbeek CJA, Spoelstra FOB, Piet AHM, Meijnen P, Bakker van der Jagt MAB, Fraikin T, Slotman BJ, van Moorselaar RJA, Lagerwaard FJ. A prospective single-arm phase 2 study of stereotactic magnetic resonance-guided adaptive radiation therapy for prostate cancer: early toxicity results. Int J Radiat Oncol Biol Phys. 2019;105(5):1086–94.
44. Hehakaya C, Vanneste BG, Grutters JP, Grobbee DE, Verkooijen HM, Frederix GW. Early health economic analysis of 1.5 T MRI-guided radiotherapy for localized prostate cancer: decision analytic modelling. Radiother Oncol. 2021; https://doi.org/10.1016/j.radonc.2021.05.022.
45. Apolle R, Brückner S, Frosch S, Rehm M, Thiele J, Valentini C, Lohaus F, Babatz J, Aust DE, Hampe J. Utility of fiducial markers for target positioning in proton radiotherapy of oesophageal carcinoma. Radiother Oncol. 2019;133:28–34.
46. Fukada J, Hanada T, Kawaguchi O, Ohashi T, Takeuchi H, Kitagawa Y, et al. Detection of esophageal fiducial marker displacement during radiation therapy with a 2-dimensional on-board imager: analysis of internal margin for esophageal cancer. Int J Radiat Oncol Biol Phys. 2013;85:991–8.
47. Schaake EE, Belderbos JSA, Buikhuisen WA, Rossi MMG, Burgers JA, Sonke J-J. Mediastinal lymph node position variability in non-small cell lung cancer patients treated with radical irradiation. Radiother Oncol. 2012;105:150–4.
48. De Roover R, Crijns W, Poels K, Peeters R, Draulans C, Haustermans K, Depuydt T. Characterization of a novel liquid fiducial marker for multimodal image guidance in stereotactic body radiotherapy of prostate cancer. Med Phys. 2018;45(5):2205–17.
49. Rydhög JS, Mortensen SR, Larsen KR, Clementsen P, Jølck RI, Josipovic M, Aznar MC, Specht L, Andresen TL, Af Rosenschöld PM. Liquid fiducial marker performance during radiotherapy of locally advanced non small cell lung cancer. Radiother Oncol. 2016;121(1):64–9.
50. Rydhög JS, Perrin R, Jølck RI, Gagnon-Moisan F, Larsen KR, Clementsen P, de Blanck SR, Persson GF, Weber DC, Lomax T. Liquid fiducial marker applicability in proton therapy of locally advanced lung cancer. Radiother Oncol. 2017;122(3):393–9.

51. Langenhuijsen JF, van Lin EN, Kiemeney LA, van der Vight LP, McColl GM, Visser AG, Witjes JA. Ultrasound-guided transrectal implantation of gold markers for prostate localization during external beam radiotherapy: complication rate and risk factors. Int J Radiat Oncol Biol Phys. 2007;69(3):671–6. https://doi.org/10.1016/j.ijrobp.2007.04.009. Epub 2007 May 23
52. Fawaz ZS, Yassa M, Nguyen DH, Vavassis P. Fiducial marker implantation in prostate radiation therapy: complication rates and technique. Cancer Radiother. 2014;18(8):736–9. https://doi.org/10.1016/j.canrad.2014.07.160. Epub 2014 Oct 16
53. Ghadjar P, Fiorino C, Af Rosenschöld PM, Pinkawa M, Zilli T, van Der Heide UA. ESTRO ACROP consensus guideline on the use of image-guided radiation therapy for localized prostate cancer. Radiother Oncol. 2019;141:5–13.
54. Loh J, Baker K, Sridharan S, Greer P, Wratten C, Capp A, Gallagher S, Martin J. Infections after fiducial marker implantation for prostate radiotherapy: are we underestimating the risks? Radiat Oncol. 2015;10(1):1–5.
55. Kwint M, Conijn S, Schaake E, et al. Intra thoracic anatomical changes in lung cancer patients during the course of radiotherapy. Radiother Oncol. 2014;113:392–7.
56. Nyeng TB, Nordsmark M, Hoffmann L. Dosimetric evaluation of anatomical changes during treatment to identify criteria for adaptive radiotherapy in oesophageal cancer patients. Acta Oncol. 2015;54:1467–73.
57. Jin P, Hulshof MC, de Jong R, van Hooft JE, Bel A, Alderliesten T. Quantification of respiration-induced esophageal tumor motion using fiducial markers and four-dimensional computed tomography. Radiother Oncol. 2016;118:492–7.
58. Møller DS, Poulsen PR, Hagner A, Dufour M, Nordsmark M, Nyeng TB, Mortensen H, Lutz CM, Hoffmann L. Strategies for motion robust proton therapy with pencil beam scanning of esophageal cancer. Int J Radiat Oncol Biol Phys. 2021; https://doi.org/10.1016/j.ijrobp.2021.04.040.
59. Møller DS, Alber M, Nordsmark M, Nyeng TB, Lutz CM, Hoffmann L. Validation of a robust strategy for proton spot scanning for oesophageal cancer in the presence of anatomical changes. Radioth Oncol. 2019;131:ca45–50.
60. Gaur P, Sepesi B, Hofstetter WL, et al. Endoscopic esophageal tumor length: a prognostic factor for patients with esophageal cancer. Cancer. 2011;117:63–9.
61. Muijs CT, Beukema JC, Pruim J, et al. A systematic review on the role of FDG-PET/CT in tumour delineation and radiotherapy planning in patients with esophageal cancer. Radiother Oncol. 2010;97:165–71.
62. Wang B, Liu C, Lin C, et al. Endoscopic tumor length is an independent prognostic factor in esophageal squamous cell carcinoma. Ann Surg Oncol. 2012a;19:2149–58.
63. Wang YC, Hsieh TC, Yu CY, Yen KY, Chen SW, Yang SN, Chien CR, Hsu SM, Pan T, Kao CH, Liang JA. The clinical application of 4D 18F-FDG PET/CT on gross tumor volume delineation for radiotherapy planning in esophageal squamous cell cancer. J Radiat Res. 2012b;53:594–600.
64. Oliver JA, Venkat P, Frakes JM, Klapman J, Harris C, Montilla-Soler J, Dhadham GC, Altazi BA, Zhang GG, Moros EG, Shridhar R, Hoffe SE, Latifi K. Fiducial markers coupled with 3D PET/CT offer more accurate radiation treatment delivery for locally advanced esophageal cancer. Endosc Int Open. 2017;5:E496–504.
65. Gwynne S, Spezi E, Wills L, et al. Toward semi-automated assessment of target volume delineation in radiotherapy trials: the SCOPE 1 pretrial test case. Int J Radiat Oncol Biol Phys. 2012;84:1037–42.
66. Jin P, Hulshof MCCM, van Wieringen N, Bel A, Alderliesten T. Interfractional variability of respiration-induced esophageal tumor motion quantified using fiducial markers and four-dimensional cone-beam computed tomography. Radiother Oncol. 2017;124:147–54.
67. Schmidt ML, Hoffmann L, Møller DS, Knap MM, Rasmussen TR, Folkersen BH, Poulsen PR. Systematic intrafraction shifts of mediastinal lymph node targets between setup imaging and radiation treatment delivery in lung cancer patients. Radiother Oncol. 2018;126:318–24.

68. Worm ES, Høyer M, Fledelius W, Hansen AT, Poulsen PR. Variations in magnitude and directionality of respiratory target motion throughout full treatment courses of stereotactic body radiotherapy for tumors in the liver. Acta Oncol. 2013;52:1437–44.
69. Jin P, van der Horst A, de Jong R, van Hooft JE, Kamphuis M, van Wieringen N, et al. Marker-based quantification of interfractional tumor position variation and the use of markers for setup verification in radiation therapy for esophageal cancer. Radiother Oncol. 2015;117:412–8.
70. Doi Y, Murakami Y, Imano N, Takeuchi Y, Takahashi I, Nishibuchi I, et al. Quantifying esophageal motion during freebreathing and breath-hold using fiducial markers in patients with early-stage esophageal cancer. PLoS One. 2018;13:e0198844.
71. Poulsen PR, Worm ES, Hansen R, Larsen LP, Grau C, Høyer M. Respiratory gating based on internal electromagnetic motion monitoring during stereotactic liver radiation therapy: first results. Acta Oncol. 2015;54:1445–52.
72. Bouchard M, McAleer MF, Starkschall G. Impact of gastric filling on radiation dose delivered to gastroesophageal junction tumors. Int J Radiat Oncol Biol Phys. 2010;77:292–300.
73. Warren S, Partridge M, Bolsi A, Lomax AJ, Hurt C, Crosby T, et al. An analysis of plan robustness for esophageal tumors: comparing volumetric-modulated arc therapy plans and spot scanning proton planning. Int J Radiat Oncol Biol Phys. 2016;95:199–207.
74. Yu J, Zhang X, Liao L, Li H, Zhu R, Park PC, et al. Motion-robust intensity-modulated proton therapy for distal esophageal cancer. Med Phys. 2016;43:1111–8.
75. Hoffmann L, Alber M, Jensen MF, Holt MI, Møller DS. Adaptation is mandatory for intensity-modulated proton therapy of advanced lung cancer to ensure target coverage. Radiother Oncol. 2017;122:400–5.
76. Schmidt MA, Panek R, Colgan R, Hughes J, Sohaib A, Saran F, Murray J, Bernard J, Revell P, Nittka M, Leach MO, Hansen VN. Slice Encoding for Metal Artefact Correction in magnetic resonance imaging examinations for radiotherapy planning. Radiother Oncol. 2016;120(2):356–62. https://doi.org/10.1016/j.radonc.2016.05.004. Epub 2016 May 21
77. Lin SH, et al. Randomized phase IIB trial of proton beam therapy versus intensity-modulated radiation therapy for locally advanced esophageal cancer. J Clin Oncol. 2020a;38(14):1569–79.
78. Lin SH, Hobbs BP, Verma V, Tidwell RS, Smith GL, Lei X, Corsini EM, Mok I, Wei X, Yao L, Wang X, Komaki RU, Chang JY, Chun SG, Jeter MD, Swisher SG, Ajani JA, Blum-Murphy M, Vaporciyan AA, Mehran RJ, Koong AC, Gandhi SJ, Hofstetter WL, Hong TS, Delaney TF, Liao Z, Mohan R. Randomized phase IIB trial of proton beam therapy versus intensity-modulated radiation therapy for locally advanced esophageal cancer. J Clin Oncol. 2020b;38:1569–79.
79. Ling TC, Slater JM, Nookala P, Mifflin R, Grove R, Ly AM, et al. Analysis of intensity-modulated radiation therapy (IMRT), proton and 3D conformal radiotherapy (3D-CRT) for reducing perioperative cardiopulmonary complications in esophageal cancer patients. Cancers. 2014;6:2356–68.
80. Dang A, Kupelian PA, Cao M, Agazaryan N, Kishan AU. Image-guided radiotherapy for prostate cancer. Transl Androl Urol. 2018;7(3):308.
81. Foster RD, Pistenmaa DA, Solberg TD. A comparison of radiographic techniques and electromagnetic transponders for localization of the prostate. Radiat Oncol. 2012;7(1):1–7.
82. Olsen JR, Noel CE, Baker K, Santanam L, Michalski JM, Parikh PJ. Practical method of adaptive radiotherapy for prostate cancer using real-time electromagnetic tracking. Int J Radiat Oncol Biol Phys. 2012;82(5):1903–11.
83. James J, Cetnar A, Dunlap NE, Huffaker C, Nguyen VN, Potts M, Wang B. Validation and implementation of a wireless transponder tracking system for gated stereotactic ablative radiotherapy of the liver. Med Phys. 2016;43(6 Part1):2794–801.
84. Worm ES, Høyer M, Hansen R, et al. A prospective cohort study of gated stereotactic liver radiation therapy using continuous internal electromagnetic motion monitoring. Int J Radiat Oncol Biol Phys. 2018;101:366–75.
85. Skouboe S, Poulsen PR, Muurholm CG, et al. Simulated real-time dose reconstruction for moving tumors in stereotactic liver radiotherapy. Med Phys. 2019;46:4738–48.

86. Zhu X, Bourland JD, Yuan Y, Zhuang T, O'Daniel J, Thongphiew D, Wu QJ, Das SK, Yoo S, Yin FF. Tradeoffs of integrating real-time tracking into IGRT for prostate cancer treatment. Phys Med Biol. 2009;54(17):N393.
87. Fiorino C, Valdagni R, Rancati T, Sanguineti G. Dose-volume effects for normal tissues in external radiotherapy: pelvis. Radiother Oncol. 2009;93(2):153–67. https://doi.org/10.1016/j.radonc.2009.08.004. Epub 2009 Sep 16
88. Michalski JM, Gay H, Jackson A, Tucker SL, Deasy JO. Radiation dose-volume effects in radiation-induced rectal injury. Int J Radiat Oncol Biol Phys. 2010;76(3 Suppl):S123–9. https://doi.org/10.1016/j.ijrobp.2009.03.078. Erratum in: Int J Radiat Oncol Biol Phys. 2019;104(5):1185.
89. Bastasch MD, Teh BS, Mai WY, McGary JE, Grant WH 3rd, Butler EB. Tolerance of endorectal balloon in 396 patients treated with intensity-modulated radiation therapy (IMRT) for prostate cancer. Am J Clin Oncol. 2006;29(1):8–11.
90. van Lin ENT, Hoffmann AL, van Kollenburg P, Leer JW, Visser AG. Rectal wall sparing effect of three different endorectal balloons in 3D conformal and IMRT prostate radiotherapy. Int J Radiat Oncol Biol Phys. 2005;63(2):565–76.
91. Smeenk RJ, Louwe RJ, Langen KM, et al. An endorectal balloon reduces intrafraction prostate motion during radiotherapy. Int J Radiat Oncol Biol Phys. 2012;83(2):661–9.
92. Smeenk RJ, van Lin EN, van Kollenburg P, Kunze-Busch M, Kaanders JH. Anal wall sparing effect of an endorectal balloon in 3D conformal and intensity-modulated prostate radiotherapy. Radiother Oncol. 2009;93(1):131–6.
93. Jaccard M, Lamanna G, Dubouloz A, Rouzaud M, Miralbell R, Zilli T. Dose optimization and endorectal balloon for internal pudendal arteries sparing in prostate SBRT. Phys Med. 2019;61:28–32.
94. Dubouloz A, Rouzaud M, Tsvang L, et al. Urethra-sparing stereotactic body radiotherapy for prostate cancer: how much can the rectal wall dose be reduced with or without an endorectal balloon? Radiat Oncol. 2018;13(1):114.
95. Teh BS, Lewis GD, Mai W, Pino R, Ishiyama H, Butler EB. Long-term outcome of a moderately hypofractionated, intensity-modulated radiotherapy approach using an endorectal balloon for patients with localized prostate cancer. Cancer Commun (Lond). 2018;38(1):11.
96. Wortel RC, Heemsbergen WD, Smeenk RJ, et al. Local protocol variations for image-guided radiation therapy in the multicenter dutch hypofractionation (HYPRO) trial: impact of rectal balloon and MRI delineation on anorectal dose and gastrointestinal toxicity levels. Int J Radiat Oncol Biol Phys. 2017;99(5):1243–52.
97. Deville C, Both S, Bui V, et al. Acute gastrointestinal and genitourinary toxicity of image-guided intensity-modulated radiation therapy for prostate cancer using a daily water-filled endorectal balloon. Radiat Oncol. 2012;7:76.
98. van Lin EN, Kristinsson J, Philippens ME, et al. Reduced late rectal mucosal changes after prostate three-dimensional conformal radiotherapy with endorectal balloon as observed in repeated endoscopy. Int J Radiat Oncol Biol Phys. 2007;67(3):799–811.
99. D'Amico AV, Manola J, McMahon E, et al. A prospective evaluation of rectal bleeding after dose-escalated three-dimensional conformal radiation therapy using an intrarectal balloon for prostate gland localization and immobilization. Urology. 2006;67(4):780–4.
100. Elsayed H, Bolling T, Moustakis C, Muller SB, Schuller P, Ernst I, et al. Organ movements and dose exposures in teletherapy of prostate cancer using a rectal balloon. Strahlenther Onkol. 2007;183:617–24.
101. de Leon J, Jameson MG, Rivest-Henault D, Keats S, Rai R, Arumugam S, Wilton L, Ngo D, Liney G, Moses D, Dowling J, Martin J, Sidhom M. Reduced motion and improved rectal dosimetry through endorectal immobilization for prostate stereotactic body radiotherapy. Br J Radiol. 2019;92(1098):20190056.
102. Nicolae A, Davidson M, Easton H, et al. Clinical evaluation of an endorectal immobilization system for use in prostate hypofractionated stereotactic ablative body radiotherapy (SABR). Radiat Oncol. 2015;10:122.

103. Vanneste BGL, Buettner F, Pinkawa M, Lambin P, Hoffmann AL. Ano-rectal wall dose-surface maps localize the dosimetric benefit of hydrogel rectum spacers in prostate cancer radiotherapy. Clin Transl Radiat Oncol. 2018;(14):17–24. https://doi.org/10.1016/j.ctro.2018.10.006.
104. Pinkawa M, Corral NE, Caffaro M. Application of a spacer gel to optimize three-dimensional conformal and intensity-modulated radiotherapy for prostate cancer. Radiother Oncol. 2011;100(3):436–41.
105. Prada PJ, Fernández J, Martinez AA, de la Rúa A, Gonzalez JM, Fernandez JM, Juan G. Transperineal injection of hyaluronic acid in anterior perirectal fat to decrease rectal toxicity from radiation delivered with intensity-modulated brachytherapy or EBRT for prostate cancer patients. Int J Radiat Oncol Biol Phys. 2007;69(1):95–102.
106. Melchert C, et al. Interstitial biodegradable balloon for reduced rectal dose during prostate radiotherapy: results of a virtual planning investigation based on the pre- and post-implant imaging data of an international multicenter study. Radiother Oncol. 2013;106(2):210–4.
107. Noyes WR, Hosford CC, Schultz SE. Human collagen injections to reduce rectal dose during radiotherapy. Int J Radiat Oncol Biol Phys. 2012;82(5):1918–22.
108. Mok G, Benz E, Vallee JP, Miralbell R, Zilli T. Optimization of radiation therapy techniques for prostate cancer with prostate-rectum spacers: a systematic review. Int J Radiat Oncol Biol Phys. 2014;90(2):278–88.
109. Quinn TJ, Daignault-Newton S, Bosch W, Mariados N, Sylvester J, Shah D, Gross E, Hudes R, Beyer D, Kurtzman S, Bogart J, Hsi RA, Kos M, Ellis R, Logsdon M, Zimberg S, Forsythe K, Zhang H, Soffen E, Francke P, Mantz C, DeWeese T, Gay HA, Michalski J, Hamstra DA. Who benefits from a prostate rectal spacer? secondary analysis of a phase III trial. Pract Radiat Oncol. 2020;10(3):186–94.
110. Karsh LI, Gross ET, Pieczonka CM, Aliotta PJ, Skomra CJ, Ponsky LE, Nieh PT, Han M, Hamstra DA, Shore ND. Absorbable hydrogel spacer use in prostate radiotherapy: a comprehensive review of phase 3 clinical trial published data. Urology. 2018;115:39–44.
111. Uhl M, Herfarth K, Eble MJ, Pinkawa M, van Triest B, Kalisvaart R, Weber DC, Miralbell R, Song DY, DeWeese TL. Absorbable hydrogel spacer use in men undergoing prostate cancer radiotherapy: 12-month toxicity and proctoscopy results of a prospective multicenter phase II trial. Radiat Oncol. 2014;9:96.
112. Pinkawa M, Berneking V, Schlenter M, Krenkel B, Eble MJ. Quality of life after radiation therapy for prostate cancer with a hydrogel spacer: 5-year results. Int J Radiat Oncol Biol Phys. 2017;99(2):374–7.
113. Whalley D, Hruby G, Alfieri F, Kneebone A, Eade T. SpaceOAR hydrogel in dose-escalated prostate cancer radiotherapy: rectal dosimetry and late toxicity. Clin Oncol (R Coll Radiol). 2016;28(10):e148–54.
114. Chapet O, Decullier E, Bin S, Faix A, Ruffion A, Jalade P, Fenoglietto P, Udrescu C, Enachescu C, Azria D. Prostate hypofractionated radiation therapy with injection of hyaluronic acid: acute toxicities in a phase 2 study. Int J Radiat Oncol Biol Phys. 2015;91(4):730–6.
115. Vanneste BGL, van De Beek K, Lutgens L, Lambin P. Implantation of a biodegradable rectum balloon implant: tips, tricks and pitfalls. Int Braz J Urol. 2017;43(6):1033–42.
116. Bertolaccini L, Lyberis P, Manno E. Lung sealant and morbidity after pleural decortication: a prospective randomized, blinded study. J Cardiothorac Surg. 2010;28(5):45.
117. Cosgrove GR, Delashaw JB, Grotenhuis JA, et al. Safety and efficacy of a novel polyethylene glycol hydrogel sealant for watertight dural repair. J Neurosurg. 2007;106:52–8.
118. Garasic JM, Martin L, Anderson RD. Acute evaluation of the Mynx vascular closure device during arterial re-puncture in an ovine model. J Invasive Cardiol. 2009;21:283–5.
119. Hamstra DA, Mariados N, Sylvester J, et al. Continued benefit to rectal separation for prostate radiation therapy: final results of a phase III trial. Int J Radiat Oncol Biol Phys. 2017;97(5):976–85.
120. Mariados N, Sylvester J, Shah D, et al. Hydrogel spacer prospective multicenter randomized controlled pivotal trial: dosimetric and clinical effects of perirectal spacer application in men undergoing prostate image-guided intensity-modulated radiation therapy. Int J Radiat Oncol Biol Phys. 2015;92(5):971–7.

121. Hamstra DA, Mariados N, Sylvester J, et al. Sexual quality of life following prostate intensity-modulated radiation therapy (IMRT) with a rectal/prostate spacer: Secondary analysis of a phase 3 trial. Pract Radiat Oncol. 2018;8(1):e7–e15.
122. Volpi N, Schiller J, Stern R, Soltés L. Role, metabolism, chemical modifications and applications of hyaluronan. Curr Med Chem. 2009;16(14):1718–45.
123. George E. Intra-articular hyaluronan treatment for osteoarthritis. Ann Rheum Dis. 1998;57(11):637–40.
124. Patino MG, Neiders ME, Andreana S, Noble B, Cohen RE. Collagen as an implantable material in medicine and dentistry. J Oral Implantol. 2002;28(5):220–5.
125. Faerber GJ, Richardson TD. Long-term results of transurethral collagen injection in men with intrinsic sphincter deficiency. J Endourol. 1997;11(4):273–7.
126. Levy Y, Paz A, Yosef RB, Corn BW, Vaisman B, Shuhat S, Domb AJ. Biodegradable inflatable balloon for reducing radiation adverse effects in prostate cancer. J Biomed Mater Res B Appl Biomater. 2009;91(2):855–67. https://doi.org/10.1002/jbm.b.31467.
127. Vanneste BGL, van Wijk Y, Lutgens LC, et al. Dynamics of rectal balloon implant shrinkage in prostate VMAT: influence on anorectal dose and late rectal complication risk. Strahlenther Onkol. 2018a;194(1):31–40.
128. Vanneste BGL, Van Limbergen EJ, van de Beek K, van Lin E, Lutgens LC, Lambin P. A biodegradable rectal balloon implant to protect the rectum during prostate cancer radiotherapy for a patient with active Crohn disease. Tech Innov Patient Support Radiat Oncol. 2018b;6:1–4.
129. Wolff RF, Ryder S, Bossi A, Briganti A, Crook J, Henry A, Karnes J, Potters L, de Reijke T, Stone N, Burckhardt M, Duffy S, Worthy G, Kleijnen J. A systematic review of randomised controlled trials of radiotherapy for localised prostate cancer. Eur J Cancer. 2015;51(16):2345–67.
130. Hutchinson RC, Sundaram V, Folkert M, Lotan Y. Decision analysis model evaluating the cost of a temporary hydrogel rectal spacer before prostate radiation therapy to reduce the incidence of rectal complications. In: Urologic oncology: seminars and original investigations. Amsterdam: Elsevier; 2016.
131. Levy JF, Khairnar R, Louie AV, Showalter TN, Mullins CD, Mishra MV. Evaluating the cost-effectiveness of hydrogel rectal spacer in prostate cancer radiation therapy. Pract Radiat Oncol. 2019;9(2):e172–9.
132. Vanneste BG, Pijls-Johannesma M, Van De Voorde L, et al. Spacers in radiotherapy treatment of prostate cancer: is reduction of toxicity cost-effective? Radiother Oncol. 2015;114(2):276–81.
133. Vanneste BG, Hoffmann AL, van Lin EN, Van De Voorde L, Pinkawa M, Lambin P. Who will benefit most from hydrogel rectum spacer implantation in prostate cancer radiotherapy? A model-based approach for patient selection. Radiother Oncol. 2016a;121(1):118–23.
134. Vanneste B, Van Limbergen EJ, van Lin EN, van Roermund JGH, Lambin P. Prostate cancer radiation therapy: what do clinicians have to know? Biomed Res Int. 2016b;2016:6829875.
135. van Wijk Y, Vanneste BGL, Jochems A, Walsh S, Pinkawa M, Lambin P. Development of an iso-toxic model integrating validated genetic markers of toxicity and tumour control probability: a multifactorial decision support system for prostate cancer radiotherapy to support the decision to place an implantable rectum spacer. Acta Oncol. 2018;28:1–7.
136. van Wijk Y, Vanneste BGL, Walsh S, van der Meer S, Ramaekers B, van Elmpt W, Pinkawa M, Lambin P. Development of a decision support system for an implantable rectum spacer during prostate cancer radiotherapy: comparison of dose, toxicity and cost-effectiveness. Radiother Oncol. 2017;125(1):107–12.

11 Artificial Intelligence in Radiation Oncology: A Rapidly Evolving Picture

Harini Veeraraghavan and Joseph O. Deasy

11.1 Introduction

Artificial intelligence (AI) has emerged as a powerful technology with widespread applications in diverse areas ranging from autonomous cars to medical decision support. In essence, AI technologies work by integrating many quantitative clues together to provide probabilistic guidance to real-world problems, such as "Is this skin abnormality cancerous?" [1] or "Is the fetus in the breech or normal position for birth?" [2]. Medical applications of AI, particularly using the techniques of deep learning, are growing. Deep learning is a statistical machine-learning approach and a subfield of AI. Deep learning methods employ several layers of convolutional filters represented as a neural network to compute a very large number of features. The appropriate set of features is learned from the data and specific to the learning problem. A primer of deep learning for radiologists is available in [3]. Deep learning is particularly amenable to learning from large imaging datasets, and the deployed classifiers allow fast, real-time, objective, and automated analysis. However, AI is a general technology, and we will briefly mention other aspects of radiation oncology we expect will be impacted. The reader should also be aware that reviews of the impact of AI in RO have also been recently published elsewhere [4–6].

Radiation oncology arguably uses the highest level of automation not only in cancer care but also across medicine generally. The need for automation to ensure accurate targeting of cancer while ensuring patient safety, and the increased reliance on image guidance for image-guided radiation treatments, has made AI and deep learning particularly relevant for radiation oncology. AI undoubtedly has the potential to disrupt and transform the treatment paradigm in radiation oncology, as well

H. Veeraraghavan (✉) · J. O. Deasy
Department of Medical Physics, Memorial Sloan Kettering Cancer Center, New York, NY, USA
e-mail: veerarah@mskcc.org; DeasyJ@mskcc.org

E. G. C. Troost (ed.), *Image-Guided High-Precision Radiotherapy*,
https://doi.org/10.1007/978-3-031-08601-4_11

as other fields in medicine. In this chapter, we will review the current state of the art in the advances of AI techniques with respect to radiation oncology and the anticipated, though uncertain, impact of AI. Emphasis will be placed on applications that rely on the analysis of images, as the clinical impact is imminent and likely transformative, in particular, automated tissue segmentation for normal tissues but also for tumors. The ability to extend auto-segmentation to cone-beam images, at the time of treatment, in particular, will allow for more accurate setup, better dose-accumulation estimates, and possibly smaller margins, perhaps leading to a true "AI-guided-RT." Before diving further into AI applications, we briefly discuss the general basis of AI.

11.2 What Is AI?

Artificial intelligence (AI) is a branch of computer science that is concerned with developing techniques to enable computer algorithms to capture and emulate intelligent human behavior [7], ultimately aiming for better-than-expert performance and greater consistency. AI considered as a whole cover both deductive (or top-down) reasoning and inductive (or bottom-up) reasoning. An overarching goal in the field of AI is to ultimately combine the versatility of bottom-up inductive reasoning via machine-learning techniques with top-down deductive reasoning to produce a rationally processing intelligent agent informed by cause and effect. We are currently far from this ideal goal, although many AI systems have demonstrated fit-for-purpose abilities to better account for complicated details compared to human operators.

Deductive learning, i.e., explanation-based learning, consists of algorithms for extracting provably correct knowledge. These methods typically combine a pre-specified knowledge, often represented as a set of established rules, to solve problems. For each observed training example, an explanation of how the examples satisfy the target concept can thus be derived from the knowledge domain, which can then be used, for example, to distinguish relevant from irrelevant features [8]. Two core requirements for these methods are a sufficient knowledge base and an efficient approach to sort through the knowledge base rules, constraining the possible solutions until the problem is solved. Deductive reasoning is used by the player, for example, to solve the puzzle game of fukoshiti. The knowledge base can be, for example, a database or an ontology consisting of rules of facts in the specific domain and represented as predicates (Fig. 11.1). An advantage of this style of learning is that inferences made from the specific observations are always supported by the rules (ontology). Hence, the conclusions are guaranteed to always be true, or at least consistent with the knowledge base. However, the key obstacle is usually the development of a comprehensive knowledge ontology, which may require significant domain expertise and effort for construction. In addition, as the size of the ontology grows, more efficient search methods are required for searching through the knowledge base.

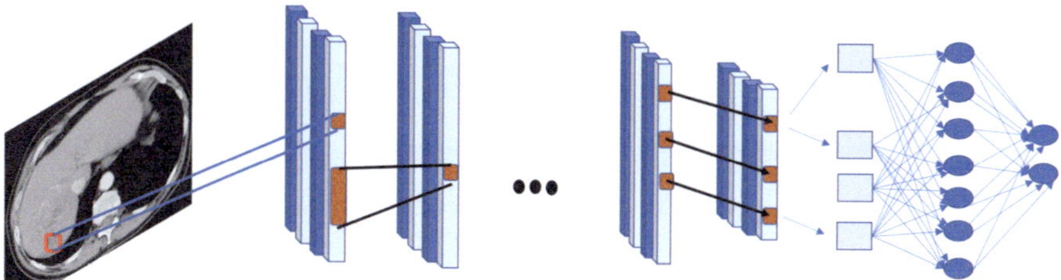

Fig. 11.1 Example schematic of a deep convolutional neural network. The network may consist of layers for generating new image representations as feature maps using convolutional layers, pooling layers to down-sample feature maps, and fully connected layers to combine feature activations to produce classification

Inductive learning or bottom-up reasoning methods are more amenable to using general big data streams and are more prevalent in modern machine learning. These methods including deep (many layered) neural networks that aim to classify samples. Figure 11.1 shows an example schematic of a deep neural network used for classification. A deep network may consist of several convolutional layers, fully connected layers, and pooling layers for processing the images in various scales and image features. Models can be learned from general off-the-shelf network architectures found to be effective in several problems, followed by a training process, in which the network weights are adjusted to improve prediction performance on a set of available examples ("the training set"). The goal of course is to perform well on new unseen user data, called generalization, and AI papers typically include performance tests on set-aside data not used for training [9]. Deep learning methods extend standard machine-learning methods by combining a large number of linear and non-linear image filter functions, for example edge detection, or mean intensity over a small 2 × 2 region, etc. These filters are arranged in layers, referred to as a convolution neural network (CNN), building new feature maps that effectively project the pixels of the original image into a space, whose dimensions consist of the many different calculation routes created in the network. In this high-dimensional space, it is typically more feasible to find an effective classification rule. Hence, deep learning solves the problem of deriving an appropriate representation of the data by extracting representations that are expressed in terms of other nested representations of the data. Increasing the depth of the network, or nesting of these representations, affords larger flexibility and increases the capacity of these methods in modeling highly nonlinear functions that are difficult to solve by lower-dimensional modeling approaches.

The rest of this chapter will therefore focus on deep learning methods and their applications.

As a result of the deep learning revolution, AI has evolved from tackling problems that are "intellectually difficult for humans" to solving every-day problems

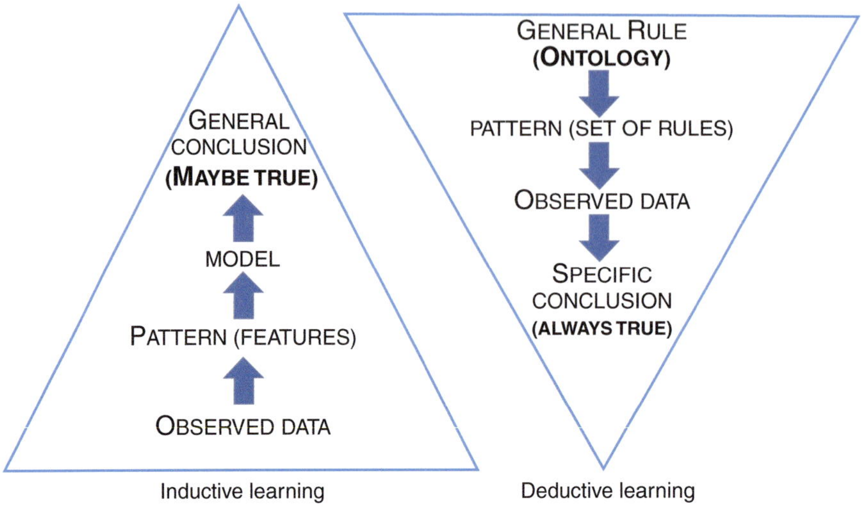

Fig. 11.2 Inductive and deductive approaches to artificial intelligence machine learning

that humans solve intuitively [10]. The widespread use and success of inductive learning techniques come from their ability to learn from massive amounts of underlying data without requiring any pre-built knowledge base, thereby eliminating the need for significant domain expertise and knowledge engineering effort to bootstrap the learning process (Fig. 11.2). Importantly, once learned, these methods are fast and therefore capable of producing real-time inference.

Importantly, one potential disadvantage of these methods is the inductive bias especially when the size of the training datasets is not sufficiently large or is not fully representative of all the variabilities occurring in the domain, as further discussed below. Inductive bias is employed by all learning methods to achieve convergence. This is the process whereby learning methods restrict the shape of hypothesis space so that only some hypotheses are preferred over others. It is possible, however, to combine deductive inference with inductive learning (described below) to produce high-quality logistical plans (not RT plans) in real time [11].

Nevertheless, inductive learning methods eliminate the need for building a large knowledge base/rule base of the domain. Deep learning methods go a step further and eliminate the need for "feature engineering," wherein the design of appropriate set of quantitative features and image filtering (or processing methods) to extract those features are no longer needed. Feature engineering requires not only extensive domain expertise but also an intimate knowledge of the image analysis and computational methods in the fields of computer vision. The deep learning revolution, of great value to all the commercial technology giants, has spawned a large number of open source and useful tools that have helped accelerate adoption of deep learning in medical research. Hence, deep learning has made AI accessible to the broader biomedical research community and will lead, in our view, to significant advances in the field of radiation oncology.

The rest of this chapter will therefore focus on deep learning methods and their applications.

11.3 Why Is Deep Learning Important for Radiation Oncology?

Deep learning methods are bringing about a transformative change in radiation oncology data processing as these methods have shown tremendous success in analyses involving images [5]. Radiation oncology is of course a highly technology-driven field. With the adoption of in-room imaging for image-guided radiation therapy [12], and the advances in in-treatment-room-imaging, including cone-beam computed tomography (CBCT; Chap. 4) [13, 14], more advanced and precise treatments such as adaptive radiotherapy [15, 16] are becoming feasible. There is a need for greater automation not only to improve the efficiency of the treatment planning and treatment delivery process, but also to aid clinicians in identifying the best course of treatment and adapting treatment as and when is necessary. Higher automation will reduce variability, and possibly treatment toxicities, while providing opportunities to escalate doses to more-precisely targeted tumor structures.

Thus, radiation oncology can benefit from the advances in deep learning and AI not only in the space of analyzing images for improving accuracy and efficiency of delineating tumors and organs for radiation treatment planning [17–24], but also in other areas of radiation oncology including automated dose prediction, outcomes prediction, and enabling MR-guided treatments through synthetic CT generation [25, 26].

11.4 Application Areas for Deep Learning in Radiation Oncology

We will focus on the most mature applications of AI/deep learning in radiation oncology, including image segmentation, artifact reduction, and MR-based synthetic CT generation for MR applications. However, we will briefly touch as well on other areas of clinical impact we expect to emerge in the next 5 years.

11.4.1 Image Segmentation for Treatment Planning

Image segmentation involves learning on voxel-level data, and clinical segmentations are often available for normal organs. Thus, deep learning methods have been developed and applied even on moderately sized datasets, especially for segmenting normal organs. This is feasible because image segmentation effectively trains the classifier on many small patches in the training image, labeled as inside or outside a labeled region. As a result, a large number of CNNs have already been developed for image segmentation. A majority of these focus on segmenting CT images, while a few recent methods have also developed methods for the more challenging CBCT images. Although MRI has better soft-tissue contrast than CT and CBCT images, the challenge with using MRI for segmentation is the lack of sufficiently large training sets.

Besides the relative technological ease of implementing deep learning methods for segmentation, segmentation in radiation oncology is also beneficial due to the dependency of image-guided treatments on the segmentation of targets and various organs at risk for conformal beam shaping. Automated segmentations are more repeatable than manual delineations [18] and reduce manual editing times [27]. As discussed further below, segmentation remains a primary bottleneck in adaptive radiation treatments and lack of precise and accurate delineations are one of the major sources of setup and treatment uncertainties in radiation therapy [15, 28].

11.4.2 Computed Tomography and Cone-Beam Computed Tomography Segmentation

Computed tomography and CBCT are the commonly used imaging modalities for planning and monitoring radiation treatments. Although CBCT imaging is acquired routinely, it is predominantly used for monitoring large setup errors and for making positional adjustments, often "by eye." Recent advance in deep learning has allowed researchers to make some progress toward CBCT segmentation. We discuss some of the most common approaches used for CT and CBCT segmentation.

Table 11.1 shows some of the representative methods developed for the different organ sites for CT and CBCT images. Methods [24, 29, 32–34, 36] often employ or build upon [18] well-known architectures such as the U-net [37]. Other commonly used networks include the VGG [30, 38] and deepLab [39] architecture used for prostate organs at risk [40] as well as heart sub-structure segmentation [41].

However, as individual architectures are often developed for a specific problem, these may not yield the best possible performance and often require extensive fine-tuning to achieve reasonable performance. In short, special architectures and learning procedures, tuned for the purpose at hand, can often perform better than generic architectures. Developing new architectures is a major area of research. Notable examples of such methods include [22, 29, 31, 34, 35, 42]. For example, a specialized architecture for preserving small structures, e.g., the esophagus [22], has been shown to be more effective than standard methods. The problem of detecting and segmenting small tumors was also handled in [42] and more recently in [43] by a special architecture called a multiple resolution residual network, where the network layers make use of residual connections arising from all image resolutions. Approaches have also been developed to handle the issue of low soft-tissue contrast and resolution in some CT images by deriving better feature representations from images using squeeze–excitation blocks [29] and self-attention formulations [21]. An advantage of self-attention methods [21] is that spatially separated image content, that can inform local segmentation, can be extracted, which in turn helps segmentation. For example, the inferred location of the mandible helps better localize

Table 11.1 Representative deep learning methods applied to radiation oncology for CT datasets

Method	Location	Approach summary
[17]	Head and neck: cord, mandible, parotid glands, submandibular glands, larynx, pharynx, eye globes, optic nerves, and optic chiasm	2D patch-based U-net for individual organs
[29]	Head and neck: brain stem, optic chiasm, mandible, optic nerves, parotid glands, submandibular glands	3D whole CT U-net combining squeeze and excitation layers
[30]	Head and neck: brain stem, larynx, eye globes, lens, mandible, oral cavity, mastoid, spinal cord, parotid gland, optic nerve	2D organ detection followed by Unet segmentation network
[31]	Gross tumor volume	3D patch densely connected network
[24]	Head and neck: brain stem, larynx, oral cavity, esophagus, esophageal sphincter, pharyngeal constrictor, cricopharynx, parotid glands, submandibular glands	3D patch-based Unet
[21]	Head and neck: parotid glands, submandibular glands, spinal cord, mandible	2D Unet with self-attention module
[32]	Head and neck: parotid glands, submandibular glands, spinal cord, mandible	3D patch-based Unet
[22]	Lung: heart, esophagus, trachea, aorta	2D sharp-mask Unet to focus on small organs, e.g., esophagus
[33]	Lung: heart, esophagus, spinal cord, and lungs	Two-stage 3D Unet for localization and segmentation
[34]	Lung: heart, esophagus, spinal cord, lungs	U-net GAN based segmentation network; fully convolutional discriminator loss distinguishes whether segmentation is from expert or algorithm
[18]	Pelvis: prostate, femoral head, bladder, rectum	3DUnet consisting of organ localization with boundary losses
[35]	Pelvis: bladder, rectum, prostate	Pseudo-MRI generated through a cycleGAN trained with paired image sets is used for segmentation

parotid gland contours. Figure 11.3 shows an example of a self-attention-based segmentation derived using our approach [21], along with the dose volume histogram (DVH) compared between this method and a standard U-net segmentation of head and neck organs. As seen, this method more closely approximates the expert-derived DVH.

The method for HN organ-at-risk (OAR) segmentation has been implemented in our clinic for routine segmentation using a in-house developed software pipeline, called the Ensemble of Voxelwise Attributors (EVA). The EVA pipeline (shown in Fig. 11.4) consists of file watchers and listeners to automatically detect when DICOM images become available for analysis, as well as when segmented results are available for storage. The file watchers and listeners interface with the

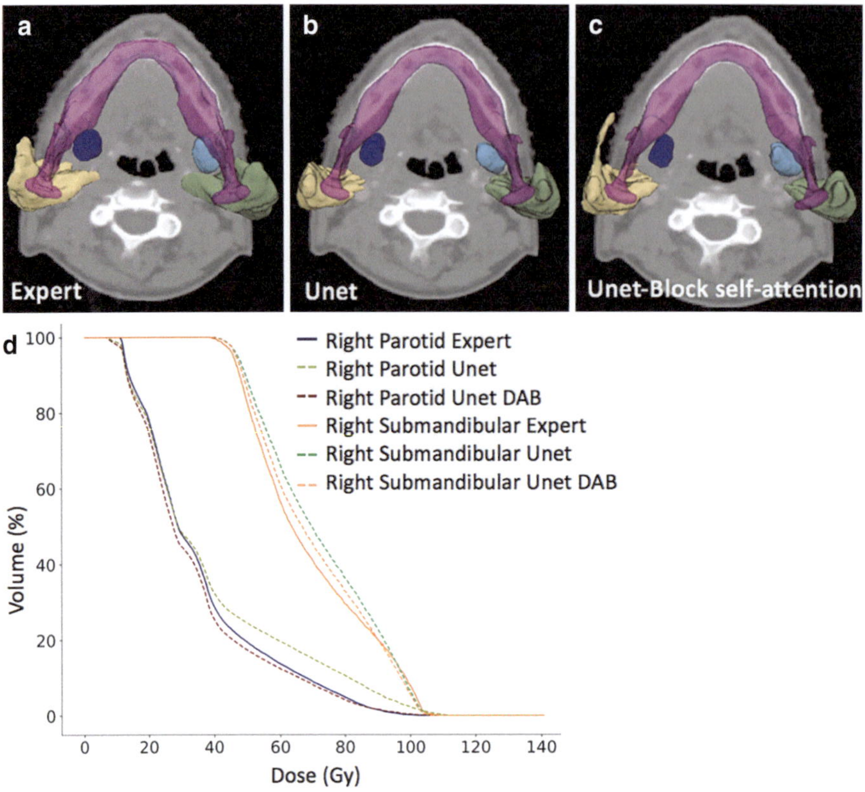

Fig. 11.3 Comparison of segmentations of multiple OARs on head and neck CT produced by an expert, standard U-net, and the Unet DAB method [21]. The three-dimensional volume representation also shows the lateral horn of the right parotid that was captured by the Unet DAB method. The DVH curves show close agreement between expert and the Unet DAB method

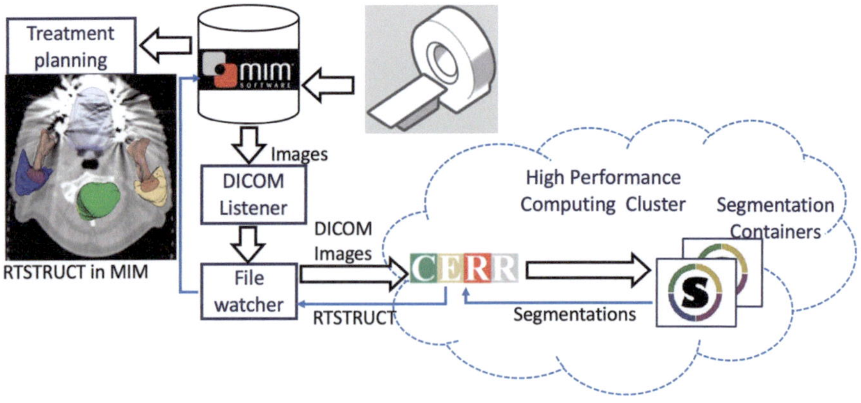

Fig. 11.4 The ensemble of voxel-wise attributors (EVA) pipeline used for routine deep learning segmentation for radiation treatments at MSK

commercial MIM software, which stores the DICOM images and results for visualization and storage and the high-performance computing clusters where the deep learning methods are executed. The appropriate deep learning method for a given disease site is automatically invoked based on DICOM headers with required preprocessing, post-processing, and conversion to RT structs handled by our in-house developed and open-source CERR software. The EVA pipeline has been used to analyze more than 300 HN cancer patients since May 2020. Automated segmentations have also reduced user effort in editing (parotids of 54.5%, submandibular glands of 56%, mandible of 59%, cord of 74%, brain stem of 70%, and oral cavity of 51%), measured on a randomly sampled subset of 71 cases.

Another approach to improve inference on low soft-tissue contrast images such as CTs is to use the more informative modality of MRI to derive more informative features [20, 35, 44, 45]. Effectively, the MRI information informs the interpretation of geometry and features in the target CT images that cannot be learned from CT-only datasets. We have developed this approach extensively. Work in [35] learned a model to synthesize a pseudo-MRI from CT images using subject paired sets of CT and MRI training sets. The work in [45] goes a step further and shows how unpaired CT and MRI image sets can be used together. A key advantage of this approach is that MRI datasets are seldom available on the same patients as a CT dataset, and just as importantly, one often has a much larger CT dataset available.

11.4.3 Magnetic Resonance Imaging Segmentation for MR-Guided Radiation Therapy

Magnetic resonance imaging, due to its better soft-tissue contrast, has become the cutting edge for treatment planning and for in-room image-guided adaptive radiation treatments [46]. However, a fundamental problem with using MRI for radiation therapy is the lack of robust auto-segmentation tools. As this modality is new for radiation oncology, implementing deep learning for MRI has a different issue stemming from the lack of sufficiently large training sets. Recent work has addressed this issue through cross-modality learning. Commonly used approaches leverage a labeled dataset in a different modality such as CT to segment on the MRI using the cycleGAN [47] method. Examples of this approach include knee segmentation from MRI [48], cardiac image segmentation [49], and MRI-based liver segmentation [50]. Improved architectures address the issue of poor image transformation especially between highly different modalities, i.e., CT and MRI, by using constraints on the geometry of the segmented structures [20, 44, 51], deep supervision losses [35]. However, a problem with these modality transformation-based techniques is the difficulty to model the appearance of the target MRI modality. Geometric constraints help to preserve the shape of the various structures, but modeling the appearance (textures) within such structures is difficult. Furthermore, as MRI has multiple sequences available, training using the standard cross-modality adaptation techniques would require training separate one-to-one modality transformation network for every sequence. In our recent work [52], we developed a new approach for better preserving the appearance of the various segmented organs by combining the segmentation probability maps with the images as a joint distribution by the discriminator [52]. We also developed a one-to-many modality transformation and unsupervised abdomen segmentation approach using a single network [53].

In summary, the number of methods and the application of deep learning methods for medical image segmentation in radiotherapy are rapidly growing. It is notable that advances particularly in the area of developing novel architectures and losses (cost functions to guide improvements) are done in disease sites with well-curated open-source datasets. As seen on Table 11.1, the number of methods developed for head and neck and lung is much higher than the methods developed for other disease sites. Open-source datasets may have a disadvantage in terms of the number of available cases, but they are nevertheless extremely useful resources. Often, such datasets are provided from multiple institutions [54], with the segmentations carefully verified [55], sometimes with multiple raters. More importantly, such datasets provide a common benchmark reference to evaluate new methods against existing methods and improve upon those methods.

11.5 Toward AI-Guided Radiotherapy

Deep learning methods have particularly demonstrated feasibility regarding tissue segmentations. A key future application of deep learning methods will be the extension to in-room cone-beam CT (CBCT) and MRI-guided analysis in real time for patient setup and monitoring. For example, the ability to estimate the position of the esophagus and the gross tumor volume together, on a per-fraction basis, in real time during standard X-ray fraction delivery for lung radiotherapy, could enable significantly better sparing esophageal sparing and smaller target volumes in general. The same principle holds true, of course, across the body. In addition to the improved use of CBCT data, these tools will enable better tracking of tumor changes over a course, thereby supporting improved dose-accumulation mapping, adaptive therapy, and generally more limited treatment margins. The potential normal tissue damage that could be avoided through this program is massive. An envisioned AI-guided RT workflow as depicted in Fig. 11.5 could become practical and clinically widespread with advances in AI segmentation and image registration methods.

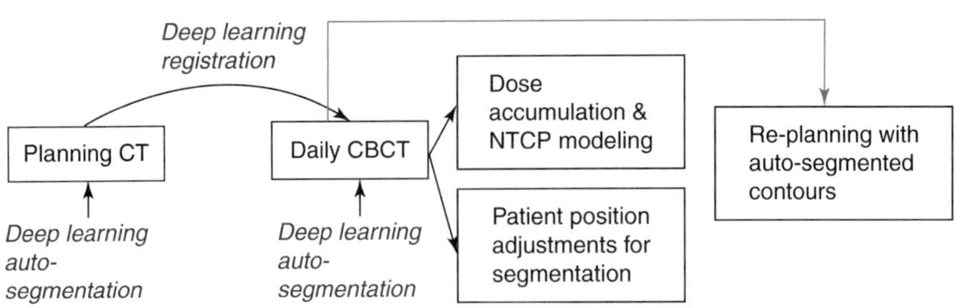

Fig. 11.5 AI-Guided Radiation Treatment (AIGRT) workflow for more precise radiotherapy

Image fusion or registration is a frequently used as a critical step in radiation therapy. Image registration is a process of bringing two images such as a planning CT image and a current image of the day (e.g., CBCT image) into alignment. Accurate volumetric image registration can quantify geometric changes in the anatomy during treatment, localize and monitor patient motion, and assess tumor and normal organ response during and post-radiation treatment. The fusion is typically accomplished by deformably warping a moving image into a target image. Image registration is thus essential for image guidance in adaptative therapy [28], tumor motion tracking [56], and dose accumulation [57, 58]. Shrinkage is known to vary spatially and also varies between some tumors even of the same histology and site [59]. Such differences in dynamic treatment response, if they can be captured accurately, could potentially be used to further characterize whether treatment is proceeding effectively, as expected, or alternatively for adapting or altering treatment [28, 60]. Deep learning provides a new toolbox, compared to standard grid-based methods, or mechanical simulation methods, to possibly improve the accuracy of derived deformations, including local tissue shrinkage [61].

One of the biggest advantageous of using deep learning methods for performing registration is the computational speed, which is typically 1 min or less due to the efficient convolution architectures. However, the problem of training deep learning methods for performing registration is the difficulty in obtaining examples with known deformation vector fields (DVF). Deep registration methods have handled this issue by employing either unsupervised learning, wherein the ground truth is not available, or through self-supervised learning mechanisms, wherein the errors are estimated based on image similarity metrics computed from the features derived using the deep network from the underlying data. These self-derived deep metrics are more easily applicable to inter-modality registrations (such as CT and MRI, CT and noisy CBCT) than commonly used metrics like the modality independent descriptors (or MIND), mutual information, and mean square metrics. For example, in [62], training used aligned pairs of image patches from target and moving images, with the transformations (scaling, rotation, translation) varied for both the image pairs. The network was optimized to accurately classify whether the image patches were subjected to the same or different transformations. The work in [63] used paired sets of MR and ultrasound images of prostate gland for registration with a network predicting the registration error, computed as a misalignment of the surface points of the prostate gland.

Deep learning registration methods often predict the registration transformation functions by directly estimating the deformation vector fields (DVF) from the images. The image to be registered is then resampled to the reference image grid using the DVF. An advantage of methods such as in [64–66] is that only one pass of through the network is required to estimate the DVF, unlike standard registration methods that require iterative optimization, and making these methods capable of producing registrations rapidly. This clearly is very attractive for real-time motion management radiation treatments. Also, as the registration network is trained in an unsupervised way, there is no need for a ground truth DVF. Instead, the network backpropagation errors are calculated directly by measuring the dissimilarity between the warped moving and target image using standard registration metrics such as mutual information or normalized cross-correlation.

In addition to using image dissimilarities to compute the registration, works such as in [67], used the insight that structures of interest are more stable and easier to use as anchors to stabilize registration. In other words, agreement between segmentations was used as the loss (goodness) metric. In addition, a spatial transformer network was used to deform the images and used to compute similarity between the deformed and the target image such that the whole training could be performed without having ground truth deformation vector fields. Other work [68, 69] has shown that combining segmentation with registration improves registration performance.

Image registration using deep learning is therefore an active and promising area of research and has many applications including multi-modal image registration for improved image guidance for radiation therapy, radiation treatment planning for leveraging other imaging modalities, and dose-accumulation studies for studying response and complications from radiation therapy.

11.6 Quality Assurance

Finally, manual assessment of plan quality can be made more efficient and less prone to user variabilities by incorporating machine learning. Previously, random forest-based methods have been shown to be useful in assessing contour quality of organs at risk [70]. These techniques could be further improved by employing deep learning methods. Bayesian deep learning methods can be leveraged to model the uncertainty in segmentation [71]. Newer approaches employ noise regularized training to model the uncertainty in segmentation [72]. Such techniques can be used to improve not only the performance of the network to unseen noise variations in the data but also provide a voxel-wise uncertainty estimate, which can be useful both for contour quality assessment, but may also be incorporated into the planning method. AI can also be used more generally in QA, to monitor other data such as machine performance and plan characteristics to identify issues that need human focus [73].

11.7 Obstacles for AI and Deep Learning

Despite the obvious potential of AI methods in oncology in general and radiation oncology in particular, it is important to keep in mind current limitations of AI, including the following: the reasoning used in deep learning models is obscure [74]; inherent vulnerability to inter-cohort differences being "over-learned," resulting in biased answers [75]; the potential for highly uncertain answers when some aspects of the analysis sample are different from the training data [76]; the often minor improvements in prediction accuracy over more transparent, and simpler, methods [77, 78]; and relatedly, the problem that inductive AI methods, such as deep learning, suffer from a "lack of common sense," due to a lack of a basic background knowledge or rules and valid deductive processes [79]. Another obstacle to the acceptance of AI is that a process to modify models, in particular target volume models, is needed. This clearly requires capturing segmentation contour modifications for later model retraining. Just as importantly, the impact of deployed AI tools must be studied to understand the positive and possibly negative impacts [80]. Despite these caveats, progress has been especially clear in the areas of image analysis, where data and training information are adequate. We briefly expand on data requirements and the issue of generalizability below.

11.7.1 Data Size Limitations

Despite the tremendous success of deep learning in radiation oncology, there are fundamental challenges that still remain for deep learning in this field. First and foremost is the data size limitation. This is because data collection is highly time-consuming, as the "ground truth" creation requires experts and is time-consuming and laborious. Second, due to the difficulty and skill required for interpreting medical images, there is no "ground truth" but only expert interpretations. Interpretations vary between experts and even for the same expert, creating an insurmountable problem for any machine learning to learn an accurate representation of the structures of interest for segmentation. Learning an algorithm that accommodates for all these variabilities is extremely difficult.

Third and finally, deep learning on small datasets leads to the problem of overfitting. Overfitting is a problem when the model exactly or very closely fits the training data such that its performance on unseen testing data degrades. This is particularly problematic for parameter heavy deep learning networks. Their large capacity can essentially allow them to memorize the training sets, ultimately leading to poor performance on the testing datasets. The field of deep learning has developed many strategies for "regularizing" answers where data are inadequate, in an attempt to reduce the likelihood of an absurd result. Hence, good regularization constraints are crucial to prevent over-generalization. The most effective way of handling over-fitting is to expand the training set by generating fake, yet realistic, data through transformations of available data, a process called augmentation. Approaches have used cross-modality information [20, 44, 53] for data augmentation and to improve accuracy [35, 45]. Physics-based data augmentation strategies have also been used to generate data using physically realistic processes known to underlie the data generation process [81].

11.7.2 Generalizability on Unseen Data and Concept Drift

Another common issue for most deep learning methods is concept drift, wherein the deep learning method trained on images obtained from a certain protocol produces very poor performance on testing data that may be acquired from a different imaging protocol or a different scanner. For example, accuracies have been shown to drop when testing of deep learning method was done on images acquired with no or different CT contrasts [82].

Handling concept drift, also known as domain adaptation, critical to generalizability, is an active area of research in computer vision and medical image analysis. Several promising approaches are being developed including the use of feature-level adaptation methods that essentially train an algorithm to extract features that are invariant across domains [83]. However, it is important to keep this issue in mind when commissioning deep learning algorithms in the clinic.

11.8 Other Areas in RO Likely to be Impacted by AI

Undoubtedly, radiation oncology will be impacted in other areas by AI, including image-based prognosis, treatment response prediction, and treatment response classification at follow-up. Other AI/machine-learning applications will emerge to support general oncology treatment decisions regarding the specific drug needed for a specific tumor that will integrate bioinformatics, statistical learning, and AI methods. Most of these applications will mature at a slower rate than image segmentation applications, due to the difficulty in assembling the huge datasets required, given that for these other applications, each subject (or lesion) represents just one learning instance. For example, AI is emerging as a key method of predicting phenotypes, including radiation treatment response, based on the germline (normal) genotype. The primary input is a genome-wide single nucleotide polymorphism (point of population genetic variability in the genetic code). We have developed and used machine-learning-based methods to build patient-specific risk prediction models for multiple endpoints, including late rectal bleeding, erectile dysfunction [84], and urinary toxicity [85], all following prostate radiotherapy, and radiation-induced breast cancer in young (40 years or younger) breast cancer patients [86]. Other applications of machine learning on genomes to predicting phenotypes have recently been reviewed [87, 88]. Likewise, the field of radiomic signatures of disease type and prognosis is likely to be enriched by using non-linear features derived using deep learning. For example, transfer learning from a network learned on non-radiological images has successfully been used to predict breast cancer phenotypes, although the incremental improvement was modest [89]. Another recent application used deep learning to classify head and neck lymph nodes according to risk of extra capsular extension [90]. Yet another recent paper on lung cancer showed the potential to automatically identify lung tumor recurrence following radiotherapy [91]. It seems likely that the line between radiomic signatures and deep learning will become blurred as more deep learning filters are used as radiomic features [92, 93]. Eventually, another set of applications will emerge eventually that individualize drug choices based on biopsy lesion transcriptomics and sequencing, combining bioinformatics, advanced mathematical/topological approaches, and machine learning [94]. Finally, we are likely to see machine-learning approaches applied to genomics merged with image-based information ("radiogenomics" in the radiological phenotype sense) to create RO decision tools. For example, "Would successful treatment of these multiple metastases be likely to extend survival?" These applications are further away from clinical use and will take longer to develop and to validate, but ultimately will be impactful.

Despite the apparent value of AI approaches, there are many applications in radiation oncology, including treatment planning algorithms [95], predicting tumor response [96, 97], or normal tissue morbidity [98], where more transparent and mechanistic approaches are likely to be just as predictive but more scientifically helpful. In some cases, mechanistic models might be linked with AI-driven methods to merge the two approaches [99, 100]. In cases where the signal has a clear low-dimensional signature, AI approaches are unlikely to be needed or helpful.

11.9 Conclusion

AI methods can emerge anywhere that precisely measured high-dimensional data can be used to drive clinical processes or treatment decisions. Success in deep learning and machine learning will undoubtedly provide another jump forward in radiation oncology, with improvements in consistency, efficiency, and dose-delivery accuracy. An area of immediate improvement is the deployment, by multiple groups and vendors, of auto-segmentation tools. Despite still frequently needing some human expert alterations, such tools still improve efficiency but most importantly improve consistency far past the consistency attainable among experts. We therefore expect deployment of these tools to actually improve outcomes, if only incrementally. Extending auto-segmentation to on-treatment images (in particular, CBCTs) to improve setup and dose-accumulation accuracy provides an exciting opportunity to increase confidence in delivered dose and to reduce margins ("AI-guided-RT"). Other exciting applications of AI will require the development of quantitative imaging endpoints representing normal tissue damage or tumor status and are in development. In addition, AI methods will allow for the more effective integration of normal tissue genomics and, at some future point, integration of imaging, bioinformatics, and tumor genomics. This is an exciting picture, but many challenges remain in dataset construction, generalizability, hidden biases, comprehensive validity testing, and even competition from non-AI methods.

References

1. Du-Harpur X, et al. What is AI? Applications of artificial intelligence to dermatology. Br J Dermatol. 2020;183(3):423–30.
2. van den Heuvel TLA, et al. Combining automated image analysis with obstetric sweeps for prenatal ultrasound imaging in developing countries. Cham: Springer International Publishing; 2017.
3. Chartrand G, et al. Deep Learning: a primer for radiologists. Radiographics. 2017;37(7):2113–31.
4. Huynh E, et al. Artificial intelligence in radiation oncology. Nat Rev Clin Oncol. 2020;17(12):771–81.

5. Thompson RF, et al. Artificial intelligence in radiation oncology: a specialty-wide disruptive transformation? Radiother Oncol. 2018;129(3):421–6.
6. Bibault J-E, Giraud P, Burgun A. Big data and machine learning in radiation oncology: state of the art and future prospects. Cancer Lett. 2016;382(1):110–7.
7. Russell S, Norvig P. Artificial Intelligence: a modern approach. In: Pearson series in Artificial Intelligence. 4th ed. London: Pearson; 2020. p. 1136.
8. Mitchell T. Machine learning. 1st ed. London: McGraw-Hill; 1997. p. 414.
9. Raschka S. Model evaluation, model selection, and algorithm selection In: Machine learning; 2018. arXiv:1811.12808.
10. LeCun Y, Bengio Y, Hinton G. Deep learning. Nature. 2015;521:436.
11. Borrajo D, Veloso M. Lazy incremental Learning of control knowledge for efficiently obtaining quality plans. Artif Intell Rev. 1997;11(1):371–405.
12. Jaffray DA. Image-guided radiotherapy: from current concept to future perspectives. Nat Rev Clin Oncol. 2012;9(12):688–99.
13. Purdie TG, et al. Respiration correlated cone-beam computed tomography and 4DCT for evaluating target motion in stereotactic lung radiation therapy. Acta Oncol. 2006;45(7):915–22.
14. Li T, et al. Four-dimensional cone-beam computed tomography using an on-board imager. Med Phys. 2006;33(10):3825–33.
15. Sonke JJ, Aznar M, Rasch C. Adaptive radiotherapy for anatomical changes. Semin Radiat Oncol. 2019;29(3):245–57.
16. Kavanaugh J, et al. Anatomical adaptation—early clinical evidence of benefit and future needs in lung cancer. Semin Radiat Oncol. 2019;29(3):274–83.
17. Ibragimov B, Xing L. Segmentation of organs-at-risks in head and neck CT images using convolutional neural networks. Med Phys. 2017;44(2):547–57.
18. Balagopal A, et al. Fully automated organ segmentation in male pelvic CT images. Phys Med Biol. 2018;63(24):245015.
19. Dolz J, et al. Interactive contour delineation of organs at risk in radiotherapy: clinical evaluation on NSCLC patients. Med Phys. 2016;43(5):2569.
20. Jiang J, et al. Cross-modality (CT-MRI) prior augmented deep learning for robust lung tumor segmentation from small MR datasets. Med Phys. 2019;46(10):4392–404.
21. Jiang J, Sharif E, Um H, Berry S, Veeraraghavan H. Local block-wise self attention for normal organ segmentation; 2019. arXiv preprint.
22. Trullo R, et al. Segmentation of organs at risk in thoracic CT images using a SHARPMASK architecture and conditional random fields. Proc IEEE Int Symp Biomed Imaging. 2017;2017:1003–6.
23. Hoang Duc AK, et al. Validation of clinical acceptability of an atlas-based segmentation algorithm for the delineation of organs at risk in head and neck cancer. Med Phys. 2015;42(9):5027–34.
24. van Rooij W, et al. Deep Learning-based delineation of head and neck organs at risk: geometric and dosimetric evaluation. Int J Radiat Oncol Biol Phys. 2019;104(3):677–84.
25. Emami H, et al. Generating synthetic CTs from magnetic resonance images using generative adversarial networks. Med Phys. 2018;45(8):3627–36.
26. Klages P, et al. Patch-based generative adversarial neural network models for head and neck MR-only planning. Med Phys. 2020;47(2):626–42.
27. Lustberg T, et al. Clinical evaluation of atlas and deep learning based automatic contouring for lung cancer. Radiother Oncol. 2018;126(2):312–7.
28. Sonke JJ, Belderbos J. Adaptive radiotherapy for lung cancer. Semin Radiat Oncol. 2010;20(2):94–106.
29. Zhu W, et al. AnatomyNet: deep learning for fast and fully automated whole-volume segmentation of head and neck anatomy. Med Phys. 2019;46(2):576–89.
30. Liang S, et al. Deep-learning-based detection and segmentation of organs at risk in nasopharyngeal carcinoma computed tomographic images for radiotherapy planning. Eur Radiol. 2019;29(4):1961–7.

31. Guo Z, et al. Gross tumor volume segmentation for head and neck cancer radiotherapy using deep dense multi-modality network. Phys Med Biol. 2019;64(20):205015.
32. Nikolov S, et al. Deep learning to achieve clinically applicable segmentation of head and neck anatomy for radiotherapy. CoRR; 2018. abs/1809.04430.
33. Feng X, et al. Deep convolutional neural network for segmentation of thoracic organs-at-risk using cropped 3D images. Med Phys. 2019;46(5):2169–80.
34. Dong X, et al. Automatic multiorgan segmentation in thorax CT images using U-net-GAN. Med Phys. 2019;46(5):2157–68.
35. Dong X, et al. Synthetic MRI-aided multi-organ segmentation on male pelvic CT using cycle consistent deep attention network. Radiother Oncol. 2019;141:192–9.
36. Elmahdy MS, et al. Robust contour propagation using deep learning and image registration for online adaptive proton therapy of prostate cancer. Med Phys. 2019;46(8):3329–43.
37. Ronneberger O, Fischer P, Brox T. U-net: convolutional networks for biomedical image segmentation. In: Medical image computing and computer assisted intervention. Berlin: Springer International Publishing; 2015.
38. Liu S, Deng W. Very deep convolutional neural network based image classification using small training sample size. In *2015 3rd IAPR Asian Conference on Pattern Recognition (ACPR)*; 2015.
39. Chen LC, et al. DeepLab: semantic image segmentation with deep convolutional nets, Atrous convolution, and fully connected CRFs. IEEE Trans Pattern Anal Mach Intell. 2018;40(4):834–48.
40. Elguindi S, et al. Deep learning-based auto-segmentation of targets and organs-at-risk for magnetic resonance imaging only planning of prostate radiotherapy. Phys Imaging Radiat Oncol. 2019;12:80–6.
41. Haq R, et al. Cardio-pulmonary substructure segmentation of radiotherapy computed tomography images using convolutional neural networks for clinical outcomes analysis. Phys Imaging Radiat Oncol. 2020;14:61–6.
42. Jiang J, et al. Multiple resolution residually connected feature streams for automatic lung tumor segmentation from CT images. IEEE Trans Med Imaging. 2019;38:134–44.
43. Um H, et al. Multiple resolution residual network for automatic thoracic organs-at-risk segmentation from CT. arXiv e-prints; 2020. arXiv:2005.13690.
44. Jiang J, et al. Tumor-aware, adversarial domain adaptation from CT to MRI for lung cancer segmentation. Med Image Comput Comput Assist Interv. 2018;11071:777–85.
45. Jue J, et al. Integrating cross-modality hallucinated MRI with CT to aid mediastinal lung tumor segmentation. Med Image Comput Comput Assist Interv. 2019;11769:221–9.
46. Kupelian P, Sonke JJ. Magnetic resonance-guided adaptive radiotherapy: a solution to the future. Semin Radiat Oncol. 2014;24(3):227–32.
47. Zhu J-Y, Park T, Isola P, Efros AE. Unpaired image-to-image translation using cycle-consistent adversarial networks. In *IEEE Intl Conf computer vision*. IEEE; 2017.
48. Liu F. SUSAN: segment unannotated image structure using adversarial network. Magn Reson Med. 2019;81(5):3330–45.
49. Chartsias A, Joyce T, Dharmakumar R, Tsaftaris SA. Adversarial image synthesis for unpaired multi-modal cardiac data. In: Simulation and synthesis in medical imaging. Berlin: Springer; 2017.
50. Zhao J, et al. Tripartite-GAN: synthesizing liver contrast-enhanced MRI to improve tumor detection. Med Image Anal. 2020;63:101667.
51. Zhang Z, Yang L, Zheng Y. Translating and segmenting multimodal medical volumes with cycle- and shape-consistency generative adversarial network. In *2018 IEEE/CVF Conference on Computer Vision and Pattern Recognition*; 2018
52. Jiang J, et al. PSIGAN: Joint probabilistic segmentation and image distribution matching for unpaired cross-modality adaptation based MRI segmentation; 2020. arXiv:2007.09465.
53. Jiang, J., Veeraraghavan H. Unified cross-modality feature disentangler for unsupervised multi-domain MRI abdomen organs segmentation; 2020. arXiv:2007.09669.

54. Yang J, et al. CT images with expert manual contours of thoracic cancer for benchmarking auto-segmentation accuracy. Med Phys. 2020;47(7):3250–5.
55. Raudaschl PF, et al. Evaluation of segmentation methods on head and neck CT: auto-segmentation challenge 2015. Med Phys. 2017;44(5):2020–36.
56. Gendrin C, et al. Monitoring tumor motion by real time 2D/3D registration during radiotherapy. Radiother Oncol. 2012;102(2):274–80.
57. Chetty IJ, Rosu-Bubulac M. Deformable registration for dose accumulation. Semin Radiat Oncol. 2019;29(3):198–208.
58. Nobnop W, et al. Evaluation of deformable image registration (DIR) methods for dose accumulation in nasopharyngeal cancer patients during radiotherapy. Radiol Oncol. 2017;51(4):438–46.
59. Belfatto A, et al. Kinetic models for predicting cervical cancer response to radiation therapy on individual basis using tumor regression measured in vivo with volumetric imaging. Technol Cancer Res Treat. 2016;15(1):146–58.
60. Zhang P, et al. Predictive treatment management: incorporating a predictive tumor response model into robust prospective treatment planning for non-small cell lung cancer. Int J Radiat Oncol Biol Phys. 2014;88(2):446–52.
61. Zhang Y, et al. Incorporating biomechanical modeling and deep learning into a deformation-driven liver CBCT reconstruction technique. In: SPIE Medical Imaging, vol. 10948. Bellingham: SPIE; 2019.
62. Simonovsky M, et al. A deep metric for multimodal registration. Cham: Springer International Publishing; 2016.
63. Haskins G, et al. Learning deep similarity metric for 3D MR-TRUS image registration. Int J Comput Assist Radiol Surg. 2019;14(3):417–25.
64. Eppenhof KAJ, Pluim JPW. Pulmonary CT registration through supervised learning with convolutional neural networks. IEEE Trans Med Imaging. 2019;38(5):1097–105.
65. de Vos BD, et al. A deep learning framework for unsupervised affine and deformable image registration. Med Image Anal. 2019;52:128–43.
66. Yang X, et al. Quicksilver: fast predictive image registration - a deep learning approach. NeuroImage. 2017;158:378–96.
67. Balakrishnan G, et al. VoxelMorph: a learning framework for deformable medical image registration. IEEE Trans Med Imaging; 2019.
68. Qin C, et al. Joint Learning of motion estimation and segmentation for cardiac MR image sequences. Cham: Springer International Publishing; 2018.
69. Beljaards L, et al. A cross-stitch architecture for joint registration and segmentation in adaptive radiotherapy; 2020. arXiv e-prints. arXiv:2004.08122.
70. McIntosh C, Svistoun I, Purdie TG. Groupwise conditional random forests for automatic shape classification and contour quality assessment in radiotherapy planning. IEEE Trans Med Imaging. 2013;32(6):1043–57.
71. Gal Y, Islam R, Ghahramani Z. Deep bayesian active learning with image data; 2017. p. 1183–1192.
72. Baumgartner CF, et al. PHiSeg: capturing uncertainty in medical image segmentation. Cham: Springer International Publishing; 2019.
73. Valdes G, et al. IMRT QA using machine learning: a multi-institutional validation. J Appl Clin Med Phys. 2017;18(5):279–84.
74. Marcus G. Deep learning: a critical appraisal; 2018. arXiv:1801.00631.
75. Adeli E, et al. Representation learning with statistical independence to mitigate bias; 2019. arXiv:1910.03676.
76. Zhang L, et al. Generalizing deep Learning for medical image segmentation to unseen domains via deep stacked transformation. IEEE Trans Med Imaging. 2020;39(7):2531–40.
77. Herrmann M, et al. Large-scale benchmark study of survival prediction methods using multi-omics data. Brief Bioinform. 2021;22(3):bbaa167.
78. Luo Y, et al. Balancing accuracy and interpretability of machine learning approaches for radiation treatment outcomes modeling. BJR|Open. 2019;1(1):20190021.

79. Brockman J. Possible minds: twenty-five ways of looking at AI. London: Penguin Group; 2019.
80. Crawford K, Calo R. There is a blind spot in AI research. Nature. 2016;538(7625):311–3.
81. Leung KH, et al. A physics-guided modular deep-learning based automated framework for tumor segmentation in PET. Phys Med Biol. 2020;65:245032.
82. Tang X, et al. Whole liver segmentation based on deep learning and manual adjustment for clinical use in SIRT. Eur J Nucl Med Mol Imaging. 2020;47:2742–52.
83. Kamnitsas K, et al. Unsupervised domain adaptation in brain lesion segmentation with adversarial networks. In: Information processing in medical imaging. Berlin: Springer International Publishing; 2017.
84. Oh JH, et al. Computational methods using genome-wide association studies to predict radiotherapy complications and to identify correlative molecular processes. Sci Rep. 2017;7:43381.
85. Lee S, et al. Machine learning on a genome-wide association study to predict late genitourinary toxicity after prostate radiation therapy. Int J Radiat Oncol Biol Phys. 2018;101(1):128–35.
86. Lee S, et al. Machine learning on genome-wide association studies to predict the risk of radiation-associated contralateral breast cancer in the WECARE study. PLoS One. 2020;15(2):e0226157.
87. Nicholls HL, et al. Reaching the end-game for GWAS: machine learning approaches for the prioritization of complex disease loci. Front Genet. 2020;11:350.
88. Ho DSW, et al. Machine learning SNP based prediction for precision medicine. Front Genet. 2019;10:267.
89. Huynh B, Li H, Giger M. Digital mammographic tumor classification using transfer learning from deep convolutional neural networks. J Med Imaging. 2016;3(3):034501.
90. Kann BH, et al. Multi-institutional validation of deep Learning for pretreatment identification of extranodal extension in head and neck squamous cell carcinoma. J Clin Oncol. 2020;38(12):1304–11.
91. Mattonen SA, et al. Detection of local cancer recurrence after stereotactic ablative radiation therapy for lung cancer: physician performance versus radiomic assessment. Int J Radiat Oncol Biol Phys. 2016;94(5):1121–8.
92. Afshar P, et al. From handcrafted to deep-Learning-based cancer Radiomics: challenges and opportunities. IEEE Signal Process Mag. 2019;36(4):132–60.
93. Avanzo M, et al. Machine and deep learning methods for radiomics. Med Phys. 2020;47(5):e185–202.
94. Vaidya P, et al. RaPtomics: integrating radiomic and pathomic features for predicting recurrence in early stage lung cancer. In: SPIE Medical Imaging, vol. 10581. Bellingham: SPIE; 2018.
95. Zarepisheh M, et al. Automated intensity modulated treatment planning: the expedited constrained hierarchical optimization (ECHO) system. Med Phys. 2019;46(7):2944–54.
96. Chen J, et al. A mathematical model for predicting the changes of non-small cell lung cancer based on tumor mass during radiotherapy. Phys Med Biol. 2019;64(23):235006.
97. Jeong J, et al. Modeling the cellular response of lung cancer to radiation therapy for a broad range of fractionation schedules. Clin Cancer Res. 2017;23(18):5469–79.
98. Thor M, et al. Toward personalized dose-prescription in locally advanced non-small cell lung cancer: validation of published normal tissue complication probability models. Radiother Oncol. 2019;138:45–51.
99. Peng GCY, et al. Multiscale modeling meets machine learning: what can we learn? Arch Computat Meth Eng. 2021;28:1017–37.
100. Gaw N, et al. Integration of machine learning and mechanistic models accurately predicts variation in cell density of glioblastoma using multiparametric MRI. Sci Rep. 2019;9(1):10063.

Part III

Outcome Evaluation

Multi-Modality Imaging for Prediction of Tumor Control Following Radiotherapy

12

Daniela Thorwarth

12.1 Introduction

In recent years, several clinical studies have shown the value of multi-modality imaging for the assessment and prediction of tumor control (TC) following radiotherapy (RT) [1–3]. Often, anatomical and additionally functional imaging techniques such as computed tomography (CT), positron emission tomography (PET), and magnetic resonance imaging (MRI) are used to acquire imaging biomarkers, which are prognostic for treatment outcome in terms of TC after RT in different tumor entities [4]. Multi-modality imaging is defined as a combination of imaging modalities using different techniques, and physical principles to visualize different functional and molecular properties of the same organ or tumor. In contrast, multi-parametric imaging may also include different image formation processes, contrast principles and analysis strategies within the same imaging modality, such as T1-weighted, T2-weighted, diffusion-weighted (DW), and dynamic contrast-enhanced (DCE) imaging, which are different contrast forming mechanisms under the roof of MRI. TC is defined as the prediction of the absence of a detectable or symptomatic tumor after the end of therapy or at a preset interval thereafter, e.g., 3 months. Consequently, TC can be interpreted as the probability of cure for one individual patient among a larger cohort of patients. Depending on the exact definition, TC can either be expressed as a fraction of patients being controlled after a certain time or as a link between the time until recurrence is detected, thus additionally involving a temporal component.

D. Thorwarth (✉)
Section for Biomedical Physics, Department of Radiation Oncology, University of Tübingen, Tübingen, Germany
e-mail: Daniela.thorwarth@med.uni-tuebingen.de

E. G. C. Troost (ed.), *Image-Guided High-Precision Radiotherapy*,
https://doi.org/10.1007/978-3-031-08601-4_12

The aim of defining models for tumor control prediction based on multi-modal, multi-parametric imaging data is to improve classical outcome models involving clinical factors such as tumor stage, tumor volume, patient age, radiation dose, etc., by local, functional, and temporal components to gain specificity and sensitivity. The ultimate goal of functional imaging-based prediction models is to have a robust, three-dimensional (3D) basis for future patient-specific RT interventions for improving the individual probability of cure by a personalized RT approach [1]. However, robust and reliable TC prediction models require quantitative imaging measures as input variables [5]. Such quantitative imaging biomarkers (QIB) are essential for reliable response modeling and subsequent therapeutic interventions on those models and QIBs in the future. According to the imaging biomarker roadmap by O'Connor et al. [6], TC prediction models can only be designed for QIBs, which have passed a first translational gap from biomarker discovery toward a technical and early clinical validation in terms of assessment of measurement precision in so-called validation trials. Consequently, for every QIB proposed for prediction of TC following RT, a technical validation assessing repeatability and reproducibility should be carried out before large clinical trials are started, in which the biological validation and clinical effectiveness of such QIBs are tested [7].

Prediction of TC following RT can be performed in two different ways. Most studies intend to identify an imaging biomarker from multi-modal imaging, which allows stratification of patients into responders and non-responders to RT. With such binary prediction model, subsequent RT interventions can only be population-based such as modifying the radiation dose for one group compared to the other group. However, to guide the radiation dose prescription based on QIB values in 3D, imaging-response models linking QIB values to a certain level of expected TC are necessary [8].

This chapter will discuss the technical prerequisites for multi-modality imaging to be used for outcome prediction and response assessment following RT in clinical practice. Mathematical details on model generation and fitting will be discussed in Chap. 15. Furthermore, this chapter will provide an overview on multi-modality imaging techniques and QIB used for response prediction following RT in recent studies covering different tumor entities.

12.2 Technical Requirements for the Use of Quantitative Imaging Biomarkers to Predict Radiotherapy Outcome

In light of the great potential of multi-modality imaging and especially QIBs for TC prediction, it is important to consider some technical and also clinical aspects of multi-modality imaging techniques before starting clinical imaging trials and interventional studies. According to the imaging biomarker roadmap by O'Connor et al. [6], a number of aspects need to be ensured before a quantitative imaging biomarker can cross the first translational gap from biomarker discovery to early clinical studies which are necessary for initial prediction models of TC.

12.2.1 Availability

An essential prerequisite for potential QIBs to be used for TC prediction following RT is a broad clinical availability. Only imaging modalities which are widely available, easy to use, and cost-effective have proven clinical value for response assessment in radiation oncology in the past. Examples for multi-modality imaging techniques used for clinical response assessment and also to train prognosis models are CT, [^{18}F]-fluorodeoxyglucose (FDG) PET, anatomical MRI (T1- and T2-weighted), and also DWI [2–4]. In contrast, other imaging modalities such as hypoxia PET (e.g., FMISO, FAZA, HX4, see Chap. 2), proliferation PET (FLT, see Chap. 2), DCE-MRI, or magnetic resonance spectroscopy (MRS) did not yet pass the second translational gap toward routine clinical usage [6]. Even though promising studies in small cohorts were published by individual centers, those modalities were not translated to larger multi-center trials, due to absence of broad availability, lack of funding, or methodologically too complex application or analysis strategies.

12.2.2 Technical Characteristics of Imaging Systems

Depending on the mode of response prediction, which can either be a probability of predicted risk for relapse or additionally the identification of high-risk regions in 3D inside the primary tumor volume, different technical characteristics of imaging systems and data sets are important to be considered.

One essential aspect of each imaging modality is the spatial and geometrical resolution. Spatial differentiation of high-risk areas can only be done using a grid size adapted to the resolution of the imaging modality. For CT and anatomical MRI, the spatial resolution is in the order of mm. In contrast, for functional MRI such as DWI or DCE and for PET, the spatial resolution lies in the order of 4–6 mm. Further essential characteristics to be considered for response prediction are geometric accuracy and signal-to-noise ratio (SNR). If imaging data, which is acquired to predict TC, shall subsequently be used to guide the creation of response-adapted RT plans, geometrical accuracy of the underlying imaging modality is of crucial importance. Especially for MRI, geometrical accuracy has to be checked carefully regarding two aspects: the imaging sequence and eventually also on a patient individual basis. The effective SNR of an imaging technique is an important factor with respect to reproducibility of the biomarker assessment. Generally, image acquisition protocols need to be carefully optimized to yield optimal SNR levels for imaging biomarker studies [9].

12.2.3 Measurement Precision and Accuracy

Repeatability and reproducibility are related measures expressing the precision of measurement of an imaging experiment [6, 10]. Repeatability refers to the precision, with which a measurement can be repeated regarding the same experiment performed multiple times using the same equipment (scanner, analysis software, etc.) within a short time frame. Such test–retest measurements should be carried out using phantom and more importantly also patient imaging data. To assess the measurement precision of an imaging technique, the repeatability of these replicate measurements can be quantified by estimating the within-subject standard deviation *w*SD

$$wSD = \sqrt{\frac{1}{N}\sum_{i=1}^{N}\sigma_i^2}$$

Here, σ_i^2 refers to the within-subject variance determined from a series of n replicate measurements in N different subjects. For a classical test–retest scenario with only $n = 2$ replicate measurements per subject, the variance simplifies to $\sigma_i^2 = d_i^2 / 2$ where d_i is the difference of the two observations. The measurement error can be quoted as *w*SD, whereas the repeatability coefficient RC according to [11, 12] is given by

$$RC = 1.96\sqrt{2\,wSD^2}$$

The repeatability coefficient represents the least significant difference between two repeated measurements taken under ideal conditions at a confidence level of 95%.

According to [9], for cases where the repeatability varies with the magnitude of the imaging biomarker measurement, the within-subject coefficient of variation *w*CV should be calculated as

$wCV = \sqrt{\frac{1}{N}\sum_{i=1}^{N}\frac{\sigma_i^2}{\mu_i^2}}$ where μ_i denominates the mean measurement value for each of the N subjects. Similarly, the percent relative repeatability coefficient RC_{rel} can be determined by

$$RC_{rel} = 1.96\sqrt{2\,wCV^2}$$

RC_{rel} can be interpreted as the cut-point where a change in the measured imaging signal can be considered real with a confidence of 95% and not a measurement error.

A further method to assess the repeatability of multiple measurements is the Bland–Altman analysis [11] with the determination of limits of agreement (LoA) of repeated measurements and visualization using Bland–Altman plots [12]:

$$LoA = [b - RC, b + RC]$$

Here, the bias b is defined by the mean difference of measurements. Further, it is important to mention that the width of RC is not directly dependent on the sample size of a repeatability experiment, but depends mainly on the number of subjects included [12].

The consistency of repeated measures relative to the total variability of the population can be assessed by determination of the intra-class correlation coefficient ICC, defined as

$$\mathrm{ICC} = \frac{\sigma_B^2}{\sigma_B^2 + \sigma_i^2}$$

where σ_B is the between-subject variance in the sampled population [12, 13].

In contrast, reproducibility refers to repeated measurements carried out at different institutions using different equipment, software, and operators to ensure the quantitative nature of parameter assessment, such as the apparent diffusion coefficient (ADC) in DW-MRI or the standardized uptake value (SUV) in PET imaging. In this context, a technical bias of the biomarker is present if the value determined via multi-modal imaging systematically differs from its real value [6].

12.2.4 Standardized Acquisition and Analysis

To ensure a high level of data comparability in multi-center settings, reproducibility is mainly assessed in dedicated phantom studies, as specified, e.g., in guidelines of the quantitative imaging biomarker alliance (QIBA) [14, 15] or the European Association of Nuclear Medicine (EANM) [16, 17]. Hence, for multi-center trials involving multi-parametric imaging accreditation of imaging procedures and analysis workflows is recommended based on phantom and patient measurements before study recruitment can be started.

In addition, a number of guidelines have been published to communicate best-practice imaging standards for MRI, functional MRI, and also PET in order to ensure maximum data compatibility with other centers and comparability of results with published literature. Such guidelines exist for PET imaging [18] and also for MRI [19, 20] to be used for RT purposes, such as treatment planning, response monitoring or control prediction, and response-adapted treatment planning [21].

12.3 Quantitative Imaging Biomarkers for TC Prediction Following RT

Over the last years, a number of different clinical studies have investigated the value of multi-modal and multi-parametric imaging for prediction of TC following RT. In addition to classical outcome indicators, such as stage, tumor volume, etc., mainly measures derived from functional MRI and PET have been proposed as QIBs for RT response prediction. Other studies have proposed combined QIBs from PET/MRI or were based on Radiomics analyses using CT and PET imaging data, mainly.

12.3.1 Magnetic Resonance Imaging

Values of apparent diffusion coefficient (ADC) derived from DW-MRI have been shown in many studies to be predictive for TC following RT. Several studies have investigated the potential of using ADC for RT response prediction in head and neck cancer (HNC) [2, 22–25]. Also in other tumor sites, such as cancer of the uterine cervix [26], brain tumors [27, 28], as well as rectal cancer [3, 29], ADC has been identified as potentially powerful QIB for RT outcome prediction. Other studies have reported changes of ADC values assessed in the first 1–2 weeks during the course of fractionated RT as prognostic imaging biomarkers [30]. For DW-MRI, repeatability coefficients of ADC assessment have been reported to be approximately 11% in brain [31, 32], around 26% for liver tumors [33, 34], and 47% for examinations of the prostate [35, 36].

For prostate cancer, multi-parametric MRI consisting of T2-weighted anatomical imaging, DW- and DCE-MRI has been shown to detect regions of recurrent tumor [37–39].

Similarly, also DCE-MRI has been proven to have prognostic value with respect to outcome after RT in different tumor sites, such as in HNC [40, 41], cervix cancer [42], and rectal cancer [3]. Dedicated studies investigated the measurement accuracy of DCE-MRI and reported repeatability coefficients for the parameter K_{trans} of approximately 21% in brain tumors and 56% for prostate examinations, respectively [43, 44].

12.3.2 Positron Emission Tomography

In the last years, a multitude of studies has shown the potential of FDG PET as QIB for TC prediction following RT. In HNC, for different metrics derived from FDG PET imaging, such as maximum, peak, or mean standardized uptake value (i.e., SUV_{max}, SUV_{peak}, or SUV_{mean}), correlations to outcome after RT were demonstrated to be prognostic to RT outcome [45]. FDG PET uptake was shown to be a major prognostic factor for RT success in non-small-cell lung cancer (NSCLC) [46]. Only a few studies assessed repeatability and reproducibility of FDG PET imaging so far. In NSCLC, percent relative repeatability coefficients for SUV_{max} and SUV_{peak} of approximately 30% were reported by Weber et al. [47]. Similar results were found by Nygard et al. [48] who reported a relative repeatability coefficient of 32.4% for total lesion glycolysis based on an iso-contour of 50% SUV_{max}. For ovarian cancer, RC_{rel} values of 16.3 and 17.3% were reported from a test–retest study for SUV_{mean} and SUV_{max}, respectively [49].

In addition, hypoxia PET imaging using different radiotracers, such as [^{18}F]-FMISO, [^{18}F]-FAZA, [^{18}F]-EF5, or [^{18}F]-HX4, was reported to show significant correlation with TC following RT in HNC as well as in NSCLC [8, 50–54]. As typically SNR is quite low for hypoxia PET, different PET-derived metrics, such as SUV_{max}, SUV_{mean}, tumor-to-blood-ratio (TBR), tumor-to-muscle-ratio (TMR), and kinetic analysis of dynamic PET data, were proposed by different groups as QIBs for RT response prediction. Also, for hypoxia PET imaging, relative changes of hypoxia metrics detected early during fractionated treatment relative to assessments before the start of RT have been identified as potential QIBs [51, 55]. Despite low SNR of hypoxia PET, studies investigating the repeatability of hypoxia metrics derived from PET imaging using dedicated hypoxia tracers have demonstrated reasonable accuracy. For FMISO PET, ICC values of 0.959 and 0.965 were reported for SUV_{max} and TMR, respectively [56]. In a recent test–retest study, hypoxia PET using EF5 showed relative repeatability coefficients of 15%, 17% and 10% for SUV_{mean}, SUV_{max}, and TMR, respectively [57]. Similar values for RC_{rel} were found by Zegers et al. [58] with 15% (SUV_{mean}), 17% (SUV_{max}), and 17% (TBR_{max}).

12.3.3 Combined PET/MR

Since the clinical introduction of multi-modal imaging using hybrid devices, such as combined PET/MRI, the added value of combining those modalities for better outcome prediction after RT has been investigated. Several studies have shown that combining QIBs from PET and MRI may considerably improve the prognostic power compared to a single imaging modality in different tumor entities such as HNC [59–61], cervical cancer [62, 63], and brain tumors [64]. Most studies investigate the combination of previously proposed QIB from PET and MRI. For example, Cao et al. found that MRI-defined QIBs, especially blood volume-related parameters derived from DCE-MRI, added predictive value to clinical variables and compared favorably with FDG PET imaging markers [60]. Similarly, Martens et al. [61] reported in their study a predictive value for RT failure, loco-regional recurrence, and death of both DW-MRI and FDG PET parameters. But combining SUV_{max} and ADC_{max} resulted in an even better prediction of treatment failure compared to single parameter assessment.

12.3.4 Radiomics

In addition to hypothesis-driven biomarker studies aiming to identify single well-described QIBs based on a biological rationale for RT outcome modeling, more and more research in the field of multi-modal imaging for outcome modeling following RT is performed using Radiomics approaches. Radiomics is a mathematical approach which characterizes patterns and statistical quantities in the image domain allowing for data-driven, un-biased searches of imaging biomarkers that might be correlated to outcome after RT.

The first Radiomics studies proposing models for TC prediction after therapy were based purely on CT imaging [65, 66]. Since then, FDG PET/CT Radiomics was demonstrated to allow for improved RT outcome prediction with respect to CT-only Radiomics especially in NSCLC [67–69] but also in HNC [70]. Similar to QIB studies performed on the value of PET and MRI for RT outcome modeling, also Radiomics models were shown to be more powerful when using imaging data acquired during the second week of treatment [71].

Technically, Radiomics biomarker research is challenging with respect to reproducibility and standardization, as a lot of different mathematical steps are required during implementation which may cause high variability on the resulting data and models. Schwier et al. [72, 73] have investigated different implementations and reported that many Radiomics features were highly sensitive to processing parameters. Zwanenburg et al. [74] proposed image perturbation in order to assess repeatability of Radiomics features as an alternative to test-retest experiments, whereas another study assessed Radiomics repeatability measures from comparison of PET/MRI and PET/CT data [75]. Due to the high level of variation caused by different implementations of Radiomics pipelines, only Radiomics features which are acquired and computed in a validated and standardized way should be integrated into models for TC prediction following RT [76].

Recently, also in Radiomics research, the added value of using data input from multi-modality imaging was acknowledged by several studies [62, 63, 70].

12.4 Radiotherapy Interventions Based on QIB Prediction Models

The ultimate goal of defining prognostic and predictive models based on QIBs in radiation oncology is the need for personalized radiotherapy, which might be realized via QIB-guided RT interventions. Hence, functional or biological RT interventions imply the prescription of higher or lower radiation dose levels to certain tumor areas based on readings from multi-modality imaging. Consequently, imaging parameters used for individualized dose prescriptions need to be quantitative [5]. This motivates the need for QIB research and clinical studies in radiation oncology [21].

QIB-based RT interventions can essentially be realized in two different ways. If imaging biomarkers, such as Radiomics analysis do not provide any spatial information, but only a numerical risk for relapse after RT, adaptations in radiation dose levels need to be prescribed to the whole gross tumor volume. In contrast, if QIBs derived from multi-modality imaging are coming with a quantitative and also 3D spatial information, spatially and at the same time response-adapted RT interventions, such as dose painting, can be applied [77, 78]. To realize dose painting treatment plans, dedicated dose prescription functions have to be defined [79–81]. Such dose prescription functions may be directly derived from TC models by virtue of their definition as a function of QIBs [8]. Using TC models or probability maps of tumor presence as an input for dose painting treatments, repeatability needs to be verified for the whole process chain in order to make sure that such individualized RT approaches are consistent and feasible despite small day-to-day variations [82].

To date, no clinical gold standards for QIB TC models exist in radiation oncology. Most studies so far are mono-centric and suffer from small sample sizes and are thus purely hypothesis generating. Referring to the imaging biomarker roadmap by O'Connor et al. [6], most imaging biomarker studies in radiation oncology are still in the first phase of biomarker discovery. To pass the translational gap toward biomarker validation, single- and multi-center studies are required to provide technical validation in test–retest and reproducibility studies and also external clinical validation in multi-center trials. Data of those validation studies may be used in the future to train validated models for TC prediction following RT based on QIBs which may in a third phase then be used as a basis for RT interventions.

In order to realize QIB-driven RT interventions with the aim of higher cure rates and/or lower side effects of high-precision RT, robust and reproducible TC models relating QIB and outcome following RT need to be established. Such models require imaging biomarkers with high sensitivity and specificity, but also a wide clinical availability of those multi-modality imaging techniques and pragmatic, easy-to-use analysis strategies. Only widely available multi-modality imaging techniques, such as DW-MRI or FDG PET, may provide large enough data sets for future paradigm-changing response-adapted RT.

References

1. Baumann M, Krause M, Overgaard J, Debus J, Bentzen SM, Daartz J, et al. Radiation oncology in the era of precision medicine. Nat Rev Cancer. 2016;16:234–49.
2. Martens RM, Noij DP, Ali M, Koopman T, Marcus JT, Vergeer MR, et al. Functional imaging early during (chemo)radiotherapy for response prediction in head and neck squamous cell carcinoma; a systematic review. Oral Oncol. 2019;88:75–83.
3. Pham TT, Liney GP, Wong K, Barton MB. Functional MRI for quantitative treatment response prediction in locally advanced rectal cancer. Br J Radiol. 2017;90:20151078.
4. Thorwarth D. Functional imaging for radiotherapy treatment planning: current status and future directions-a review. Br J Radiol. 2015;88:20150056.
5. van der Heide UA, Thorwarth D. Quantitative imaging for radiation oncology. Int J Radiat Oncol Biol Phys. 2018;102:683–6.
6. O'Connor JP, Aboagye EO, Adams JE, Aerts HJ, Barrington SF, Beer AJ, et al. Imaging biomarker roadmap for cancer studies. Nat Rev Clin Oncol. 2017;14:169–86.
7. van Houdt PJ, Saeed H, Thorwarth D, Fuller CD, Hall WA, McDonald BA, et al. Integration of quantitative imaging biomarkers in clinical trials for MR-guided radiotherapy: conceptual guidance for multicentre studies from the MR-linac consortium imaging biomarker working group. Eur J Cancer. 2021;153:64–71. https://doi.org/10.1016/j.ejca.2021.04.041.
8. Thorwarth D, Welz S, Monnich D, Pfannenberg C, Nikolaou K, Reimold M, et al. Prospective evaluation of a tumor control probability model based on dynamic (18)F-FMISO PET for head and neck cancer radiotherapy. J Nucl Med. 2019;60:1698–704.
9. Shukla-Dave A, Obuchowski NA, Chenevert TL, Jambawalikar S, Schwartz LH, Malyarenko D, et al. Quantitative imaging biomarkers alliance (QIBA) recommendations for improved precision of DWI and DCE-MRI derived biomarkers in multicenter oncology trials. J Magn Reson Imaging. 2019;49:e101–e21.
10. Kessler LG, Barnhart HX, Buckler AJ, Choudhury KR, Kondratovich MV, Toledano A, et al. The emerging science of quantitative imaging biomarkers terminology and definitions for scientific studies and regulatory submissions. Stat Methods Med Res. 2015;24:9–26.
11. Bland JM, Altman DG. Measurement error. BMJ. 1996;313:744.
12. Raunig DL, McShane LM, Pennello G, Gatsonis C, Carson PL, Voyvodic JT, et al. Quantitative imaging biomarkers: a review of statistical methods for technical performance assessment. Stat Methods Med Res. 2015;24:27–67.
13. Sullivan DC, Obuchowski NA, Kessler LG, Raunig DL, Gatsonis C, Huang EP, et al. Metrology standards for quantitative imaging biomarkers. Radiology. 2015;277:813–25.
14. Perfusion, diffusion and flow-MRI biomarker committee. QIBA profile: diffusion-weighted magnetic resonance imaging (DWI). Public comment draft. QIBA; 2019.
15. Padhani AR, Liu G, Koh DM, Chenevert TL, Thoeny HC, Takahara T, et al. Diffusion-weighted magnetic resonance imaging as a cancer biomarker: consensus and recommendations. Neoplasia. 2009;11:102–25.

16. Boellaard R, O'Doherty MJ, Weber WA, Mottaghy FM, Lonsdale MN, Stroobants SG, et al. FDG PET and PET/CT: EANM procedure guidelines for tumour PET imaging: version 1.0. Eur J Nucl Med Mol Imaging. 2010;37:181–200.
17. Boellaard R, Delgado-Bolton R, Oyen WJ, Giammarile F, Tatsch K, Eschner W, et al. FDG PET/CT: EANM procedure guidelines for tumour imaging: version 2.0. Eur J Nucl Med Mol Imaging. 2015;42:328–54.
18. Thorwarth D, Beyer T, Boellaard R, de Ruysscher D, Grgic A, Lee JA, et al. Integration of FDG-PET/CT into external beam radiation therapy planning: technical aspects and recommendations on methodological approaches. Nuklearmedizin. 2012;51:140–53.
19. Keenan KE, Biller JR, Delfino JG, Boss MA, Does MD, Evelhoch JL, et al. Recommendations towards standards for quantitative MRI (qMRI) and outstanding needs. J Magn Reson Imaging. 2019;49:e26–39.
20. Kooreman ES, van Houdt PJ, Nowee ME, van Pelt VWJ, Tijssen RHN, Paulson ES, et al. Feasibility and accuracy of quantitative imaging on a 1.5 T MR-linear accelerator. Radiother Oncol. 2019;133:156–62.
21. Gurney-Champion OJ, Mahmood F, van Schie M, Julian R, George B, Philippens MEP, et al. Quantitative imaging for radiotherapy purposes. Radiother Oncol. 2020;146:66–75.
22. King AD, Mo FK, Yu KH, Yeung DK, Zhou H, Bhatia KS, et al. Squamous cell carcinoma of the head and neck: diffusion-weighted MR imaging for prediction and monitoring of treatment response. Eur Radiol. 2010;20:2213–20.
23. Kim S, Loevner L, Quon H, Sherman E, Weinstein G, Kilger A, et al. Diffusion-weighted magnetic resonance imaging for predicting and detecting early response to chemoradiation therapy of squamous cell carcinomas of the head and neck. Clin Cancer Res. 2009;15:986–94.
24. King AD, Chow KK, Yu KH, Mo FK, Yeung DK, Yuan J, et al. Head and neck squamous cell carcinoma: diagnostic performance of diffusion-weighted MR imaging for the prediction of treatment response. Radiology. 2013;266:531–8.
25. Lambrecht M, Van Calster B, Vandecaveye V, De Keyzer F, Roebben I, Hermans R, et al. Integrating pretreatment diffusion weighted MRI into a multivariable prognostic model for head and neck squamous cell carcinoma. Radiother Oncol. 2014;110:429–34.
26. Scalco E, Marzi S, Sanguineti G, Vidiri A, Rizzo G. Characterization of cervical lymph-nodes using a multi-parametric and multi-modal approach for an early prediction of tumor response to chemo-radiotherapy. Phys Med. 2016;32:1672–80.
27. Mahmood F, Johannesen HH, Geertsen P, Hansen RH. Repeated diffusion MRI reveals earliest time point for stratification of radiotherapy response in brain metastases. Phys Med Biol. 2017;62:2990–3002.
28. Karami E, Soliman H, Ruschin M, Sahgal A, Myrehaug S, Tseng CL, et al. Quantitative MRI biomarkers of stereotactic radiotherapy outcome in brain metastasis. Sci Rep. 2019;9:19830.
29. Kim S, Han K, Seo N, Kim HJ, Kim MJ, Koom WS, et al. T2-weighted signal intensity-selected volumetry for prediction of pathological complete response after preoperative chemoradiotherapy in locally advanced rectal cancer. Eur Radiol. 2018;28:5231–40.
30. Vandecaveye V, Dirix P, De Keyzer F, de Beeck KO, Vander Poorten V, Roebben I, et al. Predictive value of diffusion-weighted magnetic resonance imaging during chemoradiotherapy for head and neck squamous cell carcinoma. Eur Radiol. 2010;20:1703–14.
31. Bonekamp D, Nagae LM, Degaonkar M, Matson M, Abdalla WM, Barker PB, et al. Diffusion tensor imaging in children and adolescents: reproducibility, hemispheric, and age-related differences. NeuroImage. 2007;34:733–42.
32. Paldino MJ, Barboriak D, Desjardins A, Friedman HS, Vredenburgh JJ. Repeatability of quantitative parameters derived from diffusion tensor imaging in patients with glioblastoma multiforme. J Magn Reson Imaging. 2009;29:1199–205.
33. Deckers F, De Foer B, Van Mieghem F, Botelberge T, Weytjens R, Padhani A, et al. Apparent diffusion coefficient measurements as very early predictive markers of response to chemotherapy in hepatic metastasis: a preliminary investigation of reproducibility and diagnostic value. J Magn Reson Imaging. 2014;40:448–56.

34. Heijmen L, Ter Voert EE, Nagtegaal ID, Span P, Bussink J, Punt CJ, et al. Diffusion-weighted MR imaging in liver metastases of colorectal cancer: reproducibility and biological validation. Eur Radiol. 2013;23:748–56.
35. Gibbs P, Pickles MD, Turnbull LW. Repeatability of echo-planar-based diffusion measurements of the human prostate at 3 T. Magn Reson Imaging. 2007;25:1423–9.
36. Litjens GJ, Hambrock T, Hulsbergen-van de Kaa C, Barentsz JO, Huisman HJ. Interpatient variation in normal peripheral zone apparent diffusion coefficient: effect on the prediction of prostate cancer aggressiveness. Radiology. 2012;265:260–6.
37. Dinis Fernandes C, Ghobadi G, van der Poel HG, de Jong J, Heijmink S, Schoots I, et al. Quantitative 3-T multi-parametric MRI and step-section pathology of recurrent prostate cancer patients after radiation therapy. Eur Radiol. 2019;29:4160–8.
38. Dinis Fernandes C, Simoes R, Ghobadi G, Heijmink S, Schoots IG, de Jong J, et al. Multiparametric MRI tumor probability model for the detection of locally recurrent prostate cancer after radiation therapy: pathologic validation and comparison with manual tumor delineations. Int J Radiat Oncol Biol Phys. 2019;105:140–8.
39. Park SY, Kim CK, Park BK, Park W, Park HC, Han DH, et al. Early changes in apparent diffusion coefficient from diffusion-weighted MR imaging during radiotherapy for prostate cancer. Int J Radiat Oncol Biol Phys. 2012;83:749–55.
40. Cao Y, Popovtzer A, Li D, Chepeha DB, Moyer JS, Prince ME, et al. Early prediction of outcome in advanced head-and-neck cancer based on tumor blood volume alterations during therapy: a prospective study. Int J Radiat Oncol Biol Phys. 2008;72:1287–90.
41. Wang P, Popovtzer A, Eisbruch A, Cao Y. An approach to identify, from DCE MRI, significant subvolumes of tumors related to outcomes in advanced head-and-neck cancer. Med Phys. 2012;39:5277–85.
42. Andersen EK, Hole KH, Lund KV, Sundfor K, Kristensen GB, Lyng H, et al. Pharmacokinetic parameters derived from dynamic contrast enhanced MRI of cervical cancers predict chemoradiotherapy outcome. Radiother Oncol. 2013;107:117–22.
43. Alonzi R, Taylor NJ, Stirling JJ, D'Arcy JA, Collins DJ, Saunders MI, et al. Reproducibility and correlation between quantitative and semiquantitative dynamic and intrinsic susceptibility-weighted MRI parameters in the benign and malignant human prostate. J Magn Reson Imaging. 2010;32:155–64.
44. Jackson A, Jayson GC, Li KL, Zhu XP, Checkley DR, Tessier JJ, et al. Reproducibility of quantitative dynamic contrast-enhanced MRI in newly presenting glioma. Br J Radiol. 2003;76:153–62.
45. Min M, Lin P, Lee MT, Shon IH, Lin M, Forstner D, et al. Prognostic role of metabolic parameters of (18)F-FDG PET-CT scan performed during radiation therapy in locally advanced head and neck squamous cell carcinoma. Eur J Nucl Med Mol Imaging. 2015;42:1984–94.
46. Kohutek ZA, Wu AJ, Zhang Z, Foster A, Din SU, Yorke ED, et al. FDG-PET maximum standardized uptake value is prognostic for recurrence and survival after stereotactic body radiotherapy for non-small cell lung cancer. Lung Cancer. 2015;89:115–20.
47. Weber WA, Gatsonis CA, Mozley PD, Hanna LG, Shields AF, Aberle DR, et al. Repeatability of 18F-FDG PET/CT in advanced non-small cell lung cancer: prospective assessment in 2 multicenter trials. J Nucl Med. 2015;56:1137–43.
48. Nygard L, Aznar MC, Fischer BM, Persson GF, Christensen CB, Andersen FL, et al. Repeatability of FDG PET/CT metrics assessed in free breathing and deep inspiration breath hold in lung cancer patients. Am J Nucl Med Mol Imaging. 2018;8:127–36.
49. Rockall AG, Avril N, Lam R, Iannone R, Mozley PD, Parkinson C, et al. Repeatability of quantitative FDG-PET/CT and contrast-enhanced CT in recurrent ovarian carcinoma: test-retest measurements for tumor FDG uptake, diameter, and volume. Clin Cancer Res. 2014;20:2751–60.
50. Welz S, Paulsen F, Pfannenberg C, Reimold M, Reischl G, Nikolaou K, et al. Dose escalation to hypoxic subvolumes in head and neck cancer: A randomized phase II study using dynamic [18F]FMISO PET/CT. Radiother Oncol. 2022;171:30–36. https://doi.org/10.1016/j.radonc.2022.03.021.

51. Zips D, Zophel K, Abolmaali N, Perrin R, Abramyuk A, Haase R, et al. Exploratory prospective trial of hypoxia-specific PET imaging during radiochemotherapy in patients with locally advanced head-and-neck cancer. Radiother Oncol. 2012;105:21–8.
52. Mortensen LS, Johansen J, Kallehauge J, Primdahl H, Busk M, Lassen P, et al. FAZA PET/CT hypoxia imaging in patients with squamous cell carcinoma of the head and neck treated with radiotherapy: results from the DAHANCA 24 trial. Radiother Oncol. 2012;105:14–20.
53. Qian Y, Von Eyben R, Liu Y, Chin FT, Miao Z, Apte S, et al. (18)F-EF5 PET-based Imageable hypoxia predicts local recurrence in tumors treated with highly conformal radiation therapy. Int J Radiat Oncol Biol Phys. 2018;102:1183–92.
54. Zegers CM, Hoebers FJ, van Elmpt W, Bons JA, Ollers MC, Troost EG, et al. Evaluation of tumour hypoxia during radiotherapy using [(18)F]HX4 PET imaging and blood biomarkers in patients with head and neck cancer. Eur J Nucl Med Mol Imaging. 2016;43:2139–46.
55. Lock S, Perrin R, Seidlitz A, Bandurska-Luque A, Zschaeck S, Zophel K, et al. Residual tumour hypoxia in head-and-neck cancer patients undergoing primary radiochemotherapy, final results of a prospective trial on repeat FMISO-PET imaging. Radiother Oncol. 2017;124:533–40.
56. Okamoto S, Shiga T, Yasuda K, Ito YM, Magota K, Kasai K, et al. High reproducibility of tumor hypoxia evaluated by 18F-fluoromisonidazole PET for head and neck cancer. J Nucl Med. 2013;54:201–7.
57. Silvoniemi A, Suilamo S, Laitinen T, Forsback S, Loyttyniemi E, Vaittinen S, et al. Repeatability of tumour hypoxia imaging using [(18)F]EF5 PET/CT in head and neck cancer. Eur J Nucl Med Mol Imaging. 2018;45:161–9.
58. Zegers CM, van Elmpt W, Szardenings K, Kolb H, Waxman A, Subramaniam RM, et al. Repeatability of hypoxia PET imaging using [(1)(8)F]HX4 in lung and head and neck cancer patients: a prospective multicenter trial. Eur J Nucl Med Mol Imaging. 2015;42:1840–9.
59. Ng SH, Lin CY, Chan SC, Lin YC, Yen TC, Liao CT, et al. Clinical utility of multimodality imaging with dynamic contrast-enhanced MRI, diffusion-weighted MRI, and 18F-FDG PET/CT for the prediction of neck control in oropharyngeal or hypopharyngeal squamous cell carcinoma treated with chemoradiation. PLoS One. 2014;9:e115933.
60. Cao Y, Aryal M, Li P, Lee C, Schipper M, Hawkins PG, et al. Predictive values of MRI and PET derived quantitative parameters for patterns of failure in both p16+ and p16− high risk head and neck cancer. Front Oncol. 2019;9:1118.
61. Martens RM, Noij DP, Koopman T, Zwezerijnen B, Heymans M, de Jong MC, et al. Predictive value of quantitative diffusion-weighted imaging and 18-F-FDG-PET in head and neck squamous cell carcinoma treated by (chemo)radiotherapy. Eur J Radiol. 2019;113:39–50.
62. Lucia F, Visvikis D, Vallieres M, Desseroit MC, Miranda O, Robin P, et al. External validation of a combined PET and MRI radiomics model for prediction of recurrence in cervical cancer patients treated with chemoradiotherapy. Eur J Nucl Med Mol Imaging. 2019;46:864–77.
63. Lucia F, Visvikis D, Desseroit MC, Miranda O, Malhaire JP, Robin P, et al. Prediction of outcome using pretreatment (18)F-FDG PET/CT and MRI radiomics in locally advanced cervical cancer treated with chemoradiotherapy. Eur J Nucl Med Mol Imaging. 2018;45:768–86.
64. Lundemann M, Munck Af Rosenschold P, Muhic A, Larsen VA, Poulsen HS, Engelholm SA, et al. Feasibility of multi-parametric PET and MRI for prediction of tumour recurrence in patients with glioblastoma. Eur J Nucl Med Mol Imaging. 2019;46:603–13.
65. Aerts HJ, Velazquez ER, Leijenaar RT, Parmar C, Grossmann P, Carvalho S, et al. Decoding tumour phenotype by noninvasive imaging using a quantitative radiomics approach. Nat Commun. 2014;5:4006.
66. Parmar C, Grossmann P, Bussink J, Lambin P, Aerts H. Machine learning methods for quantitative Radiomic biomarkers. Sci Rep. 2015;5:13087.
67. Carvalho S, Leijenaar RTH, Troost EGC, van Timmeren JE, Oberije C, van Elmpt W, et al. 18F-fluorodeoxyglucose positron-emission tomography (FDG-PET)-Radiomics of metastatic lymph nodes and primary tumor in non-small cell lung cancer (NSCLC) - a prospective externally validated study. PLoS One. 2018;13:e0192859.
68. Dissaux G, Visvikis D, Da-Ano R, Pradier O, Chajon E, Barillot I, et al. Pretreatment (18)F-FDG PET/CT Radiomics predict local recurrence in patients treated with stereotactic body

radiotherapy for early-stage non-small cell lung cancer: a multicentric study. J Nucl Med. 2020;61:814–20.
69. Luo Y, McShan DL, Matuszak MM, Ray D, Lawrence TS, Jolly S, et al. A multiobjective Bayesian networks approach for joint prediction of tumor local control and radiation pneumonitis in nonsmall-cell lung cancer (NSCLC) for response-adapted radiotherapy. Med Phys. 2018;
70. Bogowicz M, Riesterer O, Stark LS, Studer G, Unkelbach J, Guckenberger M, et al. Comparison of PET and CT radiomics for prediction of local tumor control in head and neck squamous cell carcinoma. Acta Oncol. 2017;56:1531–6.
71. Leger S, Zwanenburg A, Pilz K, Zschaeck S, Zophel K, Kotzerke J, et al. CT imaging during treatment improves radiomic models for patients with locally advanced head and neck cancer. Radiother Oncol. 2019;130:10–7.
72. Schwier M, van Griethuysen J, Vangel MG, Pieper S, Peled S, Tempany C, et al. Repeatability of multiparametric prostate MRI Radiomics features. Sci Rep. 2019;9:9441.
73. Zwanenburg A. Radiomics in nuclear medicine: robustness, reproducibility, standardization, and how to avoid data analysis traps and replication crisis. Eur J Nucl Med Mol Imaging. 2019;46:2638–55.
74. Zwanenburg A, Leger S, Agolli L, Pilz K, Troost EGC, Richter C, et al. Assessing robustness of radiomic features by image perturbation. Sci Rep. 2019;9:614.
75. Vuong D, Tanadini-Lang S, Huellner MW, Veit-Haibach P, Unkelbach J, Andratschke N, et al. Interchangeability of radiomic features between [18F]-FDG PET/CT and [18F]-FDG PET/MR. Med Phys. 2019;46:1677–85.
76. Zwanenburg A, Vallieres M, Abdalah MA, Aerts H, Andrearczyk V, Apte A, et al. The image biomarker standardization initiative: standardized quantitative Radiomics for high-throughput image-based phenotyping. Radiology. 2020;295:328–38.
77. Thorwarth D, Eschmann SM, Paulsen F, Alber M. Hypoxia dose painting by numbers: a planning study. Int J Radiat Oncol Biol Phys. 2007;68:291–300.
78. Madani I, Duprez F, Boterberg T, Van de Wiele C, Bonte K, Deron P, et al. Maximum tolerated dose in a phase I trial on adaptive dose painting by numbers for head and neck cancer. Radiother Oncol. 2011;101:351–5.
79. Vogelius IR, Hakansson K, Due AK, Aznar MC, Berthelsen AK, Kristensen CA, et al. Failure-probability driven dose painting. Med Phys. 2013;40:081717.
80. Gronlund E, Johansson S, Montelius A, Ahnesjo A. Dose painting by numbers based on retrospectively determined recurrence probabilities. Radiother Oncol. 2017;122:236–41.
81. Gronlund E, Johansson S, Nyholm T, Thellenberg C, Ahnesjo A. Dose painting of prostate cancer based on Gleason score correlations with apparent diffusion coefficients. Acta Oncol. 2018;57:574–81.
82. van Schie MA, Steenbergen P, Dinh CV, Ghobadi G, van Houdt PJ, Pos FJ, et al. Repeatability of dose painting by numbers treatment planning in prostate cancer radiotherapy based on multiparametric magnetic resonance imaging. Phys Med Biol. 2017;62:5575–88.

Modelling for Radiation Treatment Outcome

13

Almut Dutz, Alex Zwanenburg, Johannes A. Langendijk, and Steffen Löck

Almut Dutz and Alex Zwanenburg shared first authorship.

A. Dutz
OncoRay—National Center for Radiation Research in Oncology, Faculty of Medicine and University Hospital Carl Gustav Carus, Technische Universität Dresden, Helmholtz-Zentrum Dresden—Rossendorf, Dresden, Germany

Helmholtz-Zentrum Dresden—Rossendorf, Institute of Radiooncology—OncoRay, Dresden, Germany
e-mail: almut.dutz@oncoray.de

A. Zwanenburg
OncoRay—National Center for Radiation Research in Oncology, Faculty of Medicine and University Hospital Carl Gustav Carus, Technische Universität Dresden, Helmholtz-Zentrum Dresden—Rossendorf, Dresden, Germany

National Center for Tumor Diseases (NCT), Partner Site Dresden, Germany: German Cancer Research Center (DKFZ), Heidelberg, Germany, Faculty of Medicine and University Hospital Carl Gustav Carus, Technische Universität Dresden, Dresden, Germany, and Helmholtz Association/Helmholtz-Zentrum Dresden - Rossendorf (HZDR), Dresden, Germany
e-mail: alexander.zwanenburg@nct-dresden.de

J. A. Langendijk
Department of Radiation Oncology, University Medical Center Groningen, University of Groningen, Groningen, The Netherlands
e-mail: j.a.langendijk@umcg.nl

S. Löck (✉)
OncoRay—National Center for Radiation Research in Oncology, Faculty of Medicine and University Hospital Carl Gustav Carus, Technische Universität Dresden, Helmholtz-Zentrum Dresden—Rossendorf, Dresden, Germany

Department of Radiotherapy and Radiation Oncology, Faculty of Medicine and University Hospital Carl Gustav Carus, Technische Universität Dresden, Dresden, Germany
e-mail: steffen.loeck@oncoray.de

E. G. C. Troost (ed.), *Image-Guided High-Precision Radiotherapy*,
https://doi.org/10.1007/978-3-031-08601-4_13

13.1 Introduction

As many types of cancer are life-threatening, tumour control has a high priority in cancer treatment. However, radical treatment is often limited by the surrounding healthy organs that may lose their functions. These relationships were already considered by Holthusen [1] who described the probability of achieving tumour control and developing normal tissue damage after radiotherapy as a function of radiation dose (Fig. 13.1). The ability to deliver a sufficient tumour dose with a tolerable level of side effects is characterised by the therapeutic window, which defines the target dose prescription as well as dose limits for organs at risk (OARs) [2]. Efforts have been made to widen the therapeutic window and to increase tumour control or to reduce the risk of side effects, e.g. by modified fractionation schemes, new technologies, or biological modulation [3]. For these efforts, statistical modelling is essential, relating patient and treatment-specific risk factors that are associated with tumour radiosensitivity or normal tissue response to defined endpoints.

Statistical models for radiation treatment outcome are becoming increasingly specific and complex. This is caused by two factors. One is the growing amount of patient-specific data that are being collected and made accessible using electronic hospital information systems. With decreasing costs, an increasing number of patients receive in-depth analyses of their tumour tissue, generating multi-omics data that may comprise thousands to millions of parameters from genomic, methylomic, proteomic, radiomic, histomic, and other analyses. In addition, longitudinal data are more commonly acquired, including repeated imaging or liquid biopsies. The second factor comprises advances in computer technology and

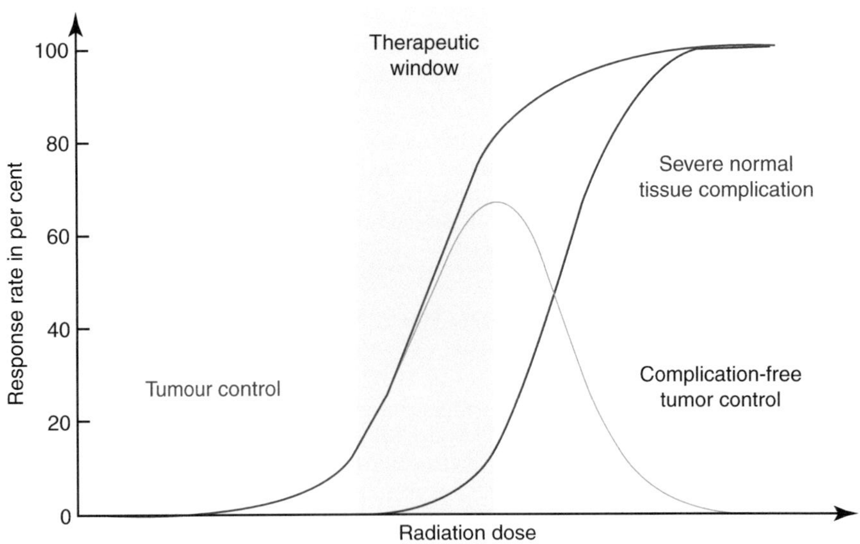

Fig. 13.1 Schematic dose–response curves for tumour control and severe normal tissue complication

machine-learning algorithms, which allow for rapid analyses of these big data and their integration in statistical models.

These developments enable new possibilities: tumour control probability (TCP) models that classify patients into groups with a different risk of treatment failure are essential for biomarker-guided interventional trials. Information from normal tissue complication probability (NTCP) models can be considered in addition to physical parameters during treatment plan optimisation in order to reduce estimated risks of complication (biological treatment plan optimisation). Moreover, predictions of NTCP models may support clinicians in identifying the optimal treatment plan among different planning options or even among different treatment modalities. Another aim that is facilitated by statistical models is adaptive radiotherapy, where radiation treatment is altered during fractionated treatment depending on tumour and normal tissue responses [4, 5].

Since the clinical application of statistical models may substantially affect the treatment of patients, the question arises, what is a good model? A good model addresses a relevant question in a reliable and reproducible manner. It is interpretable. It should either be better than the clinical standard or equivalent to it, but more efficient. Hence, not every model reported in scientific literature will find clinical application. Models may lack generalisability outside the cohort in which they were originally developed. Other models may lack reproducibility due to incomplete reporting. Again, some models may not actually address clinically relevant problems. And finally, models may require data that are too expensive or time-consuming to obtain during clinical routine. To assess these intricacies and to increase the rate of successful translation of models into clinical practice, a general understanding of statistical modelling principles and their application is essential.

In this chapter, we therefore first outline general modelling principles, comprising data types and endpoints, data pre-processing, modelling strategies, and validation procedures (Sect. 13.2). We then provide basic details on modelling tumour response and complication probabilities of normal tissue (Sect. 13.3). Finally, we present two relevant applications of outcome modelling in radiotherapy: the model-based approach for assigning patients to photon or proton-beam therapy based on NTCP models (Sect. 13.4) and radiomics analyses using medical imaging data to predict tumour control (Sect. 13.5).

13.2 Basic Modelling Principles

A model essentially describes the relationship between input variables (features) and an endpoint (outcome). In this section, we describe a modelling workflow and related approaches, see Fig. 13.2 for an overview.

13.2.1 Data

In recent years, the amount and complexity of available data in radiation oncology have increased substantially. Besides demographic, tumour or treatment-related

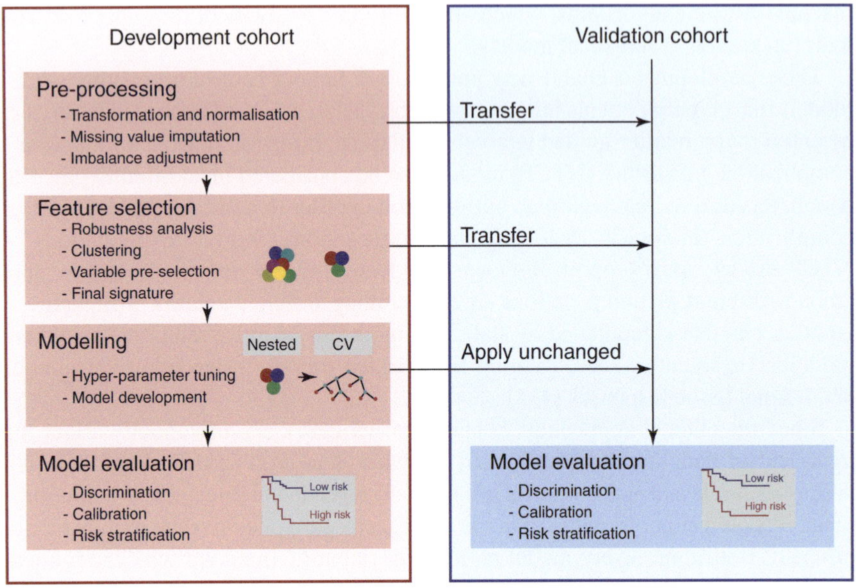

Fig. 13.2 Schematic representation of the described modelling workflow. Data are divided into two separate cohorts. The development cohort is used to create the model, which is subsequently validated on unseen data in the validation cohort. The model development process consists of several steps, including data pre-processing and feature selection, which produces additional parameters. Such parameters (e.g. scale and shift parameters for normalisation of features) are transferred to the validation cohort so that data in both cohorts are pre-processed in the same manner. *CV* cross-validation

factors, dosimetric parameters and pathological findings, increasingly complex features from the analyses of tumour tissue or liquid biopsies and from medical imaging are available. These data are used to predict specific endpoints that may be categorical (e.g. severity grades of side effects), numerical (e.g. hypoxic fraction of the tumour), or survival data (containing an event time and an event indicator, e.g. progression-free survival). Depending on the outcome type, different modelling strategies have to be applied, see Sect. 13.2.5.

The quality of a model is highly dependent on the quality of the data. In general, high-quality data must meet the following criteria:

1. **Cover Patient Heterogeneity:** The cohort used to develop the model should represent the population to which it will be applied. For example, a TCP model created using a cohort of patients with locally advanced head and neck squamous cell carcinoma (HNSCC) may not be reliable for predicting TCP of patients with early-stage HNSCC or of patients with pancreatic cancer.
2. **Completeness:** Complete data have no or very few missing feature values. Features that contain many missing values will typically fail to relate to the outcome.

3. **Uniform Labelling:** The outcome is measured in the same manner for all samples. For example, progression-free survival should be measured from the same starting date, e.g. from the start of radiotherapy or diagnosis, but not both. Likewise, follow-up should be conducted similarly for all patients and radiation-induced side effects should be reported using the same grading system and evaluation criteria.
4. **Reproducible Acquisition:** For example, tumour tissue or OARs should be segmented according to standardised clinical guidelines so that extracted parameters can be compared between patients. Imperfect reproducibility can be somewhat mitigated by ensuring that sufficient data are available to identify robust parameters.

The above requirements are generally not easy to fulfil. Covering patient heterogeneity requires a sufficient sample size in order to still detect relevant effects. Moreover, these cohorts should preferably be obtained from different institutions to allow for identifying and correcting institutional biases, e.g. due to different equipment, treatment workflows, or follow-up procedures. Uniform labelling and reproducible acquisition require standardised protocols and guidelines for prospective application and data curation for retrospective studies.

In particular, dosimetric parameters and image features depend on the delineation of OARs and target structures. This should be performed according to standardised contouring guidelines to assure uniform structures. Automated contouring may also be considered. To ensure consistent evaluation of outcomes and reduce inter-observer variability, data on side effects should be collected prospectively using standardised tests or grading systems (e.g. Common Terminology Criteria for Adverse Events [CTCAE]) by continuously trained clinical staff. Predefined long-term follow-up should be preferred, taking care to ensure the completeness of the outcome data. In addition, prospective scoring of various potential predictor variables such as patient-, disease-, and treatment-specific data is required.

Meeting these requirements can be greatly facilitated by the use of digital information systems, such as electronic health records. In addition, structured databases may link the different available clinical systems, e.g. PACS, DICOM servers, biobanks, study databases, and others. This enables standardised and structured data acquisition as well as curation and annotation of data, which in the end facilitates sharing and linking of data with other institutions and thereby the collection of larger datasets.

13.2.2 Data Analysis Strategy

The most important concern of modelling, after identifying the question and the required data, is the strategy used to analyse the data. The analysis strategy defines which data are used to develop the model, and which data are used to subsequently validate it. Validation is important because it has to be demonstrated that the model works as expected. Assessment of the model should be unbiased [6]. Before we describe different analysis strategies, it is important to consider what interrelated sources of bias may occur in an analysis:

1. **Overfitting**: Given sufficient features, models can learn to predict the outcome for development samples without error. This comes at a trade-off, as such models will typically fail to accurately predict the outcome for new samples, i.e. the model overfits the development data (Fig. 13.3). Overfitting is typically associated with increasing model complexity, i.e. the use of a large number of features relative to the sample size, or model algorithms that can capture high-dimensional data, or both. For linear regression models, ten events per feature are often recommended to prevent overfitting as a simple rule [7].
2. **Underfitting**: Underfitting is the opposite of overfitting. A model underfits when an increase in model complexity would have noticeably improved accuracy of model predictions for new samples (Fig. 13.3). Underfitting is relatively uncommon.
3. **Structural Information Leakage**: Information leakage occurs when information concerning the validation data is used during model development. As a result, the error in predictions on the validation dataset will be smaller than without leakage. Leakage occurs in many forms, e.g. the presence of identical samples in development and validation datasets or feature selection based on the combined dataset. Structural information leakage can be entirely prevented through careful data curation and appropriate methodology.
4. **Developer-Driven Information Leakage**: Developer-driven information leakage occurs when the person responsible for developing a model uses results obtained from the validation dataset, e.g. to select a particular model, tweak modelling parameters, or select important features. Developer-driven information leakage is more pernicious than structural leakage because it is difficult to prove or disprove. The best way to avoid this issue is to limit access to the validation dataset entirely until a model has been completely developed. To a lesser extent, this issue may also be addressed by registering the protocol for the modelling experiment, registering the data prior to the experiment, and automating parameter selection and other modelling steps.

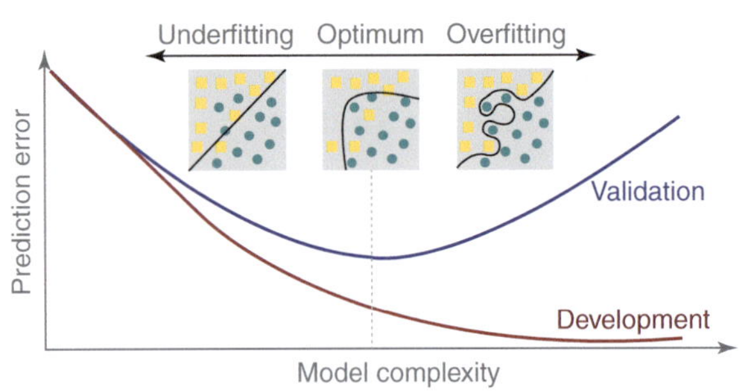

Fig. 13.3 Over- and underfitting during model development. The prediction error of the development data set (red) and the validation data set (blue) is shown as a function of model complexity. For an optimal model, the validation error has a global minimum

Four different types of analysis are described in the TRIPOD guidelines (Transparent reporting of a multivariable prediction model for individual prognosis or diagnosis) and assessed in terms of their level of evidence [8]:

Type 1: The development data used to create the model are also used to validate the model. An important limitation of this approach is the tendency to produce optimistic biases due to overfitting and information leakage.

Type 2: The available dataset is split into development and validation subsets. While the validation performance will be more realistic than for type 1 analyses, these approaches are still limited because general characteristics may be shared across development and validation sets. Hence, the model is not necessarily generalisable.

Type 3: A separate dataset is used to externally validate the model. This dataset is recruited separately, e.g. from a different study in the same institution, or from a different institution. The latter is preferable because this demonstrates model behaviour and performance in the presence of potential institutional biases.

Type 4: A model is first developed (and published) and then applied to a new dataset. Type 4 analyses provide the most reliable assessment of model performance, as it avoids information leakage.

Type 3 and 4 analyses represent external validation. Models should preferably be assessed using these analyses as the results tend to be more representative of actual model performance. For model development, we moreover recommend splitting the development dataset into internal development and validation subsets, e.g. using repeated (stratified) cross-validation. The internal validation subsets can be used to evaluate whether a model would over- or underfit by comparing model errors between the subsets. Therefore, they can be used to guide the choice for different modelling parameters, e.g. to choose a particular modelling algorithm or a signature of features included in the model.

13.2.3 Data Pre-Processing

Before models can be created, data should be pre-processed. This typically includes steps such as transformation, normalisation, and missing value imputation [9]. Though there is no fixed approach to pre-processing, we propose the following.

First, features and samples that have a large fraction (e.g. >10%) of missing values as well as constant features can be removed. Several modelling algorithms assume that numerical features follow a normal distribution. Hence, the remaining features can be power-transformed to make them follow a normal distribution more closely. A typical transformation is logarithmic transformation, but Box-Cox [10] or Yeo-Johnson power transformations [11] offer a more flexible approach.

Normalisation is used to ensure that each numerical feature has a similar value range, as modelling algorithms can be sensitive to features with greatly varying value ranges. Common methods are standardisation, which centres values at 0 by subtracting the mean value and scales their range by dividing by the standard deviation, and rescaling, which limits feature values to a [0,1] or [−1,1] interval by dividing a feature by the range of its values.

Normalisation is also a common preliminary step to batch normalisation. These methods are used to reduce technical sources of variation between the samples (batch effects), e.g. due to different imaging devices or protocols [12, 13]. All normalisation methods that can be used over the entire data set, can also be employed for batch normalisation, e.g. standardisation [14] or the ComBat algorithm [15]. However, batch normalisation may obfuscate or enhance batch effects due to actual differences in patient outcome between cohorts.

Remaining missing values may cause statistical issues and some modelling algorithms will fail to work if they are present. Therefore, they need to be addressed. One method is simply omitting all samples with missing values. However, this may bias results and leads to the loss of other, perhaps more relevant, information [16]. It is generally better to impute missing data, for which various methods exist [17, 18].

Another issue that may be addressed during pre-processing is imbalance in outcome classes. For example, low-grade radiotoxicity is generally more prevalent than high-grade toxicity. As a consequence, a model that predicts the probability of side effects may overemphasise the more frequent low-grade toxicity (majority class) and be insensitive to the rare high-grade toxicity (minority class). Balancing the outcome classes mitigates this issue, which requires either undersampling the majority class or oversampling the minority class [19, 20]. Both undersampling and oversampling have disadvantages. Undersampling is at the expense of removing samples, whereas oversampling requires the generation of synthetic data. The SMOTE [21] and ADASYN [22] algorithms are commonly used for oversampling. Class imbalances, however, may also be considered outside of pre-processing, e.g. through modelling algorithms that can handle class imbalance [23, 24].

13.2.4 Feature Selection

In modern clinical datasets, the number of features can well exceed the number of samples. However, only some of these features will be important for the outcome. We can make the modelling process more efficient by first excluding non-reproducible features, further reducing the dimensionality of the problem, and only then determining the importance of the remaining features.

In particular, in datasets where the number of features exceeds the number of samples considerably, some features may be highly dependent on the specific experimental conditions and are thus not reproducible in repeated experiments or by other centres. Such features should be excluded. For example, through repeated measurements, it has been established that radiomics features computed from medical imaging have varying degrees of reproducibility [25]. Feature reproducibility may be identified from the literature, by performing repeated measurements, through the use of phantom data, or perturbation of image data in case of radiomics [26]. Sometimes it is not possible to assess robustness and care should be taken in the interpretation of the obtained results.

Dimensionality reduction may be approached by projecting the actual feature space to a lower-dimensional feature space, e.g. by principal component analysis or linear discriminant analysis [27]. As an alternative, unsupervised clustering algorithms may be applied to remove highly correlated features. Such features carry essentially the same information and are thus redundant. Moreover, the presence of redundant features may lead to correlation bias [28]. Hence, such features can be replaced by a single cluster feature [29, 30]. Clusters are formed by computing the similarity between pairs of features using certain metrics, such as Spearman's rank correlation coefficient (for numerical features) or McFadden's pseudo R^2 (for any feature type), as input to cluster algorithms [31]. Each cluster can then be represented by a single feature, e.g. the central feature, a meta-feature such as the mean value across all features in the same cluster or the feature that is most strongly related to the outcome.

The remaining features are used in feature selection, aiming to identify the most important features that show the strongest association with the endpoint and should be incorporated into a model [32–34]. However, feature selection results may be sensitive to the underlying dataset [35, 36]. To improve the stability of results, feature selection can be repeated using resampled subsets of the data [37–39]. Feature importance in each subset is then aggregated over the ensemble of subsets to obtain an ensemble feature importance [40]. The final number of included features (signature size) can be determined during hyperparameter optimisation, which is described in the next section. Some modelling algorithms, such as LASSO regression [41] and model-based boosting [42, 43], perform feature selection internally. Still, such algorithms may benefit from filtering irrelevant features and removing redundant ones.

13.2.5 Model Training

Modelling algorithms try to learn the relationship between features and the outcome. Hundreds of algorithms have been devised [44] and their applicability may depend on the type of the considered outcome, see Table 13.1. We generally recommend starting with the use of simple algorithms such as generalised linear models [52] or algorithms based on the least absolute shrinkage and selection operator [41]. The models created by such algorithms are easily understood and reported, and they can be used as baseline models. Given sufficient samples, more complex algorithms such as random forests [53] and extreme gradient boosting [54] may produce models that give better results.

Complex algorithms are characterised by the presence of many model hyperparameters, such as the number of decision trees in a random forest or the learning rate in extreme gradient boosting. However, even simple models have one or more hyperparameters, such as the signature size. Hyperparameters need to be provided manually or determined from the data through an optimisation process. An advantage of automatic optimisation is that it avoids manual bias. Grid search is a common method that samples the hyperparameter space at specified positions, and trains and evaluates a model at each position. This works well for simple models

Table 13.1 Common models and metrics for model discrimination based on categorical, numerical, and survival endpoints

	Categorical endpoint	Numerical endpoint	Survival endpoint
Example models	Logistic regression Support vector machines Neural networks Random forest	Linear regression Random forest Neural networks	Cox regression Boosted-tree regression Survival random forest
Discrimination metrics	Area under the receiver operating characteristic curve (AUC) [45]	Mean-squared error	Concordance Index [46]
	Balanced accuracy [47]	Root-mean-squared error	Censoring-Corrected Concordance Index [48]
	Brier score [49]	Explained variance	Integrated Brier Score [51]
	Matthews correlation coefficient [50]	Median absolute error	
	Sensitivity		
	Specificity		

with few hyperparameters. For high-dimensional hyperparameter spaces, a grid search is no longer efficient. Random search [55] or sequential model-based optimisation [56, 57] is more efficient alternatives. The optimal model hyperparameters are then used to create a final model from the available development samples.

13.2.6 Model Evaluation and Interpretation

Model evaluation shows whether a model has acceptable performance characteristics and whether it generalises well. Models are evaluated on validation samples, e.g. from an external validation dataset. A comparison with development samples may moreover indicate the presence of overfitting and insufficient data heterogeneity in the development data.

There are at least three areas that should be evaluated for a model: model discrimination, model calibration, and model benefit. In addition, model stratification should be assessed for survival endpoints.

An assessment of model discrimination shows how well the model can predict the outcome of samples, and whether it discriminates better than at random. This is done by comparing the predicted outcome with the observed outcome using one or more appropriate metrics (Table 13.1). Note that many metrics for categorical endpoints, that are commonly used in clinical settings, are sensitive to class imbalances in the underlying samples, e.g. sensitivity, specificity, and accuracy [58]. These metrics should be interpreted with caution.

Even though a model may discriminate well, this does not mean that it is well-calibrated [59]. Well-calibrated models have the ability to accurately predict class probability (categorical endpoint), survival probability at a time T (survival endpoint), or value (numerical endpoint) for each sample. For example, a well-calibrated

NTCP model can be used to accurately estimate the probability of the considered radiotoxicity. A well discriminating but not well-calibrated model is capable of distinguishing between samples with and without toxicity, but the predicted probabilities do not correspond to those observed.

Another important part of model evaluation is a comparison with existing models or the clinical standard, or if these do not exist, with null or random models. If a new model is to be translated to the clinic, it should improve upon existing alternatives in terms of predictive power or cost. Additionally, clinical usefulness can be assessed using decision–curve analysis [60–62]. This analysis can be used to determine whether a model would improve decision-making.

Also, the ability of the model to stratify patients into risk groups is clinically relevant and should be assessed [63]. For this purpose, one or more thresholds are determined from the development data and used to form different risk strata. The difference between these strata can then be evaluated by an appropriate significance test [64].

The assessments discussed above only describe model characteristics. Another important aspect of modelling, one that is often overlooked, is model provenance. Many complex modelling algorithms are black boxes in practice. Understanding why an algorithm came to a certain prediction is relevant for any clinical model because it may point out particular biases or incompleteness of the model [65]. The following aspects of a model can be investigated, though this list is not final:

1. **What Is the Importance of Each Feature for the Model?** This can be answered in different ways. For example, in regression models, individual coefficients can be evaluated, e.g. odds ratios for logistic models. A model-agnostic approach expresses feature importance by comparing the discriminatory performance of the developed model between the given dataset and a dataset in which the considered feature is randomly permuted [66].
2. **How Does Each Feature Affect the Outcome?** Explaining how the outcome depends on a feature value may help to elucidate non-linear behaviour or to illustrate potential biases in the model, i.e. feature values that lead to unexpected outcome values. The relationship between a feature and the outcome may, for example, be illustrated by partial dependence plots [67] or individual conditional expectation plots [68].
3. **Which Features Are Similar?** Similar features, such as highly correlated ones, contain mostly the same information. Newly identified important features for a particular outcome should be compared for similarity with established features.

13.2.7 Model Application

After successful evaluation and potential further prospective validation, models may be applied to identify patient subgroups, for example in interventional clinical trials that test the efficacy of treatment modification. Stratified block randomisation, taking the most important confounders into account, should be preferred but may not always be applicable, as discussed in Sect. 13.4. A suitable primary endpoint and the final statistical test have to be chosen, e.g. accounting for competing risks, censored data, and patient drop-out. For sample size planning, a realistic estimate of the expected effect and variability in the primary endpoint is decisive. Monitoring should be performed following good clinical practice including site initiation, interim monitoring, and closeout. Standard operating procedures and procedures for homogenised data acquisition and storage need to be defined in case of several participating centres in order to avoid site-specific bias and missing data. Advanced biomarker-specific trial designs may enhance the success probability of the trial and combine the steps described above [69, 70].

13.3 Introduction to TCP and NTCP Models

In this section, we introduce classic TCP and NTCP models and outline their application in biological treatment plan optimisation and evaluation.

13.3.1 Poisson Model of Tumour Control Probability

Tumour control probability models are used in radiotherapy to estimate the probability of an effective tumour treatment with the planned dose. Common TCP models assume that tumour control is achieved when no single clonogenic cell of the tumour survives after irradiation. They are often based on the linear-quadratic model, which describes the surviving fraction SF of an original cell population irradiated with dose D by

$$\mathrm{SF} = e^{-\left(\alpha D + \beta D^2\right)} \tag{13.1}$$

Here, α and β are tissue-specific parameters describing the mechanisms of cell damage [71]. Combining the surviving fraction SF with the number N_0 of clonogens per tumour before irradiation, the average number of surviving clonogens per tumour $N_0 \cdot \mathrm{SF}$ is obtained. Since the elimination of cells by radiation is a random process and the probability of single cells to survive is low, TCP can be approximated by a Poisson distribution for the case of zero surviving clonogens. The standard model of tumour control is [72]

$$\mathrm{TCP} = e^{-N_0 \cdot \mathrm{SF}} \tag{13.2}$$

This function describes a sigmoidal curve increasing from 0 to 100% with increasing dose. It can be characterised by the dose TCD_{50}, at which 50% of the tumours are controlled, and by the normalised dose–response gradient (or slope) γ_{50}, defining the steepness of the TCP curve at the 50% response level. Under a single-hit assumption ($\beta = 0$), the Poisson TCP model can be quantified by [73]

$$\mathrm{TCP} = 2^{-\exp\left[\frac{2}{\ln 2}\gamma_{50}\left(1-\frac{D}{\mathrm{TCD}_{50}}\right)\right]} \tag{13.3}$$

To determine TCD_{50} and γ_{50}, clinical studies with varying prescribed dose but fixed number of fractions or dose per fraction have been conducted for several tumour entities. These parameters were tabularised, e.g. by Okunieff et al. [74]. Extensions of this model including tumour repopulation, incomplete repair, hypoxia, and non-uniform dose distributions were considered [75–77].

13.3.2 Modelling of Normal Tissue Complication Probability

NTCP models aim to predict the probability of complications based on the dose distribution in associated irradiated organs. For this purpose, the three-dimensional dose distribution is often reduced to a few simple metrics that can be derived from a dose-volume histogram (DVH). Some of the different methods for modelling clinical outcome data of retrospective patient cohorts and their dose distributions are described as follows [78].

1. **DVH-Reduction Models:** Based on the data published by Emami et al. [79], the empirical Lyman-Kutcher-Burman (LKB) model was developed. The LKB model describes the dose-response as a function of irradiated volume by reducing the DVH to a single metric to estimate model parameters for specific OARs [80–83]. The model includes TD_{50}, m and n as parameters. The parameter $TD_{50}(V)$ is the tolerance dose for uniform irradiation of a partial volume V of an OAR at which 50% of patients are likely to experience a specific toxicity. The parameter m represents the slope at the steepest part of the dose-response curve. The parameter n describes the volume effect of the investigated OAR [84]. Serially structured organs such as the spinal cord show $n \approx 0$, while parallel organs are characterised by $n \approx 1$. Taking fractional irradiation into account, the LKB-NTCP model for a uniform dose D to a volume V of an OAR is given by

$$\mathrm{NTCP_{LKB}} = \frac{1}{\sqrt{2\pi}} \int_{-\infty}^{t} \exp\left(\frac{u^2}{2}\right) \mathrm{d}u \tag{13.4}$$

$$\text{with } t = \frac{D - \mathrm{TD}_{50}(V)}{m \mathrm{TD}_{50}}, \tag{13.5}$$

and

$$\mathrm{TD}_{50}(V) = \frac{\mathrm{TD}_{50}(V_{\mathrm{OAR}})}{V^n}, \tag{13.6}$$

where V_{OAR} represents the entire volume of the considered OAR.

However, dose distributions to OARs are non-uniform. The inhomogeneous dose distribution can be reduced to a single metric that produces the same probability of a given side effect as a corresponding uniform dose distribution. Such a metric is the widely used generalised equivalent uniform dose gEUD given by

$$gEUD = \left(\sum_i v_i D_i^a \right)^{1/a} \tag{13.7}$$

where D_i is the dose defined for each dose bin i in a differential DVH. v_i is the volume in a dose bin i and a is a volume parameter that is equivalent to $1/n$. This 'homogeneous' dose can then be applied as $D = g\text{EUD}$ in the LKB model in Eq. (13.5).

2. **Tissue-Architecture Models**: These more mechanistic models are based on the functional architecture of the tissue by introducing functional subunits of an OAR. These can be anatomical substructures, such as nephrons of the kidney, or the largest cell group that still functions as long as it comprises a surviving clonogen [78]. These functional subunits can be arranged in serial or parallel order, or in a combination of both. In parallel organs, functional subunits are performing rather independently so that side effects occur after the irradiated volume exceeds a critical value. Side effects that arise from irradiation of parallel organs depend on the mean dose deposited in these organs (e.g. liver, lung, or kidney). Källman et al. [85] suggested the relative seriality model, in which an organ consists of several serial and parallel structures whose reaction is described by Poisson statistics. The volume effect is characterised by a parameter s indicating the relative seriality of the organ, i.e. the proportion of serial subunits of an organ. A serial organ is characterised by large values ($s \approx 1$) and parallel organs by small values ($s \ll 1$). Other models based on the assumption that NTCP can be determined by functional subunits are for example the critical volume model [86] or the critical element model [87].
3. **Multiple-Metric Models:** The above-mentioned models predict the complication probability for one specific side effect based on the dose to a corresponding OAR. However, some complications are caused by the irradiation of different OARs, e.g. swallowing dysfunction following the irradiation of superior pharyngeal constrictor muscle and the supraglottic larynx [88] or heart valvular dysfunction by the irradiation of heart and lung [89]. To correct for this in LKB models, an interaction gEUD variable for both OARs can be introduced [89]. Moreover, side effects may also be related to dose-independent clinical parameters, such as age, radiation technique, gender, or chemotherapy [88, 90]. Multivariable logistic regression models are appropriate to include both clinical and dosimetric parameters. They are defined by

$$\text{NTCP}_{\text{Logistic}} = \left(1 + \mathrm{e}^{-g(x)}\right)^{-1}, \tag{13.8}$$

$$\text{with } g(x) = \beta_0 + \sum_{i=1}^{p} \beta_i x_i \tag{13.9}$$

Here, β_i denote model coefficients and x_i are the p individual explanatory variables.

Example: Logistic NTCP models for acute side effects after cranial proton-beam therapy were developed and validated in independent patient cohorts treated at three different proton therapy centres, based on methodology described in Sect. 13.2 [91]. Alopecia grade ≥ 2 showed a strong association to the dose–volume parameter *D5%* of the skin in repeated cross-validation performed on the development cohort (AUC = 0.82, Fig. 13.4a). The corresponding NTCP model (Table 13.2) was applied to the two remaining validation cohorts, which showed similar AUC values (0.77 and 0.85, Fig. 13.4b). While the calibration slopes were close to one in validation, the intercept deviated from zero, possibly due to centre-specific differences in toxicity assessment (Fig. 13.4c).

13.3.3 Application: Biological Treatment Plan Optimisation and Evaluation

During the last decades, fluence modulated beam delivery techniques, such as intensity-modulated radiation therapy (IMRT) and volumetric modulated arc therapy (VMAT), successively replaced conventional 3D-conformal radiotherapy (3D-CRT). The greatest benefit of these inverse planning techniques is the multiplicity of dynamically adjustable machine parameters, allowing the creation of highly conformal treatment plans. In contrast to 3D-CRT, dose distributions in OARs can be adjusted to a much larger degree. Additionally, hardware and computing technologies evolved rapidly. Hence, more complex dose calculation algorithms could be translated into clinical routine.

To account for these developments, more and more advanced approaches for creating and evaluating treatment plans have to be designed. One of these approaches currently discussed among clinicians and medical physicists is biological treatment planning. This approach replaces the commonly used physical dose–volume parameters, which are only surrogates for biological effects, with biological measures during treatment plan optimisation and evaluation.

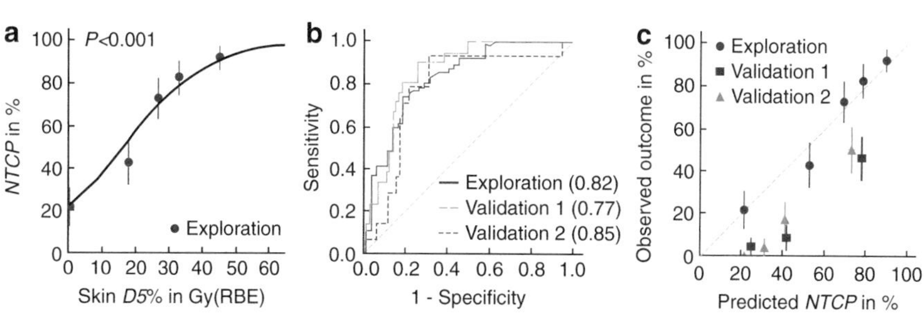

Fig. 13.4 NTCP models for acute alopecia grade ≥ 2 after cranial proton-beam therapy. (**a**) regression curve, (**b**) receiver operating characteristic curves, and (**c**) calibration plot are displayed. AUC values for each cohort are given in brackets. Data points and error bars represent mean and standard deviation of patient sets. Adapted from Dutz et al. [91]

Table 13.2 NTCP model for acute alopecia grade ≥2 after cranial proton-beam therapy, from Dutz et al. [91]

Model parameters	Model coefficients	(95% confidence interval)	p-value
Skin $D5\%$ in Gy(RBE)	0.081	(0.05 – 0.11)	<0.001
Constant	−0.94	(−2.91 to −0.27)	

RBE: relative biological effectiveness

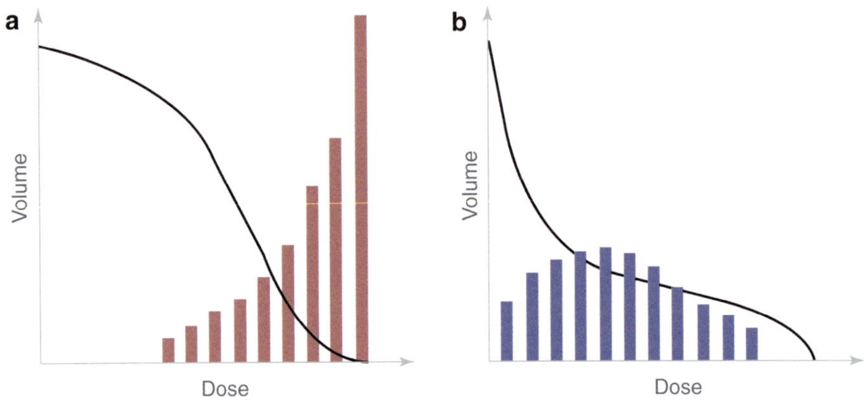

Fig. 13.5 Concept of biological optimisation for (**a**) a serial organised OAR and (**b**) a parallel organised OAR. The DVH curve is influenced by a single *g*EUD objective that achieves the same volume effect as multiple physical dose–volume objectives represented by the bars. Their different weights are expressed by the bar lengths. Adapted from [94]

For biological treatment plan optimisation, one approach is to use multivariable NTCP models directly in the objective function [92]. More common in modern treatment planning systems are optimiser functions that implement a biological objective, e.g. based on *g*EUD (Eq. 13.7), as the main optimisation parameter that adjusts the DVH curve as a whole instead of several physical dose-volume objectives [93]. For serial OARs, a high volume parameter ($a > 10$) is used to prevent dose maxima, while for parallel OARs, a low parameter value ($a = 1$) is used to reduce the mean dose [94]. In contrast to single physical dose-volume objectives (e.g. D_{max}), biological objectives influence the entire DVH curve, see Fig. 13.5.

In order to adequately apply these biological functions, the tissue-specific parameter a has to be known for all OARs. Using the relationship $a = 1/n$, it can be determined from published LKB models, e.g. in Luxton et al. [95]. Before application in clinical routine, these parameters should be calibrated on clinic-specific data. In case a cannot be calibrated, different generic initial values depending on the type of OAR (parallel or serially organised) have been recommended to be used for plan optimisation, e.g. outlined in the AAPM task group report 166 [93]. However, the use of these non-calibrated initial parameters requires an additional uncertainty analysis. For treatment plan selection and evaluation, EUD can be used to rank tentative treatment plans. Also, TCP/NTCP models can be used to make patient-specific predictions of outcome and then select a specific treatment plan. Although several dose–response models have been developed and are continuously updated, they continue to be very simplistic [96]. For some clinical situations and tumour entities, several competing models may be available. For example, the predictions of models for the same side effect but developed based on data from different tumour entities may differ (e.g. lung or heart toxicity for lung and breast cancer patients). Hence, clinicians should determine the appropriate biological models for each tumour entity, clinical setting, and radiation modality.

Some treatment planning systems may already include a library of models or model parameters with default values. However, these published models have been developed at other institutions including different patient populations, treatment planning systems, dose calculation algorithms, fractionation schemes, etc. The patient characteristics may differ substantially such that further variables may affect the considered endpoint. Thus, TCP/NTCP models used in biological plan evaluation have to be calibrated based on the institutional situation before use. This requires a comprehensive collection of outcome data and large patient cohorts. If multivariable models are to be implemented that contain additional clinical variables (e.g. comorbidities, age, or concomitant therapies), this information must also be available. Since this complex calibration for different tumour entities and OARs is not feasible for most clinics, partial biological optimisation is currently used, combining biological and physical objectives.

The main limitation of biological treatment planning lies in the uncertainties of the biological models. Due to the increasing amount of patient-specific data and the development of advanced modelling strategies, a reduction of these uncertainties seems feasible. This would allow for implementing such biological techniques widely into clinical practice in the future.

13.4 Case 1: Patient Selection for Proton-Beam Therapy: The Model-Based Approach

One example for the application of NTCP models is the patient assignment to proton-beam therapy (PBT). Although the number of operating PBT facilities is increasing worldwide, the high technical and time expenditure leads to high costs of this treatment modality. Therefore, it is important to offer PBT to those patients who may benefit most from it compared to conventional photon therapy (XRT).

Randomised controlled trials (RCT) are considered as the highest evidence for practice change in oncology. However, there are challenges in performing RCTs to compare different radiotherapy techniques or modalities. The heterogeneity between centres in terms of treatment planning systems, quality assurance, training skills, image guidance techniques, treatment adaptation, immobilisation strategies, etc., may be so pronounced that it may be difficult to generalise results from RCTs into clinical routine [97, 98]. In addition, for trials comparing PBT and XRT in terms of reduced late side effects, the considered endpoints may manifest many years after radiotherapy. Thus, results from large long-term RCTs may be obsolete as radiotherapy (and PBT in particular) is still a rapidly evolving technology [99]. To reduce the number of patients and thus the duration of the study, a proper pre-selection of eligible patients is necessary.

A feasible approach to meet these challenges and to identify patients suitable for PBT is based on comparative NTCP modelling, the so-called model-based approach [99]. In the Netherlands and Denmark, it has already been implemented in clinical practice for patients with various tumour sites, including HNSCC, non-small cell lung cancer, breast cancer, and mediastinal lymphoma. This section discusses the principles of the two-phase model-based approach as proposed by Langendijk et al. [99] and applications.

13.4.1 Principles of the Model-Based Approach

The model-based approach consists of two phases: model-based selection and validation. The first phase, in turn, comprises three steps: development and validation of NTCP models, patient-specific plan comparison, and estimation of the clinical benefit of PBT. The individual steps are explained in more detail below.

13.4.1.1 Phase α: Model-Based Selection

Patients are selected according to their reduction of side effect probabilities under PBT compared to XRT. If this reduction exceeds a given threshold, those patients will be suitable for PBT treatment. The side effect probabilities for each patient are estimated using NTCP models.

1. **Development and Validation of NTCP Models:** NTCP models have to be developed and externally validated for different entities and relevant side effects that may occur following XRT or PBT. General aspects on development and validation of NTCP models are described in Sect. 13.3.2. Most NTCP models have been derived from data of patients treated with XRT. NTCP models can already differ between various XRT techniques [88, 100, 101]. Since dose distributions of XRT and PBT may show even stronger differences, XRT-based models need to be validated on prospectively collected PBT patient data. In case of negative validation, the development of technique-specific NTCP models may become necessary. Continuous NTCP validation and updating may be implemented, for example, in the framework of a rapid learning health care system [102, 103].
2. **Individual in silico Planning Comparative Studies:** For each patient, two treatment plans are created, one with protons and the other with a state-of-the-art XRT technique. The values of the dosimetric parameters that are supposed to be important in the selected NTCP models should be reduced, if possible, during treatment planning.
3. **Estimation of the Clinical Benefit:** The in silico treatment plans and NTCP models are used to estimate the difference (ΔNTCP) in side effect probabilities between XRT and PBT:

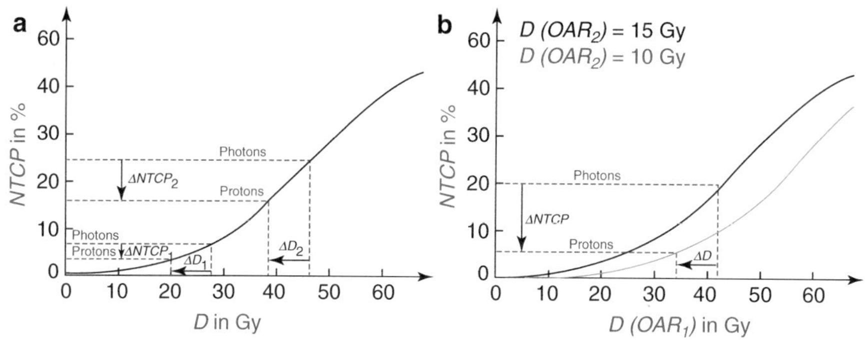

Fig. 13.6 Model-based approach according to [99]. (**a**) An equal dose difference between proton and photon treatment plan may translate into different NTCP reductions in a univariable model. (**b**) In a multivariable model including dosimetric predictors of two different OARs, the NTCP difference may be even higher if PBT is able to reduce dose to both OARs simultaneously

$$\text{''}\,\text{NTCP} = \text{NTCP}_{\text{XRT}} - \text{NTCP}_{\text{PBT}} \tag{13.10}$$

Figure 13.6a shows that a similar dose difference between a photon and a proton treatment plan may lead to different NTCP reductions, depending on the slope of the NTCP curve at the considered dose values. In a multivariable model including dosimetric predictors of two different OARs, the difference in NTCP between the proton and photon plan may be even higher if PBT is able to spare both OARs simultaneously [88], see Fig. 13.6b. A patient is finally selected for PBT if the extent of NTCP reduction in the PBT plan compared to XRT exceeds a given threshold. This threshold depends on the severity of the side effects, with lower thresholds for more severe toxicities. For toxicities of CTCAE grade 2, 3, and 4–5, the Dutch Society of Radiation Oncology suggests thresholds of 10%, 5%, and 2% points, respectively [97]. In some cases, multiple side effects are considered in the selection procedure (NTCP profiles). Here, both the NTCP difference of every single endpoint as well as the summarised NTCP difference for all considered endpoints must exceed different thresholds [97]. If the NTCP difference remains below the recommended threshold, the patient is treated with state-of-the-art XRT.

13.4.1.2 Phase β: Model-Based Clinical Evaluation

The initial hypothesis of reduced side effects after PBT compared to XRT is evaluated during model-based clinical validation. Patients who were selected for PBT during phase α are enrolled in prospective clinical evaluation studies and are treated with the proton treatment plan created during step 2. The finally observed toxicity rates of patients treated with PBT are then compared to the initially predicted proton NTCP values to detect possible shortcomings of the applied NTCP models [97]. Furthermore, it can be tested whether the observed toxicity rate following PBT is indeed lower than the estimated NTCP values for XRT (calibration in the large [104]).

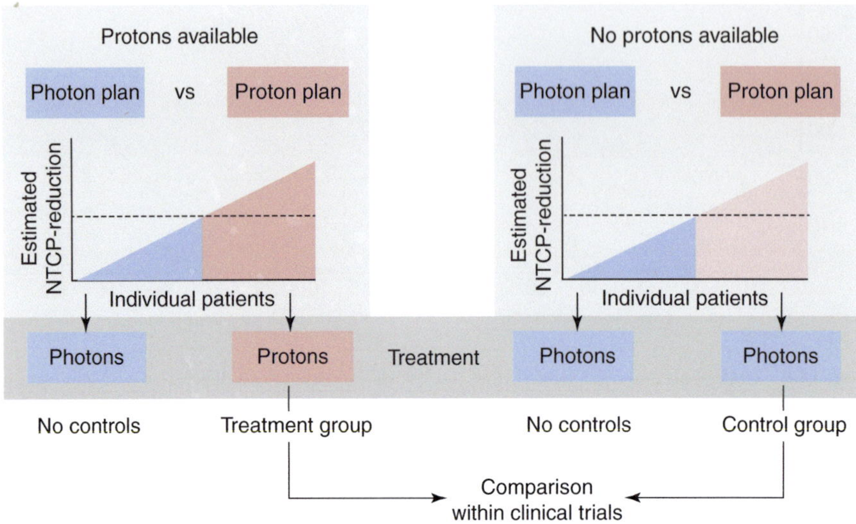

Fig. 13.7 Schematic overview of model-based clinical evaluation according to [99]

Moreover, the real outcome of PBT and XRT can be compared directly using prospectively collected patient data from cohorts treated with one of the treatment modalities (Fig. 13.7). Both patient groups of such clinical trials need to be selected according to the same selection procedure. The control group includes patients who would have been candidates for PBT but were still treated with XRT, e.g. historical cohorts [99] or patients treated in radiotherapy centres without access to PBT.

13.4.2 Application: Proton-Beam Therapy for Head and Neck Cancer

The model-based approach for patient selection for PBT has been introduced into clinical practice in some European countries. Arts et al. [105] investigated the impact of treatment accuracy, in terms of setup and range uncertainties, on the selection procedure based on a cohort of 78 patients with oropharyngeal cancer. They analysed the number of patients selected for PBT based on four NTCP models and using the above-mentioned ΔNTCP thresholds of 10% and 5% points for grade 2 and grade 3 side effects, respectively (Table 13.3). To analyse the impact of the treatment accuracy, three different planning target volume (PTV) margins for IMRT plans as well as five different setup and range robustness settings for intensity modulated proton-beam therapy (IMPT) were applied. In a setting of a 3 mm PTV margin for IMRT and 3 mm setup and 3% range error for IMPT, a total of 77% of patients were selected for PBT if the corresponding threshold was exceeded in at least one of the four NTCP models. For all models, the more robust the IMPT plans were for the same PTV margin, the fewer patients were selected for

Table 13.3 Investigated NTCP models predicting side effects following the irradiation head and neck cancer patients in the study by Arts et al. [105]

Side effect and NTCP model	Severity grade	Time after RT	Model predictors	Model type
Tube feeding dependence Wopken et al. [106]	3	6 months	Mean dose of the superior and inferior PCM, contralateral parotid, and cricopharyngeal muscle Advanced T stage Weight loss (moderate/severe) Accelerated radiotherapy Chemoradiation Radiotherapy plus cetuximab	Logistic regression model
Reduced parotid flow Dijkema et al. [107]	2	1 year	Mean dose in parotid glands	LKB model
Patient-rated problems swallowing solid food[a] Christianen et al. [88]	2	6 months	Mean dose superior PCM and supraglottic larynx Age	Logistic regression model
Patient-rated xerostomia[a] Beetz et al. [108]	2	6 months	Mean dose contralateral parotid gland Baseline xerostomia score	Logistic regression model

LKB Lyman–Kutcher–Burman; *PCM* pharyngeal constrictor muscle; *RT* radiotherapy

[a]Assessed with the head-and-neck cancer-specific quality of life questionnaire EORTC QLQ-H&N35

PBT. With the same robustness settings of the IMPT plan, more patients were selected for PBT the greater the PTV margin of the IMRT plan. The study by Arts et al. [105] showed that, in addition to the choice of an appropriate threshold for each severity grade, treatment accuracy also affects the proportion of patients selected for PBT.

13.5 Case 2: Radiomics

Medical imaging is commonly acquired prior to and during radiation treatment. It may contain information on disease diagnosis or treatment outcome and thereby improve corresponding TCP or NTCP models. It can thus enable further treatment personalisation, e.g. by selecting patients for specific treatments [109]. In a radiomics analysis, information is extracted from each image and quantitatively assessed. Radiomics draws upon mathematically well-defined ('hand-crafted') features, automated feature generation based on deep learning algorithms, or both

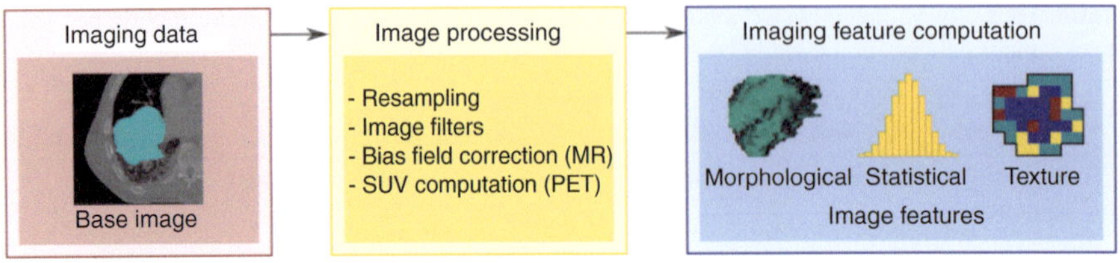

Fig. 13.8 Schematic representation of image processing and feature calculation. *MR* magnetic resonance, *SUV* standardised uptake value, *PET* positron emission tomography. Adapted from [29]

[110, 111]. Radiomics has been applied to numerous tasks in radiation oncology including TCP and NTCP modelling for several tumour entities [112–115].

13.5.1 The Radiomics Workflow

A radiomics analysis using hand-crafted features consists of several steps, as illustrated in Fig. 13.8 and explained in the following.

1. **Image Acquisition and Reconstruction:** A patient is scanned in a medical imaging device according to a specific protocol. Software, usually provided by the vendor, then converts the acquired image data into something interpretable by human readers.
2. **Segmentation:** This usually aims to characterise part of an image, e.g. the primary tumour or different OARs. Clinical experts or (semi-)automatic algorithms segment or delineate the image to identify the regions of interest (ROIs).
3. **Image Processing:** Image processing primarily harmonises images across patients. For example, voxels (3D pixels) in images of different patients are resampled to the same dimensions to decrease variability of radiomics features related to different voxel sizes in the reconstructed images [116]. Another component of image processing is the use of image filters, e.g. to remove noise or emphasise edges, blobs, or directional structures [117]. A general image processing scheme for radiomics is described by the Image Biomarker Standardisation Initiative (IBSI) [118].
4. **Radiomics Feature Computation:** After image processing, radiomics features are computed from the ROI. This generates a feature value for each image. Many common features were standardised by the IBSI, and described in their documentation [118].
5. **Modelling:** The previous steps yield radiomics feature values that are easily converted to a tabular format. The modelling component of a radiomics analysis is therefore not specific to radiomics but follows the principles described earlier in this chapter.

Radiomics based on deep learning is quite similar, but the radiomics feature computation and modelling steps are typically replaced entirely by a deep learning algorithm. Manual segmentation may not be required, as a deep learning network is capable of learning what aspects and regions of the image are of interest, given sufficient data. Some image processing is usually required because of constraints on the input of deep learning algorithms.

13.5.2 Application: Radiomics for Adaptive Treatment

One way to personalise radiotherapy is to monitor the treatment progress and adapt treatment correspondingly [4]. Treatment progress may potentially be monitored by medical imaging and its comprehensive radiomics analysis. This particular subfield of radiomics is called delta-radiomics because radiomics features are computed from images acquired at different time points [119, 120].

We have previously performed a delta-radiomics analysis to assess whether computed tomography (CT) imaging during treatment can be used to classify patients with locally advanced HNSCC into a high and a low-risk group for loco-regional recurrence [121]. We will describe this study here as an example of how radiomics could be used for adaptive treatment.

The study involved three patient cohorts, a development cohort ($n = 48$), a validation cohort ($n = 30$), and a cohort that was only used to assess the robustness of radiomics features ($n = 18$). The patients in the development and validation cohort were followed up for several years, and loco-regional recurrence was recorded. Patients in these cohorts were scanned prior to treatment (CT_0) and during the second week of treatment (CT_2). Based on the primary tumour contours, we computed 1583 radiomics features with the IBSI-compliant software MIRP [122] for every imaging dataset.

We identified 269 robust features, which we computed from CT_0 and CT_2. Furthermore, we computed the difference between the two time points, i.e. 269 delta features. The three feature sets were compared for modelling loco-regional control (LRC) in a TRIPOD type 3 survival analysis: using CT_0-features only, CT_2-features only, and the combined set including delta features. Modelling followed the steps outlined in Sect. 13.2. Features in the development cohort were pre-processed by standardisation and subsequent clustering of similar features (Spearman correlation $\rho > 0.90$). We then determined variable importance by performing feature selection using six different methods on 1000 bootstraps of the data and aggregated the feature ranks. Subsequently, we optimised model hyperparameters for six different algorithms through grid search in a cross-validation scheme. Models were then trained on 1000 bootstraps of the development cohort and combined into an ensemble model for each combination of feature selection method and learner. In total, we created 36 ensemble models, based on earlier findings that indicated that a combination of different methods should be assessed to reduce the risk of accidental findings [29]. Furthermore, it could be assessed whether an increase in model complexity justifies a decrease in model explainability by better performance.

We then validated all models in the validation dataset, see Fig. 13.9. Model performance was assessed using a concordance index (C-index; 0.5: random, 1.0

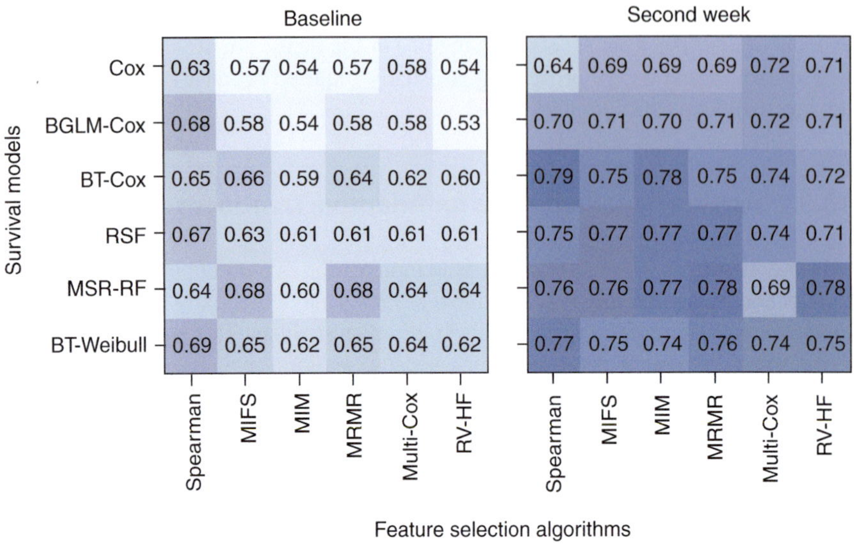

Fig. 13.9 Concordance indices of radiomics models (0.5: random, 1.0: perfect discrimination) based on treatment planning CT images (left panel) and on CT images after the second week of treatment (right panel). The performance of several survival models based on imaging features selected from different feature selection algorithms is shown for the validation cohort. For details, see [121]

perfect discrimination) [46]. Stratification into low- and high-risk groups for loco-regional recurrence was evaluated using a log-rank test. We found that models based on the CT_2 (C-index: 0.73 ± 0.04, mean ± standard deviation over all models) and combined feature sets (0.70 ± 0.05, not shown) exceeded the performance of models using CT_0 only (0.62 ± 0.04). The combined feature set ($p = 0.06$) and CT_2 only ($p = 0.005$) enabled better performance compared to CT_0.

Our results indicate that imaging obtained during treatment can be more suited to identify patients at lower or higher risk of tumour recurrence than pre-treatment imaging. Though this effect should be validated in a larger dataset, the results do show the potential for image-guided treatment adaptation. For instance, if the tumour has a very low risk of recurring, treatment may be stopped early, while in case of a high recurrence risk, the patient and clinician may choose to pursue an extended radiation treatment. In the future, such options for treatment adaptation may become available for patients with a clear prognosis based on precise and validated models.

13.6 Summary and Outlook

Due to the growing amount of patient-specific data and corresponding advances in computer technology and adapted machine-learning algorithms, models predicting tumour control or normal tissue complications are becoming increasingly complex, which in turn may allow for more accurate predictions. This brings forward new fields of application, e.g. in personalised radiotherapy, for model-based patient selection or biological treatment planning.

It is thus essential to understand the basic principles of model development and validation, which we have presented in this chapter. We outlined important aspects of data quality, data pre-processing, feature selection, model development, model evaluation, and model validation. The application of these concepts was presented for NTCP modelling within the model-based approach selecting patients for photon or proton-beam therapy and for adaptive TCP modelling based on radiomics analyses from pre-treatment and in-treatment CT imaging.

In future, data science and artificial intelligence may play a central role in the development of high-precision radiotherapy. For these developments, homogeneous patient cohorts of sufficient sample size are required. This necessitates the formation of large cooperative networks pooling their data or federated learning strategies with decentralised data storage [123]. Furthermore, data publication according to the FAIR principles [124] will ensure the continued improvement of models on radiation treatment outcome.

References

1. Holthusen H. Erfahrungen über die Verträglichkeitsgrenze für Röntgenstrahlen und deren Nutzanwendung zur Verhütung von Schäden. Strahlentherapie. 1936;57:254–69.
2. Karger CP. Klinische Strahlenbiologie. In: Schlegel W, Karger CP, Jäkel O, editors. Medizinische Physik: Grundlagen—Bildgebung—Therapie—Technik. Berlin, Heidelberg: Springer; 2018. p. 451–72.
3. Baumann M, Krause M, Overgaard J, et al. Radiation oncology in the era of precision medicine. Nat Rev Cancer. 2016;16:234–49. https://doi.org/10.1038/nrc.2016.18.
4. Ajdari A, Niyazi M, Nicolay NH, et al. Towards optimal stopping in radiation therapy. Radiother Oncol. 2019;134:96–100.
5. Beaton L, Bandula S, Gaze MN, Sharma RA. How rapid advances in imaging are defining the future of precision radiation oncology. Br J Cancer. 2019;120:779–90.
6. Zwanenburg A, Löck S. Why validation of prognostic models matters? Radiother Oncol. 2018;127:370–3.
7. van Smeden M, de Groot JA, Moons KG, et al. No rationale for 1 variable per 10 events criterion for binary logistic regression analysis. BMC Med Res Methodol. 2016;16:163.
8. Moons KGM, Altman DG, Reitsma JB, et al. Transparent reporting of a multivariable prediction model for individual prognosis or diagnosis (TRIPOD): explanation and elaboration. Ann Intern Med. 2015;162:W1–73.
9. García S, Luengo J, Herrera F. Data preprocessing in data mining. Berlin: Springer International Publishing; 2015.
10. Box GEP, Cox DR. An analysis of transformations. J R Stat Soc Series B Stat Methodol. 1964;26:211–52.
11. Yeo I, Johnson RA. A new family of power transformations to improve normality or symmetry. Biometrika. 2000;87:954–9.
12. Orlhac F, Boughdad S, Philippe C, et al. A postreconstruction harmonization method for multicenter radiomic studies in PET. J Nucl Med. 2018;59:1321–8.
13. Orlhac F, Frouin F, Nioche C, et al. Validation of a method to compensate multicenter effects affecting CT radiomics. Radiology. 2019;291:53–9.

14. Chatterjee A, Vallières M, Dohan A, et al. Creating robust predictive radiomic models for data from independent institutions using normalization. IEEE Trans Radiat Plasma Med Sci. 2019;3:210–5.
15. Johnson WE, Li C, Rabinovic A. Adjusting batch effects in microarray expression data using empirical Bayes methods. Biostatistics. 2007;8:118–27.
16. Greenland S, Finkle WD. A critical look at methods for handling missing covariates in epidemiologic regression analyses. Am J Epidemiol. 1995;142:1255–64.
17. Donders ART, van der Heijden GJMG, Stijnen T, Moons KGM. Review: a gentle introduction to imputation of missing values. J Clin Epidemiol. 2006;59:1087–91.
18. Luengo J, García S, Herrera F. On the choice of the best imputation methods for missing values considering three groups of classification methods. Knowl Inf Syst. 2012;32: 77–108.
19. He H, Garcia EA. Learning from imbalanced data. In: IEEE Transactions on Knowledge and Data Engineering; 2008. pp 1263–1284.
20. Krawczyk B. Learning from imbalanced data: open challenges and future directions. Prog Artif Intell. 2016;5:221–32.
21. Chawla NV, Bowyer KW, Hall LO, Kegelmeyer WP. SMOTE: synthetic minority oversampling technique. J Artif Intell Res. 2002;16:321–57.
22. He H, Bai Y, Garcia EA, Li S. ADASYN: adaptive synthetic sampling approach for imbalanced learning. In: 2008 IEEE International Joint Conference on Neural Networks (IEEE World Congress on Computational Intelligence); 2008. pp 1322–1328.
23. Kubat M, Holte R, Matwin S. Learning when negative examples abound. In: Machine learning: ECML-97. Berlin, Heidelberg: Springer; 1997. p. 146–53.
24. O'Brien R, Ishwaran H. A random forests quantile classifier for class imbalanced data. Pattern Recogn. 2019;90:232–49.
25. Zwanenburg A. Radiomics in nuclear medicine: robustness, reproducibility, standardization, and how to avoid data analysis traps and replication crisis. Eur J Nucl Med Mol Imaging. 2019;46:2638–55.
26. Zwanenburg A, Leger S, Agolli L, et al. Assessing robustness of radiomic features by image perturbation. Sci Rep. 2019a;9:614.
27. Cunningham JP, Ghahramani Z. Linear dimensionality reduction: survey, insights, and generalizations. J Mach Learn Res. 2015;16:2859–900.
28. Tolosi L, Lengauer T. Classification with correlated features: unreliability of feature ranking and solutions. Bioinformatics. 2011;27:1986–94.
29. Leger S, Zwanenburg A, Pilz K, et al. A comparative study of machine learning methods for time-to-event survival data for radiomics risk modelling. Sci Rep. 2017;7:13206.
30. Park MY, Hastie T, Tibshirani R. Averaged gene expressions for regression. Biostatistics. 2007;8:212–27.
31. Kaufman L, Rousseeuw PJ. Finding groups in data: an introduction to cluster analysis. Hoboken: John Wiley & Sons; 2009.
32. Guyon I, Elisseeff A. An introduction to variable and feature selection. J Mach Learn Res. 2003;3:1157–82.
33. Li J, Cheng K, Wang S, et al. Feature selection: a data perspective. ACM Comput Surv (CSUR). 2018;50:94.
34. Saeys Y, Inza I, Larrañaga P. A review of feature selection techniques in bioinformatics. Bioinformatics. 2007;23:2507–17.
35. Haury A-C, Gestraud P, Vert J-P. The influence of feature selection methods on accuracy, stability and interpretability of molecular signatures. PLoS One. 2011;6:e28210.
36. Kalousis A, Prados J, Hilario M. Stability of feature selection algorithms: a study on high-dimensional spaces. Knowl Inf Syst. 2007;12:95–116.
37. Abeel T, Helleputte T, Van de Peer Y, et al. Robust biomarker identification for cancer diagnosis with ensemble feature selection methods. Bioinformatics. 2010;26:392–8.
38. Meinshausen N, Bühlmann P. Stability selection. J R Stat Soc Series B Stat Methodol. 2010;72:417–73.

39. Saeys Y, Abeel T, Van de Peer Y. Robust feature selection using ensemble feature selection techniques. In: Daelemans W, Goethals B, Morik K, editors. Machine learning and knowledge discovery in databases. Berlin, Heidelberg: Springer; 2008. p. 313–25.
40. Wald R, Khoshgoftaar TM, Dittman D, et al. An extensive comparison of feature ranking aggregation techniques in bioinformatics. In: 2012 IEEE 13th International Conference on Information Reuse Integration (IRI); 2012. pp 377–384.
41. Tibshirani R. Regression shrinkage and selection via the Lasso. J R Stat Soc Series B Stat Methodol. 1996;58:267–88.
42. Bühlmann P, Hothorn T. Boosting algorithms: regularization, prediction and model fitting. Stat Sci. 2007;22:477–505.
43. Hofner B, Boccuto L, Göker M. Controlling false discoveries in high-dimensional situations: boosting with stability selection. BMC Bioinformat. 2015;16:144.
44. Fernández-Delgado M, Cernadas E, Barro S, Amorim D. Do we need hundreds of classifiers to solve real world classification problems? J Mach Learn Res. 2014;15:3133–81.
45. Hand DJ, Till RJ. A simple generalisation of the area under the ROC curve for multiple class classification problems. Mach Learn. 2001;45:171–86.
46. Pencina MJ, D'Agostino RB. Overall C as a measure of discrimination in survival analysis: model specific population value and confidence interval estimation. Stat Med. 2004;23:2109–23.
47. Brodersen KH, Ong CS, Stephan KE, Buhmann JM. The balanced accuracy and its posterior distribution. In: 2010 20th International Conference on Pattern Recognition; 2010. pp 3121–3124.
48. Uno H, Cai T, Pencina MJ, et al. On the C-statistics for evaluating overall adequacy of risk prediction procedures with censored survival data. Stat Med. 2011;30:1105–17.
49. Brier GW. Verification of forecasts expressed in terms of probability. Mon Weather Rev. 1950;78:1–3.
50. Matthews BW. Comparison of the predicted and observed secondary structure of T4 phage lysozyme. Biochim Biophys Acta. 1975;405:442–51.
51. Gneiting T, Raftery AE. Strictly proper scoring rules, prediction, and estimation. J Am Stat Assoc. 2007;102:359–78.
52. Nelder JA, Wedderburn RWM. Generalized linear models. J R Stat Soc Ser A. 1972;135: 370–84.
53. Breiman L. Random forests. Mach Learn. 2001;45:5–32.
54. Chen T, Guestrin C. XGBoost: a scalable tree boosting system. In: Proceedings of the 22nd ACM SIGKDD International Conference on Knowledge Discovery and Data Mining; 2016. pp 785–794.
55. Bergstra J, Bengio Y. Random search for hyper-parameter optimization. J Mach Learn Res. 2012;13:281–305.
56. Feurer M, Klein A, Eggensperger K, et al. Efficient and robust automated machine learning. In: Cortes C, Lawrence ND, Lee DD, et al., editors. Advances in neural information processing systems 28. New York: Curran Associates, Inc.; 2015. p. 2962–70.
57. Hutter F, Hoos HH, Leyton-Brown K. Sequential model-based optimization for general algorithm configuration. In: Coello CAC, editor. Learning and intelligent optimization. Berlin, Heidelberg: Springer; 2011. p. 507–23.
58. Japkowicz N, Stephen S. The class imbalance problem: a systematic study. Intell Data Anal. 2002;6:429–49.
59. Van Calster B, McLernon DJ, van Smeden M, et al. Calibration: the Achilles heel of predictive analytics. BMC Med. 2019;17:230.
60. Vickers AJ, Cronin AM, Elkin EB, Gonen M. Extensions to decision curve analysis, a novel method for evaluating diagnostic tests, prediction models and molecular markers. BMC Med Inform Decis Mak. 2008;8:53.
61. Vickers AJ, Elkin EB. Decision curve analysis: a novel method for evaluating prediction models. Med Decis Mak. 2006;26:565–74.

62. Vickers AJ, van Calster B, Steyerberg EW. A simple, step-by-step guide to interpreting decision curve analysis. Diagn Progn Res. 2019;3:18.
63. Royston P, Altman DG. External validation of a Cox prognostic model: principles and methods. BMC Med Res Methodol. 2013;13:33.
64. Mallett S, Royston P, Waters R, et al. Reporting performance of prognostic models in cancer: a review. BMC Med. 2010;8:21.
65. Doshi-Velez F, Kim B. Towards a rigorous science of interpretable machine learning; 2017. arXiv [stat.ML].
66. Fisher A, Rudin C, Dominici F. All models are wrong, but many are useful: learning a Variable's importance by studying an entire class of prediction models simultaneously. J Mach Learn Res. 2019;20:1–81.
67. Friedman JH. Greedy function approximation: a gradient boosting machine. Ann Stat. 2001;29:1189–232.
68. Goldstein A, Kapelner A, Bleich J, Pitkin E. Peeking inside the black Box: visualizing statistical learning with plots of individual conditional expectation. J Comput Graph Stat. 2015;24:44–65.
69. Antoniou M, Kolamunnage-Dona R, Jorgensen AL. Biomarker-guided non-adaptive trial designs in phase II and phase III: a methodological review. J Pers Med. 2017;7:1.
70. Lin J-A, He P. Reinventing clinical trials: a review of innovative biomarker trial designs in cancer therapies. Br Med Bull. 2015;114:17–27.
71. Joiner MC. Quantifying cell kill and cell survival. In: Joiner MC, van der Kogel A, editors. Basic clinical radiobiology. 4th ed. Boca Raton: CRC Press; 2009.
72. Bentzen SM. Dose–response relationships in radiotherapy. In: Joiner MC, van der Kogel A, editors. Basic clinical radiobiology. 4th ed. Boca Raton: CRC Press; 2009.
73. Warkentin B, Stavrev P, Stavreva N, et al. A TCP-NTCP estimation module using DVHs and known radiobiological models and parameter sets. J Appl Clin Med Phys. 2004;5:50–63.
74. Okunieff P, Morgan D, Niemierko A, Suit HD. Radiation dose-response of human tumors. Int J Radiat Oncol Biol Phys. 1995;32:1227–37.
75. Roberts SA, Hendry JH. A realistic closed-form radiobiological model of clinical tumor-control data incorporating intertumor heterogeneity. Int J Radiat Oncol Biol Phys. 1998;41:689–99.
76. Sanchez-Nieto B, Nahum AE. The delta-TCP concept: a clinically useful measure of tumor control probability. Int J Radiat Oncol Biol Phys. 1999;44:369–80.
77. Webb S, Nahum AE. A model for calculating tumour control probability in radiotherapy including the effects of inhomogeneous distributions of dose and clonogenic cell density. Phys Med Biol. 1993;38:653–66.
78. Gulliford S. Modelling of Normal tissue complication probabilities (NTCP): review of application of machine learning in predicting NTCP. In: El Naqa I, Li R, Murphy MJ, editors. Machine learning in radiation oncology: theory and applications. Cham: Springer International Publishing; 2015. p. 277–310.
79. Emami B, Lyman J, Brown A, et al. Tolerance of normal tissue to therapeutic irradiation. Int J Radiat Oncol Biol Phys. 1991;21:109–22.
80. Burman C, Kutcher GJ, Emami B, Goitein M. Fitting of normal tissue tolerance data to an analytic function. Int J Radiat Oncol Biol Phys. 1991;21:123–35.
81. Kutcher GJ, Burman C. Calculation of complication probability factors for non-uniform normal tissue irradiation: the effective volume method gerald. Int J Radiat Oncol Biol Phys. 1989;16:1623–30.
82. Kutcher GJ, Burman C, Brewster L, et al. Histogram reduction method for calculating complication probabilities for three-dimensional treatment planning evaluations. Int J Radiat Oncol Biol Phys. 1991;21:137–46.
83. Lyman JT. Complication probability as assessed from dose-volume histograms. Radiat Res Suppl. 1985;8:S13–9.
84. Gulliford SL, Partridge M, Sydes MR, et al. Parameters for the Lyman Kutcher Burman (LKB) model of Normal tissue complication probability (NTCP) for specific rectal complications observed in clinical practise. Radiother Oncol. 2012;102:347–51.

85. Källman P, Agren A, Brahme A. Tumour and normal tissue responses to fractionated non-uniform dose delivery. Int J Radiat Biol. 1992;62:249–62.
86. Niemierko A, Goitein M. Modeling of normal tissue response to radiation: the critical volume model. Int J Radiat Oncol Biol Phys. 1993;25:135–45.
87. Niemierko A, Goitein M. Calculation of normal tissue complication probability and dose-volume histogram reduction schemes for tissues with a critical element architecture. Radiother Oncol. 1991;20:166–76.
88. Christianen MEMC, Schilstra C, Beetz I, et al. Predictive modelling for swallowing dysfunction after primary (chemo)radiation: results of a prospective observational study. Radiother Oncol. 2012;105:107–14.
89. Cella L, Palma G, Deasy JO, et al. Complication probability models for radiation-induced heart valvular dysfunction: do heart-lung interactions play a role? PLoS One. 2014;9:e111753.
90. Wijsman R, Dankers F, Troost EGC, et al. Multivariable normal-tissue complication modeling of acute esophageal toxicity in advanced stage non-small cell lung cancer patients treated with intensity-modulated (chemo-)radiotherapy. Radiother Oncol. 2015;117:49–54.
91. Dutz A, Lühr A, Agolli L, et al. Development and validation of NTCP models for acute side-effects resulting from proton beam therapy of brain tumours. Radiother Oncol. 2019;130:164–71.
92. Kierkels RGJ, Korevaar EW, Steenbakkers RJHM, et al. Direct use of multivariable normal tissue complication probability models in treatment plan optimisation for individualised head and neck cancer radiotherapy produces clinically acceptable treatment plans. Radiother Oncol. 2014;112:430–6.
93. Li XA, Alber M, Deasy JO, et al. The use and QA of biologically related models for treatment planning: short report of the TG-166 of the therapy physics committee of the AAPM. Med Phys. 2012;39:1386–409.
94. Fogliata A, Thompson S, Stravato A, Tomatis S, Scorsetti M, Cozzi L. On the gEUD biological optimization objective for organs at risk in photon optimizer of eclipse treatment planning system. J Appl Clin Med Phys. 2018;19(1):106–14. https://doi.org/10.1002/acm2.12224.
95. Luxton G, Keall PJ, King CR. A new formula for normal tissue complication probability (NTCP) as a function of equivalent uniform dose (EUD). Phys Med Biol. 2008;53:23–36.
96. Niemierko A. Biological optimization. In: Bortfeld T, Schmidt-Ullrich R, De Neve W, Wazer DE, editors. Image-guided IMRT. Berlin, Heidelberg: Springer; 2006. p. 199–216.
97. Langendijk JA, Boersma LJ, Rasch CRN, et al. Clinical trial strategies to compare protons with photons. Semin Radiat Oncol. 2018;28:79–87.
98. Widder J, van der Schaaf A, Lambin P, et al. The quest for evidence for proton therapy: model-based approach and precision medicine. Int J Radiat Oncol Biol Phys. 2016;95:30–6.
99. Langendijk JA, Lambin P, De Ruysscher D, et al. Selection of patients for radiotherapy with protons aiming at reduction of side effects: the model-based approach. Radiother Oncol. 2013;107:267–73.
100. Beetz I, Schilstra C, van Luijk P, et al. External validation of three dimensional conformal radiotherapy based NTCP models for patient-rated xerostomia and sticky saliva among patients treated with intensity modulated radiotherapy. Radiother Oncol. 2012b;105:94–100.
101. Troeller A, Yan D, Marina O, et al. Comparison and limitations of DVH-based NTCP models derived from 3D-CRT and IMRT data for prediction of gastrointestinal toxicities in prostate cancer patients by using propensity score matched pair analysis. Int J Radiat Oncol Biol Phys. 2015;91:435–43.
102. Lambin P, Roelofs E, Reymen B, et al. "Rapid learning health care in oncology"—an approach towards decision support systems enabling customised radiotherapy. Radiother Oncol. 2013;109:159–64.
103. Lambin P, Zindler J, Vanneste B, et al. Modern clinical research: how rapid learning health care and cohort multiple randomised clinical trials complement traditional evidence based medicine. Acta Oncol. 2015;54:1289–300.

104. Steyerberg EW, Vickers AJ, Cook NR, et al. Assessing the performance of prediction models: a framework for traditional and novel measures. Epidemiology. 2010;21:128–38.
105. Arts T, Breedveld S, de Jong MA, et al. The impact of treatment accuracy on proton therapy patient selection for oropharyngeal cancer patients. Radiother Oncol. 2017;125:520–5.
106. Wopken K, Bijl HP, van der Schaaf A, et al. Development of a multivariable normal tissue complication probability (NTCP) model for tube feeding dependence after curative radiotherapy/chemo-radiotherapy in head and neck cancer. Radiother Oncol. 2014;113:95–101.
107. Dijkema T, Raaijmakers CPJ, Ten Haken RK, et al. Parotid gland function after radiotherapy: the combined Michigan and Utrecht experience. Int J Radiat Oncol Biol Phys. 2010;78:449–53.
108. Beetz I, Schilstra C, van der Schaaf A, et al. NTCP models for patient-rated xerostomia and sticky saliva after treatment with intensity modulated radiotherapy for head and neck cancer: the role of dosimetric and clinical factors. Radiother Oncol. 2012a;105:101–6.
109. Morin O, Vallières M, Jochems A, et al. A deep look into the future of quantitative imaging in oncology: a statement of working principles and proposal for change. Int J Radiat Oncol Biol Phys. 2018;102:1074–82.
110. Hatt M, Le Rest CC, Tixier F, et al. Radiomics: data are also images. J Nucl Med. 2019;60:38S–44S.
111. Lambin P, Leijenaar RTH, Deist TM, et al. Radiomics: the bridge between medical imaging and personalized medicine. Nat Rev Clin Oncol. 2017;14:749–62.
112. van Dijk LV, Brouwer CL, van der Schaaf A, et al. CT image biomarkers to improve patient-specific prediction of radiation-induced xerostomia and sticky saliva. Radiother Oncol. 2017;122:185–91.
113. van Dijk LV, Langendijk JA, Zhai T-T, et al. Delta-radiomics features during radiotherapy improve the prediction of late xerostomia. Sci Rep. 2019;9:12483.
114. van Dijk LV, Noordzij W, Brouwer CL, et al. 18F-FDG PET image biomarkers improve prediction of late radiation-induced xerostomia. Radiother Oncol. 2018a;126:89–95.
115. van Dijk LV, Thor M, Steenbakkers RJHM, et al. Parotid gland fat related magnetic resonance image biomarkers improve prediction of late radiation-induced xerostomia. Radiother Oncol. 2018b;128:459–66.
116. Shafiq-Ul-Hassan M, Zhang GG, Latifi K, et al. Intrinsic dependencies of CT radiomic features on voxel size and number of gray levels. Med Phys. 2017;44:1050–62.
117. Depeursinge A, Al-Kadi OS, Ross Mitchell J. Biomedical texture analysis: fundamentals, tools and challenges. Cambridge: Academic Press; 2017.
118. Zwanenburg A, Vallières M, Abdalah MA, et al. The image biomarker standardization initiative: standardized quantitative radiomics for high-throughput image-based phenotyping. Radiology. 2020;295:328–38.
119. Carvalho S, Leijenaar RTH, Troost EGC, et al. Early variation of FDG-PET radiomics features in NSCLC is related to overall survival-the "delta radiomics" concept. Radiother Oncol. 2016;118:S20–1.
120. Cunliffe A, Armato SG 3rd, Castillo R, et al. Lung texture in serial thoracic computed tomography scans: correlation of radiomics-based features with radiation therapy dose and radiation pneumonitis development. Int J Radiat Oncol Biol Phys. 2015;91:1048–56.
121. Leger S, Zwanenburg A, Pilz K, et al. CT imaging during treatment improves radiomic models for patients with locally advanced head and neck cancer. Radiother Oncol. 2019;130:10–7.
122. Zwanenburg A, Leger S, Starke S, Löck S. Medical image radiomics processor. Version 1.0URL; 2019b. https://github.com/oncoray/mirp
123. Jochems A, Deist TM, van Soest J, et al. Distributed learning: developing a predictive model based on data from multiple hospitals without data leaving the hospital—a real life proof of concept. Radiother Oncol. 2016;121:459–67.
124. Wilkinson MD, Dumontier M, Aalbersberg IJJ, et al. The FAIR guiding principles for scientific data management and stewardship. Sci Data. 2016;3:160018.

Correction to: Use of $[^{18}F]$FDG PET/CT for Target Volume Definition in Radiotherapy

Johanna E. E. Pouw, Dennis Vriens, Floris H. P. van Velden, and Lioe-Fee de Geus-Oei

Correction to:
Chapter 1 in:
E. G. C. Troost (ed.), *Image-Guided High-Precision Radiotherapy*,
https://doi.org/10.1007/978-3-031-08601-4_1

The original version of Chapter 1 was erroneously published with the incorrect name of the author Hanneke E. E. Pouw. It has been updated as Johanna E. E. Pouw.

The updated version of this chapter can be found at https://doi.org/10.1007/978-3-031-08601-4_1

E. G. C. Troost (ed.), *Image-Guided High-Precision Radiotherapy*,
https://doi.org/10.1007/978-3-031-08601-4_14

MIX
Papier aus verantwortungsvollen Quellen
Paper from responsible sources
FSC® C105338

If you have any concerns about our products,
you can contact us on
ProductSafety@springernature.com

In case Publisher is established outside the EU,
the EU authorized representative is:
Springer Nature Customer Service Center GmbH
Europaplatz 3, 69115 Heidelberg, Germany

Printed by Libri Plureos GmbH
in Hamburg, Germany